Understanding Genetics: DNA, Genes, and Their Real-World Applications

David Sadava, Ph.D.

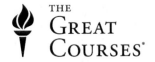

THE
GREAT
COURSES®

PUBLISHED BY:

THE GREAT COURSES
Corporate Headquarters
4840 Westfields Boulevard, Suite 500
Chantilly, Virginia 20151-2299
Phone: 1-800-832-2412
Fax: 703-378-3819
www.thegreatcourses.com

David Sadava, Ph.D.

Pritzker Family Foundation Professor of Biology
The Claremont McKenna, Pitzer, and Scripps Colleges

Professor David Sadava is the Pritzker Family Foundation Professor of Biology at Claremont McKenna, Pitzer, and Scripps, three of The Claremont Colleges. Professor Sadava graduated from Carleton University as the science medalist, with a B.S. with first-class honors in Biology and Chemistry. A Woodrow Wilson Fellow, he received a Ph.D. in Biology from the University of California at San Diego.

Following postdoctoral research at the Scripps Institution of Oceanography, he joined the faculty at Claremont, where he has twice won the Huntoon Award for Superior Teaching, as well as receiving numerous other faculty honors. He teaches undergraduate courses in general biology, biotechnology, and cancer biology, and has been a visiting professor at the University of Colorado and at the California Institute of Technology.

A visiting scientist in oncology at the City of Hope Medical Center, Professor Sadava has held numerous research grants and written more than 55 peer-reviewed scientific research papers, many with his undergraduate students as coauthors. His research concerns resistance to chemotherapy in human lung cancer, with a view to developing new, plant-based medicines to treat this disease.

He is the author or coauthor of five books, including *Plants, Genes, and Crop Biotechnology* and the recently published eighth edition of a leading biology textbook, *Life: The Science of Biology*.

Table of Contents

Understanding Genetics:
DNA, Genes, and Their Real-World Applications

Understanding Genetics:
DNA, Genes, and Their Real-World Applications

Scope:

Perhaps no branch of knowledge has been as exciting over the past 50 years as genetics, the scientific study of heredity. The DNA double helix, discovered in 1953, is one of the great icons of science in our society, rivaling the atom in its pervasiveness in our culture. Like the atom, DNA symbolizes not just scientific knowledge that in this case doubles every few years, but immense implications for humanity. Knowledge of DNA and genetics is radically impacting the two important applications of biology to human welfare—medicine and agriculture. In addition, studies of genes are changing the way we look at ourselves and the other organisms with which we share the Earth.

Lectures One through Three describe genetics as we knew it before DNA. People have long wondered how characteristics are passed on through generations. Before the mechanism of inheritance was investigated with the methods of experimental science, there were many ideas. Some scientists and philosophers thought that only the male (or female) contributed inheritance to offspring. Others proposed that, while the sexes contributed equally to the offspring, whatever it was that each contributed blended together permanently after the union of male and female. The Austrian monk and scientist Gregor Mendel put an end to these notions in 1866 when he published the results and interpretation of years of deliberate and careful experiments on pea plants. He clearly showed not only that the sexes contribute equally to offspring, but also that the genetic determinants, or genes, were particulate and retained their individuality after mating. Almost 40 years later, his results and conclusions were independently verified by other scientists. As biologists began to study life at the microscopic level, in the tiny cells that make up every organism, the genes were located in structures inside of every cell called chromosomes. Mendel and his successors, and the cell biologists looking at chromosomes, gave geneticists the tools to work out the rules of inheritance. But the exact nature of what determined inherited characteristics remained unknown.

The nature of genes and how they are arranged and expressed is described in Lectures Four through Nine. The search for what the gene really is made of quickly focused on DNA. Circumstantial evidence favored it: DNA was in the right place at the right times in the right amounts. But these were correlations—and as such are not valid scientific evidence. A set of experiments on many different organisms provided the proof that DNA was the molecule of heredity. Soon afterward, the double-helix model of DNA was described, as was the elegant way in which it duplicates itself when cells reproduce. The next issue was to determine how DNA as the gene is expressed. The information in each gene is usually expressed as a protein. These complex molecules have vital roles in the organism. They provide structure and can act as enzymes to speed up chemical transformations inside cells. With thousands of such proteins, there are thousands of genes. Coming full circle, the gene-protein relationship was described in a genetic code that is virtually universal in all life on Earth. By the end of the 20th century, biologists were able to determine the information content of every gene of an organism (the genome) and were on the way to describing the functions of these genes. Genome projects, ranging from bacteria to humans to rice plants, are accumulating information at a dizzying rate.

Lectures Ten through Fifteen describe how our knowledge of DNA and its expression can be used to manipulate it for our own purposes. The creation of gene splicing (recombinant DNA) in 1973 was an epochal event in the history of genetics. It is now possible to take any gene from any organism and transfer it to another organism or cell. We are no longer confined to breeding within a species. The applications of this technology range from coaxing bacteria to make human proteins for use as pharmaceuticals (for example, insulin) to inserting genes into "super bugs" that can clean up environmental pollutants (for example, oil spills). The development of new ways to manipulate DNA, including the rapid amplification of DNA from just a single cell, the ability to make and sequence DNA quickly and efficiently in the lab, and the ability to shut down gene expression at will have opened up new horizons in research and application that were unheard of until just recently. The well-publicized use of DNA in forensic identification is just one example.

Lectures Sixteen and Seventeen deal with evolution, the great unifying idea of biology. DNA and its expression can explain Charles Darwin's idea that there are changes in genes that create variations, some of which have an advantage for reproduction, and that natural selection results in those variants being passed on to the next generation. So there is change through time—evolution. Comparisons of organisms' DNAs are now possible, and these show clear relationships between organisms and descent with modification. DNA changes even provide an evolutionary "molecular clock" through which organisms can be related.

Lectures Eighteen through Twenty-Two describe how knowledge of DNA and genetics is leading to a new kind of medicine called molecular medicine. With increasing precision, we are gaining an understanding of what goes wrong in illness and devising specific ways of dealing with it. Genetic screening is allowing for timely interventions, before a disease caused by abnormal genes takes effect. Our understanding of how the immune system fights invaders to the body has been enhanced and harnessed. Even cancer, the great scourge of modern societies, is under intense investigation—and new therapies are either here or on the horizon. At the frontier of molecular medicine are gene therapy, in which deliberate genetic changes to human cells can be used for treatment, and cloning and stem cells, in which new tissues can be made to replace ones that are damaged. The need for these approaches is there, the potential is impressive, and both knowledge and applications are progressing.

Lectures Twenty-Three and Twenty-Four deal with agriculture, that other application of biology to human welfare. Genetics has been part of food production for thousands of years, and increasingly effective ways to breed better crops have been developed as knowledge about genetics has accumulated. This culminated in the impressive achievements of agriculture in the last 50 years, in which food production has more than kept pace with population growth. DNA and biotechnology have the potential to take this progress even further. These applications are just starting, and they include introducing specific genes to crops to make them grow better, need fewer pesticides, and produce more nutritious foods.

As with any technology that is so radically different, biotechnology has its critics, on both philosophical and practical grounds. There is great potential, but also risk. Biological scientists have opened up the "genetics bottle"; it is up to us if and how we use it.

Lecture One
Our Inheritance

Scope: Genetics is the science of heredity. It seeks to explain how the characteristics of living things are passed on from parent to offspring. Genetics is not genealogy, which describes family relationships. Nor does genetics fully explain all the characteristics of a plant or animal: The environment plays an important role. From our earliest days, humans have wondered about genetics, and when we began selectively breeding plants and animals for desirable characteristics, understanding the rules of inheritance became more important. At first, scientists thought that genetic determinants blended after mating, like inks. But later, it was shown by experiments that genetic determinants have a particulate nature, and that this is a chemical substance called DNA. These discoveries in chemical genetics have led to powerful new ways not just to understand how genes work, but to manipulate them for our purposes. These methods have real-world applications in medicine and agriculture.

Outline

I. Opening story: a "perfect crime."
    A. We begin with the story of a "perfect crime"—or so the bank robber thought. A discarded cigarette butt led to the identification of the robber as a "cold hit" because the robber's DNA was in a database, as he had been arrested previously for armed robbery. In the past he had been arrested because of his fingerprints—a phenotype, or outward expression of an inherited characteristic, or gene. This time, his genes—DNA—gave him away.
    B. There is a lot of genetics and biotechnology behind this police work. We can look at it as a series of questions:
        1. What are the rules of inheritance?
        2. How do we know that DNA is the gene, the material that is inherited?
        3. What is the basis of the differences between individuals that are inherited?
        4. How often do these differences occur, and how can that be a basis for identification?

5. How can a tiny amount of DNA on a cigarette butt be amplified for analysis in the lab?

II. Introduction to the science of genetics.

  A. Genetics is the science of heredity.

    1. When you consider the diversity of organisms on Earth, from the tiniest bacteria, invisible to the human eye; to the tallest redwood tree; to yourself; the diversity of living things is obvious.

    2. But behind this diversity is a unity at the basic chemical level.

    3. Three major ideas tie biological science together.

      a. Mechanism. Many societies have believed, and many people continue to believe, that the rules that govern life are different from the inanimate universe. They propose a "vital force" to explain this. Examples of this are the "chi" of Chinese philosophy and traditional medicine. Biological science rejects this idea, proposing instead that the same rules of physics and chemistry that govern the lifeless world (e.g., rocks, the air) govern life.

      b. Cell theory. Since the microscope was first used to visualize living things, biologists have agreed that cells are the building blocks of life (just as atoms are the building blocks of chemistry). All living things are made up of cells, and all cells come from other cells.

      c. Evolution. Organisms are related by common ancestry, and there has been and continues to be change through time, or descent with modification. In 1859, Charles Darwin proposed natural selection as a way to explain how organisms with different characteristics change through many generations.

    4. Genetics explains the rules by which characteristics, such as hair color in people, come to differ and how these differences are passed on to the next generation (inherited). The last half of the 20th century saw the nature of the genetic determinants, and how they are expressed in organisms, described in chemical terms. This is the science of molecular biology, including DNA.

  B. Genetics is not destiny or genealogy.

    1. Genetics is not destiny. Genes do not always predict what will happen in an organism. Is my hair really dark brown? Only my hairdresser knows for sure. What any person—or other organism—ends up looking like is determined by both heredity and environment.

2. Genetics is not genealogy. Genealogy deals with relationships between families of organisms: A family tree is genealogy. Genetics deals with the rules of inheritance: The patterns of inherited biological characteristics in the family are genetics.

III. A very short history of genetics.

A. People began selectively breeding other creatures for human purposes long ago.

1. The date palm was bred by ancient Egyptians 5000 years ago to improve the quality and amount of the fruit.

2. Horses were bred in the Near East and Asia 4000 years ago for speed in war and racing.

B. Deliberate breeding and human curiosity led people to ask: What are the rules of inheritance?

1. The Greek philosopher Aristotle (382–322 B.C.) proposed that the male semen had imperfect ingredients that were "organized" by the menstrual fluid during intercourse. His ideas had great influence on scientific thinking in Western cultures for over 1500 years.

2. The Dutch scientist Antonie van Leeuwenhoek in the 17th century looked at human sperm under the microscope and thought he saw little people, curled up. This was in accord with Aristotle's view.

3. Soon, other microscopists thought they saw little people curled up in the human egg cell. This set up an intellectual battle between "spermists" and "ovists" as to which gender passed on the hereditary characteristics to the offspring.

4. Careful observations from crosses by Dutch tulip breeders in the next 100 years showed that both sexes contribute equally to the inheritance of the offspring.

C. Does the genetic material blend, or is it particulate?

1. Attention turned to what happened to the genetic material when the sperm and egg cells unite.

2. Initially, plant breeders felt that the genetic determinants blended when put together in the fertilized egg: A sperm from a red-flowered tulip combining with an egg of a white-flowered tulip would often produce pink offspring. And like

inks that blend, these hereditary determinants would never be seen again in that offspring. It would pass on only the genetic determinant for pink color.

3. Blending reigned as the explanation for heredity until the late 1800s, when Gregor Mendel performed careful experiments using garden pea plants that showed that hereditary determinants were particulate. Mendel's results led to a rejection of blending.

4. Mendel's results were consistent with the idea that the genetic material is carried on particles in the cell called chromosomes; these had been discovered about the same time he did his work.

5. In the mid-20th century, the genetic material was identified as a chemical substance—DNA.

IV. The goals of this course.

A. The first goal is to understand the idea of genes as determinants of inheritance.

1. This begins with the rules of inheritance (Lectures Two and Three) and the chemical nature of genes as DNA (Lectures Four and Five).

2. This discussion is followed by the relationship between genes and their expression as some outward characteristics (Lectures Six through Nine).

B. The second goal is to learn about how our understanding of genes has led to powerful tools to manipulate them for our purposes.

1. This includes splicing genes together as recombinant DNA (Lectures Ten and Eleven) and using these tools to make products such as drugs and to clean up the environment (Lectures Twelve and Thirteen).

2. New ways to identify organisms have been devised, and these are used not only in forensics, as we described earlier, but also to study evolution—changes in organisms through time (Lectures Fourteen through Sixteen).

C. The third goal is to learn how our knowledge of genetics and tools of manipulating genes are being used in real-world applications.

1. These applications include molecular medicine (Lectures Seventeen through Twenty-Two) and genetically modified plants in agriculture (Lectures Twenty-Three and Twenty-Four).

2. These applications, while they hold great promise for improving life for people, are not without controversy.

Essential Reading:

Ricki Lewis, *Human Genetics*, 7th ed. (New York: McGraw-Hill, 2006), chap. 1.

David Sadava, Craig Heller, Gordon Orians, William Purves, and David Hillis, *Life: The Science of Biology,* 8th ed. (Sunderland, MA: Sinauer Associates; New York: W. H. Freeman and Co., 2008), pt. 3.

Supplemental Reading:

Anthony Griffiths, Susan Wessler, Richard Lewontin, William Gelbart, and David Suzuki, *An Introduction to Genetic Analysis*, 8th ed. (New York: W. H. Freeman and Co., 2007).

Edwin McConkey, *How the Human Genome Works* (Sudbury, MA: Jones and Bartlett, 2004).

Questions to Consider:

1. Consider yourself as you read through this course. Can you describe some of your characteristics that are clearly hereditary and some that are environmentally determined? What are some characteristics that are determined by a combination of the two?

2. What are some nonscientific beliefs about inheritance? Survey your nonscientist friends to find out what people think about the rules of inheritance.

Lecture One—Transcript
Our Inheritance

Welcome. In the last 50 years, genetics—the scientific study of heredity—has been among the most exciting of all areas of human knowledge. The DNA double helix first unveiled in 1953 is one of the great icons of science in our society. It rivals the atom with its whizzing electrons in its pervasiveness in our culture. Like the atom, DNA symbolizes not just scientific knowledge but immense implications for humanity. Knowledge in the field of DNA and its expression doubles every few years, radically impacting the two most important applications of biology to human welfare, namely medicine and agriculture. Studies of DNA and genes are changing how we look at ourselves as well as the other organisms with which we share the world.

I begin with a story. I'm going to begin all of my lectures with a story, hopefully to engage your interest but also to set the stage for the subject matter that follows. This is a story of a "perfect crime," or so the bank robber thought. Jim—I'm changing the name to protect the guilty—was a bank robber who had been robbing banks since he was age 18, and we meet him at age 35 when he's convicted of bank robbery in St. Louis, Missouri. It's 1990. Jim thought he had carefully planned this robbery so he could get away with it. He had learned from his previous bank robberies what to do. He came to the bank as the last customer, late in the day. He chose a branch that was out of the way. He wore a ski mask so no one would see his face. He even dyed his red hair black so people might not identify him in that way.

Well, he got away with it for about two weeks, and a couple of weeks later the police were at his door. He was nabbed by the fact that he had left a lot of fingerprints all over the bank. His fingerprints had been taken in a previous arrest and sent to the Federal Bureau of Investigation, the FBI, and stored in a large database. When the fingerprints in the bank matched Jim's, the police were at his door, and they had other evidence that led to his conviction.

He served 10 years in the penitentiary during the 1990s, and while he was there, there were two things that happened that are of interest for our story. First, he became a smoker. It's kind of boring in prison, and I guess smoking was a way to relieve the tension, whiling away the time. In addition, in 1998

Jim had his blood drawn and a blood sample sent to the FBI once again for what he was told were identification purposes. The FBI in the 1990s got permission to do blood analysis of all convicts who were in the federal penitentiary system.

Jim was released in the year 2000, and he decided to move away from the Midwest to California. It didn't take him long to once again become engaged in his vocation, namely bank robbery. Well, once again, he approached a bank late in the day. It was a small branch. It was in a small town in California. He wore a ski mask. He dyed his hair black so his red hair wouldn't show. This time he learned from his previous mistake, as he had before, and he wore surgical gloves so he wouldn't leave any fingerprints. As he was walking out of the bank with the loot, he was kind of nervous so he disposed of the gloves, in his pocket actually, and lit up a cigarette. He took a couple of puffs on his way down the street to his car and discarded the cigarette on the sidewalk. A couple of weeks later the police were at his door, and an incredulous Jim asked the police, how did you find me this time? They replied with three letters, D-N-A. You see, Jim had left some DNA on the cigarette butt, and the cigarette butt in this particular town in California was an unusual thing. In California, where I live, it's become more and more difficult to smoke anywhere in public in the last 10 years, and the reason smoking has become more difficult is that, as we'll see later on in the course, cigarette smoke damages DNA and leads to lung cancer. So, banning cigarette smoking in this particular town in all public places led to a cigarette butt being found by the police near the bank to be an unusual thing. The police said, oh, this is an out-of-towner for sure. Now, Jim left a souvenir on the cigarette butt. In his saliva that was dried up was some DNA from some of the tissue in his mouth. The police carefully took the cigarette butt, sent it to the FBI, and the FBI analyzed the DNA in the cigarette and matched it to the DNA from Jim's blood that had been collected earlier on. This was called a "cold hit." There was no other evidence that connected Jim to this crime. This was the only evidence they had that a previous bank robber was there.

Now, there are a lot of genetics questions behind the police work, and I'll phrase it in five different questions. First, what are the rules of inheritance? Second, how do we know that DNA is the genetic material that's inherited? Third, what's the basis for differences in DNA between individuals? Fourth, how often do these differences between individuals occur, and how is this the basis for identification, as was the case with Jim? And fifth, how can

DNA on a cigarette butt in a teeny, tiny amount be amplified for analysis in the lab? The answers to these and other questions will be apparent as we go through this course.

I want to introduce genetics to you in two contexts. First of all, I want to tell you about the science of genetics, and secondly, I want to give you a short history of genetics that illuminates that science. Then I'll describe what the goals of this course are.

First, an introduction to the science of genetics. Genetics is the science of heredity. When you look at the diversity of organisms on earth from the tiniest bacteria, to large redwood trees, to us, to all sorts of other creatures, behind this diversity is an amazing unity at the basic chemical level. All living things have the same basic chemistry. This leads me to an excursion into the science of biology and of genetics. There are three major ideas that hold biological science and genetics together, and those ideas are mechanism, the cell theory, and evolution.

First, mechanism. Many societies have believed, and still believe, that there is a "vital force"—that life has a different set of rules from nonliving things, that we have something different in us than in the air and rocks—and not just humans but any living thing. Think of the ideas in Chinese philosophy about an energy called the "chi." The Chinese philosophy involving the chi has led to ways to manipulate the chi. This is thought to be a life force that all living things have. So, we can manipulate the chi by doing chi kung, which is where a practitioner manipulates the chi in a person; or tai chi, where you manipulate your own chi by movement; or acupuncture, which redistributes the flow of the chi. The chi is nothing that we can lay our hands on in terms of physics and chemistry. I can't hold up a glass and say, "Here's some chi. Drink it." That's not the way it works. It's a force that we don't understand, but a force that has led to medical practices such as acupuncture.

Since the Renaissance several hundred years ago, Western science, and biology in particular, and later genetics, has believed that the same laws that govern physics and chemistry in inanimate, nonliving nature, govern life. There is no vital force. We used to think that diseases like the plague were caused by evil spirits. We know better now. We know they're caused by an infection. Many people believe that there is a vital force in some way. It's a different way of looking at life. Some people use religion for this vital force. Other people talk about the chi for this vital force. But in this course, as a biologist and as a biological scientist, I'm going to use mechanism as the way to explain life, the physics and chemistry of life.

The second idea that ties biology together is called the cell theory. No, it's not economics. It's not selling stocks. It's "cell" with a "c"—cell theory. When scientists first looked through the microscope at living tissues, they saw building blocks, which they called cells. And in 1838, two scientists named Schleiden and Schwan came up with the cell theory that has two aspects to it.

First, the cell is the unit of life. So, cell biology is all of biology. Cells exhibit all the characteristics of biological structure and function, much like the atom is the basic unit of chemistry and elementary particles, like electrons and protons, are the basis of physics. The second aspect of cell theory is that the cell is the unit of biological continuity—that all reproduction is by cell so that humans, for example, reproduce by gametes, which are the sex cells, the egg and sperm. We'll talk about cell theory later on in the course.

When I do scientific research—and my research concerns cancer, specifically lung cancer—I take cells from patients in the laboratory dish and study their mechanism. So, I'm very aware of these two aspects of mechanism and cell theory in the work that I do.

The third idea that ties biology together is evolution. Evolution is a way of relating organisms on Earth and in the past by common ancestry. It's called descent, coming down, with modification. Evolution says that organisms of a given type—worms, apes, horses—change through generations of time, many generations of time, and that the organisms on earth now are not the same as their progenitors that were on earth eons ago. There's a progression in many cases from the years ago, eons ago, types to the organisms that exist now. In the 1850s, Charles Darwin proposed a way by which the organism's changes would be selected. He called this natural selection. We'll come to that later on in the course. How organisms came to be different from one another, how the organisms that exist became different from one another, is explained by the science of heredity—genetics—as well as in the long-term evolution by natural selection.

Genetics as a science explains the rules by which characteristics come to differ and how these differences are passed on from one generation to the next. Evolution is looking at many generations. Since 1950 geneticists have focused on the nature of genetic determinants—mechanism again. We're looking at what is their nature—what is their physics and chemistry, and how they are expressed in organisms as some outward characteristic? The outward expression of characteristics is called the phenotype. The genetic material, of course, is called genes, and now we can explain these, as we'll see in the course, in chemical terms. This is the whole field of molecular biology, the science of DNA.

So, the first aspect of the science of genetics is that genetics is a science. It's a biological science, and it centers on three assumptions, three things that we work on, which are the ideas of mechanism, the idea of cell theory, and the idea of evolution. The second aspect of genetics is that genes are not destiny. Genes mean potential. The environment shapes their expression. You remember Jim. He dyed his hair black, his red hair. Well, his red hair was in the genes. His red hair was genetically inherited. He dyed it black because he didn't want people to recognize him. My wife will say, "Well, I have dark brown hair with salt and pepper. Oh yeah? Only my hairdresser knows for sure." Now, that's kind of a fun example, but keep this in mind throughout this course, and throughout your reading, and in the media, as you're exposed every day to an announcement of a new gene for X, or Y, or Z. The gene does not mean destiny. The gene doesn't mean it will be expressed. Genes just mean potential. Genes interact with one another. The gene expression interacts with the environment.

The third aspect of the science of genetics I want to bring up is what genetics is not. Again, genetics is not genealogy. Genealogy is a family tree—who begat who—relationships between families. A family tree is genealogy. Genetics deals with the rules of inheritance, the patterns of diverse characteristics that are inherited going from one generation to the next in a family.

I want to turn now to a very short history of genetics. We begin with the first selective breeding. It doesn't mean that you're domesticating an animal or plant, just growing it for your own purposes. It means you're saying this animal will cross with this animal. This plant will cross with this plant for the following genetic purposes. The first plant to be crossed deliberately is the date palm. There's evidence that the Egyptians 5000 years ago crossed one type of date palm with another for certain characteristics, for the quality and amount of fruit.

These days, dates grow still in Egypt. They also grow near where I live in Southern California in the Coachella Valley near the resort area of Palm

Springs. One of my favorite places along the road is a shack near a group of date trees where they're doing genetics. You can go in and watch a movie that is entitled *Romance and Sex Life of the Date*. Now, that's a movie a biologist would really enjoy.

The first animal to be bred deliberately was the horse, and it was bred because people wanted faster and stronger horses for war. This was done about 4000 years ago in the Near East and Asia, and this, of course, led to one king saying, "You know, I got a really fast horse through breeding," and another king saying, "Oh yeah, mine is faster." And so they began horse racing, which is the reason that I go to the race track often and take my classes to the racetrack. You know when I take your class to the race track a week later I'll get a call from a parent saying, "You took my daughter to what—to the race track?" And my response is, "Well, we're looking at a long genetic tradition here."

Now, deliberate breeding of animals and plants and human curiosity led people to ask, well, what are the rules of inheritance? What are the rules by which things are passed down from one generation to the next? The Greek philosopher Aristotle, proposed that the male semen had imperfect ingredients, he called them, that were "organized" by the menstrual fluid during intercourse. So, the male was responsible for the hereditary characteristics, and it's the female that provided some sort of environment to get these to unfold. If you take other Teaching Company courses that have to do with philosophy, as I have, you know that Aristotle, who was a terrific philosopher and a very keen observer of nature, had views that had enormous impact on Western thought for the next 1500 years after he lived.

For the next 1500 years, scientists' job was to confirm what Aristotle had said. So, in the 17th century, when the Dutch scientist Antonie van Leeuwenhoek invented the microscope for looking at human tissues and looked at human sperm under the microscope, he made a drawing of a little curled-up being, a little curled-up baby inside of the head of the sperm—he kind of squinted his eyes and saw that. We scientists try to be objective, and we try our best not to be influenced by what we're trying to see. We try to see nature as it is. Well, it's a really good example of that not happening. Van Leeuwenhoek was a terrific observer of nature. Yet he was so influenced by Aristotle that he squinted, and squinted, and squinted to try to see that little curled up baby in there that would then, of course, be organized by the menstrual fluid.

Another scientist named Graff looked at sperm in the microscope and said, I don't see any little beings in there at all. Graff looked at eggs and saw little beings inside egg cells, and so this set up an intellectual battle between "spermists" and "ovists" about which gender passed hereditary characteristics to the offspring.

Crosses by the Dutch tulip breeders—now, flowers are a big thing, especially tulips in Holland, and we'll see this several times in the course— kind of laid to rest the idea that one or the other sex was responsible for heredity. They would cross a tulip plant that gives red flowers with one that gives white flowers. They would do a genetic cross, and they would get offspring that were pink. Now if the male flower was red and the white flower was female, they got pink. If the red flower was female, and the white flower was male, the opposite cross, they still got pink. So, they came to the conclusion, no, the sexes are equal in their contribution of genetic material, hereditary material, to the offspring.

Well, the next question to ask is, okay, what happens to this genetic material, whatever it is, when the sperm and egg cells unite? Initially, plant breeders like the Dutch tulip breeders felt that the genetic determinants blended. When sperm—yes, plants have sperm—and egg—yes, plants have egg—mated, the red determinants and the white determinants disappeared completely. The offspring were pink, and you could never get the red and white back again. The idea of blending was like putting two different colored paints together. Normally, you can't separate them once they're blended together, and blending reigned as the explanation for heredity until well into the late 1800s, when Gregor Mendel, using experiments on garden pea plants, showed very clearly that the hereditary determinants were particulate. They weren't some vague thing that got destroyed and blended in the offspring, but they were discreet particles. There was a red determinant for red color and a white determinant for white color. They never disappeared. In the pink, the red and the white were still there, and you could get them out again in subsequent generations.

Now, true to the idea of mechanism, of the mechanistic explanation of life— the red, and the white, and the particulate nature of genes—led scientists to begin to look at what the nature of genetic material was. It took about the first half of the 20th century to determine what the genetic material was and is. This was done through a series of experiments on a wide variety of organisms, on model organisms as we will describe them. Model organisms are organisms that are easy to use in the laboratory. They're organisms that people can manipulate and that had genetic mutations and genetic changes that people could study.

These experiments as well as circumstantial evidence led to the identification by about the mid-20th century of DNA as the genetic material. The last half of the 20th century that brings us to the 21st century has been concerned, was concerned, and still is concerned, with how the DNA, the genetic material, is expressed as the phenotype, its outward appearance. It turns out that this expression is by molecules called proteins, which will be the subject of a later lecture, and that these proteins are molecules that determine the chemistry of the cell. So, red and white are determined ultimately by proteins that are the expression of DNA.

I now turn to the goals of this course, and there are three goals that I have in this course. The goals are first to understand the idea of genes as determinants of inheritance. My second goal is to learn about how our understanding of genes has led to powerful tools to manipulate genes for our purposes, and my third goal is to learn how our knowledge of genetics and the tools of manipulating genes—that is the first two parts of the course—are being used in real-world applications.

Now let's go into those goals in a little bit more detail in outline. First, to understand the idea of genes as determinants of inheritance—in Lectures Two and Three, I will describe what the rules of inheritance are. They were first found by Gregor Mendel, the monk I mentioned earlier, and the nature and particulate nature of these hereditary determinants was then described in terms of chromosomes: where they are located in the cell and the nucleus, which is part of the cell where the genes are located. In Lectures Four and Five, I'll describe how the mechanistic search for what the gene is in chemical terms led us to DNA, and as I mentioned, this was largely through experiments as well as some circumstantial evidence. DNA was there at the right place, in the right time, but these were dynamic experiments. I'll describe what experimental science is and how we accept evidence as being valid in experimental science. In Lectures Six through Nine, I'll describe how in the last 40 or 50 years scientists have been concerned with how genes are expressed as outward characteristics, and this will lead us to proteins and how genes are controlled in their expression.

My second goal in the course is to learn how our understanding of genes has led to powerful tools to manipulate genes for human purposes. It's a way of our mastering of nature in our own ways. This will include, in Lectures Ten and Eleven, the idea of splicing genes together: of taking a gene from an organism in the test tube in the laboratory, and another organism, and putting them together to make what is called recombinant DNA. I'll describe how this was initially quite controversial but is a remarkable advance in our ability to manipulate genes and study them. Using the tools of recombinant DNA in Lectures Twelve and Thirteen, I'll show you how people are able now to make products such as valuable pharmaceutical drugs, as well as genetically engineered bacteria, to do environmental cleanup or assist in other methods of environmental clean up, and to do mining as well.

The methods of DNA manipulation have led to ways to identify organisms such as us. So, for example, Jim, our bank robber in the opening story, in forensics was identified by his DNA. These methods also have been used to study evolution by natural selection as well as not by natural selection as you will see—changes in organisms through generations of time. That's the subject of Lectures Fourteen through Seventeen. So, the mid-part of the course is to learn an understanding of genes, the tools of manipulating them, and some of our knowledge from that.

The last goal of the course is to learn how our knowledge of genetics and the tools of manipulating genes are being used in real-world applications. The two major applications of biology to human welfare, and it is certainly true of genetics, are medicine and agriculture. So, in Lectures Eighteen through Twenty-Two, I'll describe molecular medicine. We'll see how genes and DNA are used to screen for human genetic diseases in newborns as well as adults. We'll talk about cancer as a genetic disease. We'll talk about the immune system and how we fight disease and then introduce you to new aspects of genetics and DNA, namely, gene therapy, cloning, and stem cells—molecular medicine. Lectures Twenty-Three and Twenty-Four are concerned with agriculture, and the reason for talking about agriculture last is that it's something that we take for granted. It's something that's extremely important, but we in the rich world take it for granted. Here I'll describe how traditional methods for breeding plants for higher amounts of crops produced have limitations—and these limitations are possibly able to be overcome by molecular biology and DNA manipulation.

We begin in the next lecture where modern genetics began—with Gregor Mendel. Thank you.

Lecture Two
Mendel and Genes

Scope: Gregor Mendel, a monk from what is now the Czech Republic, did the experiments and came to the conclusions that founded the modern science of genetics. As the son of a farmer, who took courses in science and mathematics at the University of Vienna, Mendel was well prepared to undertake his investigations, which occurred in 1856–1863 while he was teaching at a monastery. He wisely chose pea plants as his experimental subject, as they had clearly defined patterns of inheritance. He made careful crosses and counted the offspring plants, expressing the data mathematically. He concluded that the factors that determine inheritance, which we now call genes, are particulate and that each individual has two copies of every gene, one from each parent. Only one of these copies ends up in each sex cell (sperm or egg) to be passed on to the offspring. Genes that determine different characteristics (such as seed color and height) are inherited independently. Mendel's conclusions apply to most organisms, including humans. But since we cannot do deliberate genetic crosses as experiments, analysis of human genetics is done by pedigrees. Genes are not destiny. While genes determine the capability for a certain characteristic, the environment often has an important role in their expression.

Outline

I. Opening story.
  A. It does not take an advanced degree and a well-funded position to do important science.
    1. Gregor Mendel, who made one of the two key discoveries in genetics, was not a university professor or a member of a prestigious research institute. He was a monk and a teacher. His laboratory was not a large room with lots of equipment and a cadre of assistants. He worked alone on a small plot of land adjacent to the monastery.
    2. Nevertheless, Mendel's background prepared him to make the discoveries he did. Born in 1822 in what is now the eastern

Czech Republic, he was the son of a farmer and a mother whose father was a gardener. So he knew a lot about plants.

3. In 1843, he joined an Augustinian monastery at Brno. Assigned to teach, he was so good that the abbot sent him to the University of Vienna for further education. There he took courses in mathematics, chemistry, and biology. He learned the scientific method, which had been developed centuries before.

   a. Science begins with a hypothesis: a testable idea.

   b. A hypothesis is tested by an experiment under controlled conditions.

   c. The experiment either proves that the hypothesis is valid or not; if the latter, the hypothesis must be revised.

   d. Scientific investigations must be published so that they can be verified and extended. This takes the form of a scientific paper that is a complete description of the work. In the fields of genetics and DNA, hundreds of research papers are published every day.

4. Mendel returned to the monastery from Vienna, and from 1856 to 1863, he taught and did experimental work on garden pea plants that laid the foundation for the modern science of genetics.

5. In 1865, Mendel gave a public lecture at the local medical society on his findings and published them a year later in the society's journal. Unfortunately for science, he was "kicked upstairs" and promoted to abbot a year later, and the burden of administration precluded further investigations.

6. Also unfortunately, his paper was published in a journal that was not read by most scientists in the field, and its conclusions were so new that few would accept them.

B. Mendel's work was not appreciated until 1901, when three botanists working separately came to the same conclusions from genetics experiments that Mendel did, and then found his paper, which had just been translated from German to English.

II. Mendel performed experiments on pea plants.

A. Mendel used pea plants for several good reasons.

   1. They were easy to grow in the monastery garden.

   2. He could control which plants mated. The flowers have both male and female reproductive organs, so cutting off the

pollen-producing male organs from a plant's flowers allowed him to brush pollen from another plant onto that one, which became the female for the cross.

3. There were well-defined strains of pea plants that were true-breeding for that characteristic, or phenotype. So, true-breeding plants that formed seeds that were spherical (plump) always formed spherical seeds when crossed among each other; true-breeding plants with wrinkled seeds formed only wrinkled seeds, etc.

B. Mendel's experiments led to laws of heredity.

1. When Mendel crossed two true-breeding strains differing only in one characteristic (e.g., spherical × wrinkled), the first-generation offspring always showed just one of the two characteristics (in this case, all spherical). He called this the dominant characteristic and the one not there the recessive characteristic. There was no blending!

2. This was confirmed when he crossed the first-generation plants among themselves. He got the spherical and wrinkled plants back in the second generation!

3. Now Mendel's mathematics education came into the picture: He counted the plants in the second generation and found that there were 5474 spherical and 1850 wrinkled, a 3:1 ratio. He got this ratio with six other pairs of characteristics, such as tall and short plant height.

4. On the basis of his data, Mendel proposed that:

   a. The genetic determinants are particulate; they are not lost after fertilization.

   b. Each individual plant has two copies of the determinant (he called them "elementen," and we call them "genes"). One comes from each parent.

   c. The genes for a particular characteristic (e.g., seed shape) can exist in different forms. We call these alleles. In a true breeding plant, the two alleles were the same (e.g., two alleles that result in spherical seeds—we call them "spherical" alleles). In the first-generation plants, the two alleles were different (e.g., one "spherical" and one "wrinkled"). One allele is dominant ("round") and expressed in the offspring when it is present together with the recessive allele ("wrinkled"). But the alleles never disappear, as would be the case if there was blending.

    d.   Only one allele is passed on to the next generation in the sperm or egg. It is random which allele a particular sperm or egg contains for that characteristic. So on average, each plant in the first generation of his seed shape cross would make half of the sperm or egg cells with the "round" allele and half with the "wrinkled" allele. This is called the "law of segregation." It is a law in science because it was shown after 1900 to be general and to apply to most other organisms, not just peas.

    5.   Mendel crossed peas with two sets of differing characteristics (e.g., seed shape and height) and showed that these characteristics behaved as if they were independent of each other. This led to the law of independent assortment.

    6.   Mendelian laws of genetics follow simple laws of probability. This can be illustrated by tossing two coins. The probability of tossing one heads is 1/2. The probability of tossing two heads at once is $1/2 \times 1/2$, or 1/4.

III. Mendelian laws of genetics apply to most organisms, including humans.

    A.   Because we cannot do genetic crosses in humans to determine genes and alleles, we rely on the past—a pedigree (or genealogy with inherited characteristics). In a pedigree following a phenotype that is expressed by a dominant allele—for example, with Huntington's disease—every affected individual has one parent who is affected. Since most unusual alleles are rare, the affected parent is most likely heterozygous (one dominant and the other recessive allele). The zygote is the biological word for a fertilized egg. So there is a 50% chance of passing this allele on to a child.

    B.   In a pedigree following a phenotype that is expressed by a recessive allele, an individual must have two identical alleles (that is, be homozygous) for the recessive alleles. This is the case for albinism, for example. Again, since the unusual allele is rare, an individual with albinism must have inherited one "albinism" allele from each parent, and both parents must be carriers (they are heterozygous, but normal). Recall the two first-generation heterozygous pea plants that all had spherical seeds but when crossed among themselves produced plants with wrinkled seeds.

IV. Not all inheritance follows the Mendelian ratios.

A. In codominance (e.g., the ABO blood groups in humans), both alleles are expressed in heterozygotes.

B. The ABO blood groups also are an example of multiple (more than two) alleles for a characteristic. But note that an individual only has two alleles (e.g., AB, AO, etc.).

C. Many complex characteristics are determined by the interactions of numerous genes (e.g., height in humans).

V. Genes are not destiny. The environment plays a vital role.

Essential Reading:

Ricki Lewis, *Human Genetics*, 7th ed. (New York: McGraw-Hill, 2006), chap. 4.

Benjamin Pierce, *Genetics: A Conceptual Approach* (New York: W.H. Freeman and Co., 2005), chap. 3.

Supplemental Reading:

Anthony Griffiths, Susan Wessler, Richard Lewontin, William Gelbart, and David Suzuki, *An Introduction to Genetic Analysis*, 8th ed. (New York: W. H. Freeman and Co., 2007).

Robin Henig, *The Monk in the Garden: The Lost and Found Genius of Gregor Mendel* (Boston: Houghton-Mifflin, 2001).

Questions to Consider:

1. Draw a three-generation genealogy of your family. Now, use a single characteristic—such as blue or brown eye color, presence or absence of dimples, presence of absence of a cleft in the cheek, or presence or absence of freckles—and draw the pedigree. Can you determine whether the characteristic you chose is inherited as a dominant or recessive pattern?

2. In Labrador retrievers, coat color is determined by two interacting genes (with alleles). The B allele (dominant) produces a black coat. The b allele produces a brown coat. So what color is a Bb dog? A bb dog? A second gene, E, must be present for any color to form at all; a dog that is homozygous recessive for e (that is, has ee) is white. What is the color of a BBee dog? And a bbEe dog? If you have a lab (I do—both the scientific and canine kinds!), draw its pedigree and try to figure out its genetics.

Lecture Two—Transcript
Mendel and Genes

Welcome back. In the last lecture, I introduced the subject of genetics as a science and as history. I want to retrace our steps in genetic history back to Mendel, the real founder of modern genetics. In the story of Gregor Mendel, there's a moral, I guess, and the moral is you don't have to have an advanced degree in science and lots of federal funding to do important work in the sciences. Gregor Mendel was not a university professor. He was not a prestigious member of a research institute. This guy was a monk and a teacher. His lab was not a big room with lots of equipment and a cadre of assistants ready to do his bidding. He worked alone on a small plot of land adjacent to a monastery.

Mendel's background prepared him for the discoveries he made. He was born in 1822 in what is now the eastern Czech Republic. As the son of a farmer and a mother whose father was a gardener, Mendel knew a lot about plants. You can imagine the dinner-table conversation at the Mendel home. It was about, well, this variety of plants grows in this way; agricultural production of this plant is pretty good. So he knew a lot about plant varieties. In 1843, at 21 years old, he joined the Augustinian monastery at Brno, which is in what is now the eastern Czech Republic. Assigned to teach, Mendel was so good at it that the abbot in charge sent him to the University of Vienna for further studies. At the university, Mendel took a wide variety of courses, and for our purposes the most notable ones were math, chemistry, and biology. In addition, Mendel learned about the scientific method, which had been developed in science during the previous couple of centuries.

What is the scientific method? Science begins with a hypothesis, a testable idea. What do I mean by that? Well, let me describe research I've been doing. I have been interested, in my research, in lung cancer. I'm specifically interested in the chemotherapy or drug treatment of lung cancer. In a recent research project, I decided to investigate one of the active ingredients of green tea for possible treatment for lung cancer. My hypothesis in my experiments was not "green tea can cure lung cancer"; that's the subject of a clinical trial where you'd give it—you'd give green tea or this active ingredient—to patients. I didn't do that. I took cancer cells from patients in the laboratory. You remember cell theory, one of our three great ideas of biology—the other two being mechanism and evolution. Cell theory says that life can go on in cells, and so I took cells out of patients. My hypothesis was the active ingredient in green tea will kill cancer cells.

Now, the next step in the scientific method is to test the hypothesis by an experiment. If we phrase our hypothesis right, it kind of leads to an experiment. In my case, it leads to an experiment where I took some cancer cells, and I gave them the active ingredient of green tea, and I did a control, or untreated, group that didn't get the active ingredient and saw what happened. And my hypothesis was, of course, that the cells treated with the extract of green tea might die, and then I would study how. The next step in the scientific method is to look at the results of the experiment, and the experiment either proves the hypothesis as valid or not. And if it's not valid, the hypothesis must be revised. In my case, it was valid. I showed that the cells died. I showed an investigation of the mechanism by which they would die.

The last step in the process of science is not really part of the scientific method. We've already done the scientific method. We've proven or disproven and revised the hypothesis. The last step in science is to publish the scientific research. Science is a totally open business. You can't lie; you have to publish everything and say, "This is what I found; this is what I did; now what do you think of it?" Other people will confirm, extend, or deny what you did. This is done in what is called a scientific paper. A scientific paper has the following sections. It starts with an introduction. So in my paper, for example, that I published on green tea, I said people have been drinking green tea for years. They seem to get healthier. There are some studies on cancer patients where it seems to act as a preventative, etc. Then you describe in detail the methods. You have to describe it in enough detail that anyone with similar lab equipment to you can repeat your experiments and get the same results. It has to be totally detailed, so I had to do that.

Then you present the results, and the results in modern science are often presented formally. I can't say the cells were killed by the green tea extract compared to the untreated cells that were not treated with green tea extract. I can't say the cells were killed. I could say that in the results, but I have to present numbers—data. What percentage of the cells were killed? How long did it take? What were the other chemical things going on in the cell? Finally, at the end of the scientific paper are the conclusions. The conclusions restate the hypothesis, saying I thought green tea extract would work, and then the conclusion says yes, it worked. Then it's the only place in a scientific paper where you can begin to wax poetic and speculate. So, for example, in my paper, I speculate that the active ingredient of green tea, and green tea itself, might be useful in cancer treatment, and this might lead to clinical trials on patients.

The important thing is there has to be enough detail so anyone in the field can replicate the paper; otherwise it's useless to science. Science is not a mere description of nature; certainly not experimental science. That's natural history. Just saying, "Look, that's a pine tree," is natural history. That's okay, but an ecologist doesn't just say "Look, that's a pine tree." They say, "Where does it live? What are the relationships to other organisms? What are the relationships to other pine trees?" So it's a science of relationships rather than mere description.

Back to Mendel. Mendel returned to the monastery from the University of Vienna educated; remember he studied math, chemistry, biology, and the scientific method. From 1856 to 1863, he taught and did experimental work in the garden by the monastery using pea plants, and this work laid the foundations for the modern science of genetics. True to the scientific process, in 1865 Mendel gave a public lecture at the local medical society on his findings, and a year later published them in the society's journal. Unfortunately for science, Mendel was "kicked upstairs." He was promoted to abbot a year later. He went into administration, and the burden of administration precluded him from doing further scientific investigations. Unfortunately number two, Mendel's paper was published in a journal that wasn't read by most scientists in the field. Kind of unfortunate number three, his conclusions were so new, so novel, that few people who read the paper would accept them.

In 1901, 35 years later, three botanists (plant biologists) working separately on genetics of plants came to this same conclusion from genetics experiments that Mendel did. They found Mendel's paper, all three of them, which had just been translated from German to English. It was the great rediscovery of Mendel. Rather than bury it and say this guy is not important and we're going to ignore him, they duly recognized him, all three of them, and it's the great rediscovery of the greatness of Mendel. The English translation is an interesting sidebar of this story. English was and is the international language of science. That's just a fact. Any scientist who is serious about being involved in the flow of science worldwide publishes in English. I looked at the scientific journal I published the green tea article in recently, and the editor is French, and there were people from seven different countries publishing papers in that particular issue.

Back to Mendel's experiments. Mendel performed his experiments on pea plants, and he used pea plants for several good reasons. First of all, they were easy to grow in the garden of the monastery. That's important: to use an organism that you can handle, that's easy to grow. Second, Mendel could control which plants mated. The pea flower, the flower of the pea plant, has both male and female reproductive organs. So if Mendel cut off the male parts—the pollen is the male sex cell in a flowering plant—the pollen-producing male organs from a plant's flowers, that's going to be a female plant. Then he would take a camel's hair brush and brush pollen from another plant onto that particular one. So he could control which plant was the male and which plant was the female. You'll note from the last lecture, males and females have equal contributions in general to heredity of offspring. So Mendel had an easy-to-grow thing, and he had an easy-to-manipulate thing for the plants.

Third, there were well-defined genetic strains, genetically different pea plants, that had different phenotypes—the outward expressions of genes. They were different in a single characteristic. For example, there were plants that were tall versus short; that's the height characteristic. There were plants that gave plump spherical seeds or wrinkled seeds; that's another characteristic, seed plumpness. There were plants that gave yellow seeds or green seeds, seed color. All of these varieties that I've described, these pairs, were all true-breeding for their phenotype, for their outward appearance. So when he had a true-breeding plant that formed spherical or plump seeds, and he crossed them among each other, they always formed spherical seeds. They were true breedings; spherical gave rise to spherical. It didn't matter which plant was the male and female. So tall gave rise to tall always, short gave rise to short. These were true breedings. True-breeding wrinkled plants would cross with other wrinkled plants, and they would only form wrinkled offspring.

When Mendel crossed two true-breeding strains with each other for this single characteristic—for example, a plant that gave spherical seeds was crossed with a plant that gave wrinkled seeds (true breeding)—the offspring, the first generation offspring, always, in Mendel's experiment, showed just one of the two characteristics; in this case, "spherical" and "wrinkled." All the offspring showed spherical seeds. All the pea seeds that came out were spherical seeds. He called this characteristic the dominant characteristic; spherical was dominant to wrinkled. Now the characteristic is a phenotype; it's an outward expression. He doesn't know anything yet about genes that determine the phenotype. The one that is not appearing—the wrinkled in this case—he called the recessive characteristic.

Now when he said these things, he said, Wait a minute. There must be two characteristics in this offspring. The offspring looks spherical, but it's a carrier—it's got a spherical character and a wrinkled character. Now he was going against the current idea at the time, which was that the characters disappear, they blend; do you remember? The Dutch tulip breeders said that characters blend rather than remaining discrete particles. Mendel then performed experiments that proved that the particles were still there. He crossed his first generation plants among themselves. I guess that's called plant incest. He crossed his plants that were spherical, but he thought were carrying the characteristic for wrinkled, with other plants of the same genetic composition. And what happened? In the second generation, miraculously, he saw wrinkled plants again. Now, the blending would say you'd never see wrinkled again—or spherical, for that matter. They would have been gone in the first generation.

Now Mendel's mathematics education came into the picture. He counted the seeds of the next generation, the second generation, and he found 5474 seeds were spherical and 1850 were wrinkled. The ratio was three-quarters spherical seeds, one-quarter wrinkled seeds. Now, Mendel got this similar ratio in the second generation from six other pairs of characteristics—you know, tall and short. So when he crossed true-breeding tall with true-breeding short, all of the first generation were tall. But he said they're carriers for that short characteristic, and he got the short back one-quarter of the time in the second generation.

In science, what you try to do is repeat experiments, but you try to do it with other parameters, other characteristics, to generalize. On the basis of all of his data, Mendel made the following proposals. First, he said genetic determinants are particulate; they don't blend. You don't lose them; they're not lost after the fertilization event forms the offspring. They're always there. They're particulate; they don't blend. Second, he proposed that each individual plant has two copies of the hereditary determinant. He called these determinants "elementen"; we call them "genes." One copy, according to Mendel, came from each parent. Third, Mendel proposed that the genes for a particular characteristic like seed shape (spherical vs. wrinkled) can exist in different forms. Again, the forms would be determining sphericalness or wrinkledness. We call these different forms of genes "alleles." In a true-breeding plant, the two alleles that the plant has were the same. So for example, in a spherical plant, there were two alleles for sphericalness, we would call it, if that plant was true-breeding.

In the first generation offspring in Mendel's cross—you'll remember they were spherical but a carrier—he said the two alleles were different: one spherical allele, the other wrinkled allele. We see our terminology now. When I talk about a spherical allele, of course the allele is not, the genetic determinant is not, shaped spherically. It's a jargon term. We're saying yeah, I should say the allele that determines spherical seeds, the allele that determines wrinkled seeds. I'm not going to say that anymore. I'll just call it spherical and wrinkled with the assumption that we mean the allele that determines. Now, one allele, according to Mendel, in this pair would be dominant spherical, and it's expressed in the offspring when it's present together with the recessive allele; in this case, wrinkled. But—the important "but"—the alleles don't disappear, as would be the case if there was blending. That was fundamental, and the major contribution of Mendel.

Now for Mendel's fourth idea. Only one allele, he said, is passed on from a plant or organism to the next generation in the sperm or egg, as plants have sperm and eggs. It's random which allele a particular sperm or egg contains for that characteristic. So, on the average, each plant in the first generation of his seed shape cross—the one that was spherical and was carrying the wrinkled as well—makes half of its sperm or egg cells with the spherical allele and half with the wrinkled allele. He called this the "law of segregation." The alleles segregate when the sex cells are formed because the sex cells only carry one of the two alleles of the organism. It became a law, this law of segregation, in science because after 1900 when these three botanists rediscovered Mendel, and lots of other people did experiments, it became pretty general and applied to most other organisms, not just peas. Mendel also crossed peas with two sets of differing characteristics—for instance, seed shape and height—and these behaved as if they were independent of one another. This he called the "law of independent assortment."

Mendel's laws follow simple laws of probability. Consider two coins. I've got two coins I toss. If I toss one of them and get a head, it's half the time. Half of the time it'll be heads. If I toss the other coin, half of the time it'll be heads. So if I toss both coins, the probability of two heads at once is $1/2 \times 1/2$, or $1/4$. Let's go back to our spherical plant that was a carrier; it had a spherical allele and a wrinkled allele. One-half of its gametes, or sex cells, will have the wrinkled allele. By the same token, if it crosses with a similar plant, one-half of them will have the wrinkled allele. So the probability of getting wrinkled seeds is $1/2 \times 1/2$, or $1/4$, and that's exactly the numbers that Mendel got.

Mendel's laws apply to most organisms, including humans. We can't do genetic crosses in humans; it's unethical. So to determine genes and alleles in humans, we look at phenotypes and rely on the past. We do a pedigree. A pedigree is a genealogy with inherited characteristics. For instance, consider an unusual allele that happens to be inherited as a dominant; for example, Huntington's disease is a disease in people that is determined by an allele inherited as a dominant. That means that everyone who has Huntington's disease inherited that dominant allele from at least one of their parents, so you see that in the pedigree. For "albinism," albino, which is inherited as a recessive, everybody who is an albino inherited one allele from one of the albino recessive alleles from both parents, and so both parents are at least carriers for it. And so a physician dealing with an inherited disease and a new patient will always do a family tree, a genealogy, and then draw out the pedigree, which is the genealogy with the phenotypes as well as the genotypes. This is a way of doing genetics based on surmising. We really don't know much about the genes, but we can surmise based on the phenotypes that we see in a family tree.

Now some terms here. If the two alleles are the same in a particular organism—for example, a person who is albino inherits a recessive allele from each parent—because it's a recessive it's only expressed if both alleles are recessive. If the dominant allele for skin pigmentation is there, you have skin pigmentation. It doesn't matter if the recessive happens to be there also; the dominant supplies enough pigmentation. We call a person who has two alleles identical a "homozygote." The zygote is the fertilized egg; "homo" means the same. So a person is homozygous for a given allele if both alleles for a characteristic are the same. For example, our wrinkled seeds were homozygous for wrinkled. Our round-seeded plants that were true-breeding were homozygous for spherical rather than round; we can call it spherical. If the two alleles are different, as in the first generation of Mendel's seed cross—where the plant had one allele that gave spherical seeds, and the other allele gave wrinkled seeds—it is called "heterozygous." Homozygous and heterozygous; I'll be using these terms in the remaining part of the course.

I've talked about Mendel, Mendel's experiments on peas that were extended to other organisms, and I've described how his laws of genetics apply to humans as well. But not all inheritance is straightforward and follows what are called the Mendelian laws. You know you're a big-shot scientist when they turn your name into an adjective: Mendel to Mendelian. In codominance, both alleles—remember, we only have two—are expressed. A good example of that is what's called the ABO blood type system in humans. The ABO blood type involves three different alleles. The alleles are coding for determining A, determining B, and determining O. Now A, B, and O are chemicals on the surface of red blood cells. If a person has an A, or a B, or an O, you can detect it quite readily, especially if they're homozygous for O, or A, or B.

Here's how it works and why it's called codominance. I am a type A person. Now that doesn't mean my personality is type A; it means my blood is type A, which means on the surface of my red blood cells is this A marker, this A chemical that is genetically determined. Now A and B turn out to be codominant—they're both expressed—but both of them are dominant to O, so O is recessive. So if I am type A, it means I inherited an A from one of my parents, and the other allele I have is either A (I'm homozygous) or O, because O is recessive, and I'm heterozygous. Is that clear so far?

If you were type B, you'd have a B from one parent and either another B or an O. But if you're type AB, you inherit an A from one parent and a B from another parent, and both of them show up. That's called codominance. Both of them are expressed; there's no dominant or recessive between A and B. A person of type O blood is OO; they have an O from one parent and an O from another. They're like the plant with wrinkled seeds. They are homozygous for the recessive. This is a good example of codominance. It's also a good example of something called multiple alleles. They're not just two alleles, tall and short, spherical and wrinkled. There's three—A, B, and O—and there are many, many characteristics in many organisms that are determined by multiple alleles.

Some characteristics are determined by genes that interact, different genes and their alleles that interact. The best example of that is coat color in many animals: horses, dogs. Many, many animals have coat color that is determined by multiple alleles. For example, in Labrador retrievers, for you dog owners, there are two genes, B and E, involved to make the black pigment. When those two genes are present in their dominant form, regardless of what the other allele is—so you could have the dominant B with the recessive B or the dominant B with the dominant B; it doesn't matter. When both B and E are present, the dog is black. If only E is present as a dominant allele, and B is recessive—so we have two recessive B alleles and a dominant E allele—the dog is brown. In the cases where we have two recessive E alleles, regardless of what the other alleles are, the dog is yellow. So dominant B/dominant E, black; dominant E/recessive B, brown; and recessive E regardless of the Bs, yellow. It's a little bit more complicated than the simple genetics that Mendel had. The principles of segregation, independent assortment, that Mendel had are the same. It's just that the phenotype is more complex in its determination.

Many complex characteristics of organisms are determined by the interactions of many genes, and alleles as well; not just two. So, for example, consider height in humans. Height in humans is determined by a wide variety of genes, many genes; not a single gene, as we showed in plants, tall versus short. Actually, Mendel was lucky because in most plants, height is determined by a number of genes. I'll describe this later on when I talk about wheat plants and agricultural genetics in Lecture Twenty-Three. You can think of what some of these genes determining height in humans might be: genes that determine the length of bones, genes that determine hormones like the growth hormone, genes that determine the ability to put calcium into bones to build them, genes that determine the ability to assimilate food and build up muscles, etc. There is a complex of genes that determine a phenotype as complicated as height in a human. The genetics here gets very, very sophisticated and statistical, and so we'll talk about this later on when we talk about agricultural genetics. It's not easy and not straightforward, but still, at base, each of these allele pairs is obeying Mendel's laws.

Genes are not destiny. The environment, I have to stress—and I stressed in my previous lecture—plays a vital role. Consider again height in humans. Poor nutrition can lead to a person who is shorter than a person who has good nutrition. And as I mentioned before, my wife may say, "My hair is dark brown with salt and pepper"; my hairdresser may know my genes are different. With the particulate nature of genes established, we turn now in the next lecture to how genes fit into cells, the basic units of life. Thank you.

Lecture Three
Genes and Chromosomes

Scope: Animals and plants are made up of many cells. These units of biological structure and function have the fundamental characteristics of life, including chemical complexity, the ability to regulate what enters and leaves the cell, the ability to grow, and the capacity to reproduce. Even tiny bacteria are cells; viruses, which must infect cells to function, are not. The cell nucleus contains its genes, and cloning experiments show that a specialized cell has all of the genes for the organism of which it is a part. Within the nucleus, genes are carried on structures called chromosomes. These are duplicated before a cell reproduces. There are two chromosome sets—and two gene sets, as Mendel proposed—in every somatic (body) cell nucleus, but there is only one set in the sperm or egg cell, again, as Mendel proposed. With many more genes than chromosomes, each chromosome must carry many genes. For instance, the 24,000 genes in humans are carried on 23 chromosomes. In mammals, including humans, the X and Y chromosomes are a special pair. The X has many genes not present on the Y, which has the gene for maleness. Genes present on the X chromosome will always be expressed in males.

Outline

I. Opening story. You do not have to be a geneticist to figure out genetics.

    A. In the Jewish religion, all males must be circumcised as a symbol of their covenant with God.

    B. In the Babylonian Talmud, an ancient commentary on the Bible written about A.D. 500, the rabbis had a dilemma: Boys were bleeding to death during circumcision.

    C. The rabbis noted that the boys who bled to death were all the sons of certain mothers. It did not matter who the father was. They exempted further sons from these mothers from circumcision. They made their judgment based on observations of genetic pedigrees.

     D. We now know that the boys were dying because of the disease hemophilia, which is inherited through the X chromosome of the mother.

II. Cells carry genes.

    A. Complex organisms are made up of cells.

        1. Two kinds of pneumonia with similar symptoms can define what a cell is. The agent causing the first kind of pneumonia can be observed under a common microscope as a rod-shaped object, about 1-millionth of a meter (1 thousandth of a millimeter) across. This infectious agent, a bacterium, can grow and reproduce in a laboratory dish if supplied with simple nutrients such as sugars. It is made up of thousands of different types of chemical substances.

        2. The second type of pneumonia is caused by a much smaller agent, 1% the size of a bacterium. This infectious agent, a virus, cannot grow and reproduce on its own in the lab; it needs to infect living tissue. It is chemically simple.

        3. Bacteria are cells. Viruses are not cells.

    B. Cells are the basic building blocks of biology.

        1. All living things are made up of cells.

        2. Cells exhibit the characteristics of life: They are complex, have many chemical reactions, can determine what comes in and out, can grow, and can reproduce. While nonliving things can do some of these things, only cells can do all of them.

        3. Cells are the unit of biological continuity. Complex organisms reproduce by cells (e.g., sperm and egg). So these cells must contain genes.

    C. There are two types of cells.

        1. Those without complex internal structures are called prokaryotic (e.g., bacteria).

        2. Eukaryotic cells (e.g., liver cells) have complex internal structures for compartmentalization of functions. One of these structures is the cell nucleus.

III. The cell nucleus contains the genes.

    A. Experiments define the genetic role of the nucleus.

        1. Removal of the nucleus from a single-celled amoeba leads to cell death.

  2. Swapping of the nucleus between species of a single-celled plant called *Acetabularia* leads to the new cell having the genetic characteristics of the nucleus it received.

  3. In 1958, Frederick Steward took a specialized cell from a carrot plant, and by putting it into a special chemical environment he was able to coax the cell to act like a fertilized egg and grow into a whole plant. This cloning experiment showed that the nucleus of a specialized cell has all of the genetic determinants of the organism: It is totipotent.

 B. Genes in the nucleus are carried on large, visible structures called chromosomes that are visible during cell reproduction (also called cell division).

IV. Chromosomes carry genes.

 A. Chromosomes provide an explanation for Mendel's genetics laws.

  1. There are two copies of every chromosome in every nonsex cell (also called somatic cells).

  2. When cells divide, the chromosomes reproduce prior to separation so that each of the two new cells gets a full set of the original chromosomes.

  3. There is only one copy of each chromosome pair in the sex cells (gametes).

 B. Specific genes have been linked to specific chromosomes.

  1. The full set of chromosomes with genes is the genome. Because there are thousands of genes (humans have 24,000) and few chromosomes (humans have 23 pairs) there must be many genes on each chromosome. The genome is like a library: The chromosomes are its volumes, and the genes are paragraphs.

  2. In mammals, including humans, the X and Y chromosomes are an exception to the rule that chromosomes come in complete pairs. The X has many genes, but the Y has only a few, most notably the gene that determines male sex. So any person with a Y chromosome is a male.

  3. Males have only one copy of most genes carried on the X chromosome (they are not on the Y). So any recessive allele on the X chromosome will be expressed in males. In females, a dominant gene on the other X chromosome would mask the expression of the recessive allele.

4. The most common form of hemophilia (see opening story) and red-green colorblindness are caused by recessive alleles carried on the X chromosome. So these characteristics are much more common in males than in females.

5. For the majority of human characteristics whose genes are carried on nonsex chromosomes (also called autosomes), there is no preferential sex distribution.

6. Primary sex, the formation of sperm or eggs, is determined genetically by the presence of a gene called SRY on the Y chromosome.

7. Secondary sex, the appearance of male or female body parts such as developed breasts, body hair, muscular development, etc., is also genetically determined, but by a different set of genes. In this case, the genes involved are responsible for hormone signaling involving such familiar hormones as testosterone (males) and estrogen (females).

Essential Reading:

Benjamin Pierce, *Genetics: A Conceptual Approach* (New York: W. H. Freeman and Co., 2005), chap. 4.

David Sadava, Craig Heller, Gordon Orians, William Purves, and David Hillis, *Life: The Science of Biology*, 8th ed. (Sunderland, MA: Sinauer Associates; New York: W. H. Freeman and Co., 2008), chap. 10.

Supplemental Reading:

Martin Brookes, *Fly: The Unsung Hero of 20th-Century Science* (New York: HarperCollins, 2001).

Matt Ridley, *Genome: The Autobiography of a Species in 23 Chapters* (New York: HarperCollins, 2006).

Questions to Consider:

1. The cloning of Dolly the sheep involved transferring the nucleus of a specialized sheep cell (the donor) into a sheep egg cell (recipient) whose nucleus had been removed. Following chemical stimulation, the egg acted like it had been fertilized and divided to form an embryo. The embryo was surgically implanted into a foster mother (surrogate) and grew to a lamb, Dolly. Was Dolly genetically identical to the donor, recipient, or surrogate? What does this result indicate about the genetic capacity of the nucleus?

2. If cells are the unit of life, where did the first cells on Earth come from? Two scientific ideas are that they came from another place in the solar system (life may have existed on other planets and/or their moons) or that cellular life evolved from chemicals on Earth. Which of these ideas is most intellectually and emotionally satisfying to you?

Lecture Three—Transcript
Genes and Chromosomes

Welcome back. The subjects of this lecture are genes and chromosomes. In the last lecture, I described how the nature of genes as particles was first defined by Mendel and was later shown to be true in all other organisms. Now, we define the gene further in terms of its particulate nature.

My opening story concerns people who weren't geneticists, weren't scientists, weren't even doctors and who figured out some genetics. It's an old story—a very old story. In the Jewish religion, all males must be circumcised as a symbol of their covenant with their God. In the Old Testament, the first story of this was with Abraham, the founder of the Jewish religion, and it was later codified in the book of Exodus with Moses. As in almost all religions, scholars spend a lot of time trying to figure out what the ancient texts mean, and the Jewish religion is no exception. There have been many, many commentaries written by rabbis, the Jewish teachers or ministers, about the Old Testament. One of the most remarkable is the Babylonian Talmud. The Babylonian Talmud is a commentary on the Old Testament, the five books of Moses, and this commentary was written in pieces from about 400 B.C. to about A.D. 200. Now, let's picture what's happening here. Here are Jews wandering around out in the dessert with their Ark of the Covenant trying to figure out what God was really telling them in these texts. In one passage, the rabbis have a dilemma. Boys are bleeding to death when they are infants and they are circumcised. What's going on? Well, the boys have to be circumcised. Otherwise, they're not going to be admitted into the Jewish religion, but dying is not a good idea. What the rabbis note in this Biblical commentary was that the boys who bled to death were all the sons of certain mothers. Now, in those days, you may know, women had children virtually every year during their reproductive lives. Many children would die in infancy because of infectious disease or other reasons. They were essentially producing a lot of kids.

The boys dying, as I mentioned, were all the sons of certain mothers. That is, the mother would have one boy that died, and then she might have a normal boy, a girl, and then she might a couple of years later have another boy that died. Records were being kept by the rabbis of this. So, the rabbis decided to create some rules for circumcision in the case of the boys that were dying. That is, they looked at the pedigrees of these children. They didn't actually draw out the pedigrees. They described them in their biblical commentary, and what they described was that if a woman even remarried, she still would oddly produce some children who had this obvious disease of bleeding to death.

So, they decided that after a woman had more than two sons who bled to death, all further sons were exempt. They were the only males who were ever exempt from this circumcision rite. And it didn't matter who she was married to; it seemed to be passed through the mother. They described in this passage a series in which there were two sisters, both of whom had sons who died. In this instance, they said, if two sisters have sons that die, both of their sons will be exempt from circumcision. Without knowing anything about genes and chromosomes, these rabbis, working probably 2000 years ago trying to figure out what God was telling them in their Bible, had described a genetic disease called hemophilia and had described a type of inheritance called sex linkage, or X-chromosome linkage.

Now, today we know all about this particular disease. In fact, through biotechnology, as I'll describe later on in the course, the missing phenotype—that is the chemical that's missing in the children who have hemophilia—has been purified and manufactured by biotechnology. Now, it's very unusual for someone to die of this bleeding disease. You can just give this child, or an adult who has hemophilia, the mystery blood clotting factor, and that's what it turns out to be. These are called the hemophilia rules. So, you really don't have to be a scientist or a geneticist to figure out genetics. You could just be a theologian trying to figure out what your God is telling you.

I want to talk about the particulate nature of genes now, and first I'll describe how cells carry genes and what cells are. Then we'll begin to narrow it down. Where are the genes in the cell? Well, they're in the cell nucleus, so I'll describe what the cell nucleus is and how we know the nucleus carries the genes. Finally, I'll even narrow it more to describe how chromosomes inside the nucleus carry the genes. So, you see we're going from organism, to cell, to nucleus, to chromosome. Remember, mechanism is one of the major ideas of biology. We're not giving up, saying, "Genes are mysterious. They're part of the vital force, so we'll stop there." We're saying, "There is a chemical or physical explanation. We'll keep looking for it."

What's a cell? Well, I described earlier on in cell theory that complex organisms are made up of cells. Remember, that's another one of the major ideas of biology besides mechanism and evolution. I'll define cells by looking at a human disease, an infectious disease: pneumonia. You may be familiar with what pneumonia is. Many people still die of pneumonia every year even in hospitals. Pneumonia begins with chills and fever and a cough. It's obviously a disease of the lungs, and in that cough is, well, we'll call it phlegm. We'll call it sputum. That's a fancy word. How about that? That's the medical term, sputum, for the gunk that you cough up when you have pneumonia. Let's use a medical term, and we can impress people rather than calling it gunk.

Now, how do we find out how pneumonia is transmitted? Well, it's pretty clear. We find out by looking at the pattern of transmission, and what you find is it's transmitted when one person sneezes on another. So, droplets of the sputum are in the air, and some of those droplets end up being breathed in. Whatever the organism is that's infecting a person and causing the disease is in that sputum, and then it gets inside the other person, and that's how it spreads. How do we identify the causative agent? Identifying causative agents that are very small, microscopic, is the province of a field of biology called microbiology, and the founder of modern microbiology lived in the 19th century. He was a German named Robert Koch. Robert Koch came up with a series of experiments that would provide evidence that an infective agent causes a disease. Just knowing that the infective agent is there is not enough. You have to perform a dynamic series of experiments. Biology as a science doesn't do well with correlations. Correlations are more the province of advertising, right? You'll be happy if you have this car. Happiness and car go together. Or politics—the economy is bad because of this politician. That's not necessarily cause and effect. That's two events happening at the same time. That's a correlation. Just because an infective agent is present with the disease, it doesn't necessarily indicate that it causes the disease. For the cause we have to do science, and science means experiment.

Robert Koch proposed his postulates, or experimental scheme, and his experimental scheme is in four parts—isolate, infect, symptoms, and repeat. Isolate means you go into the sputum, and you isolate your suspected organism, whatever it is. It might be a bacterium or a protozoan or some other organism—isolate. Then, infect—what you do now is you do an experiment where you infect some creature. Now, in human diseases, we can't infect a human with what we expect to be a disease-causing agent. That's unethical science. We would never think of doing that. So, we use animal models, and this is where animal research turns out to be extremely important. It's the only way to find out if an agent is infective and if that agent will infect an animal. We have to make sure that it's possible. Then we allow the infection to proceed, and now we look for the third aspect of Koch—remember, isolate, infect—symptoms. We look for the same symptoms, in this case pneumonia, in the animal and see that the animal has a disease similar to the human disease. Finally, repeat, which means we re-isolate the suspected disease-causing agent from the animal, and we repeat with a second animal—isolate, infect, symptoms, and repeat. This series of experiments has gone on for infective agents since Robert Koch's time.

If you look at pneumonia, there are two different kinds of organisms that we can isolate, and their behavior and their chemistry and their biology are very different. Yet they both cause pneumonia. The first type of organism is very small. You can't see it with the naked eye. In fact, it's a rod-shaped or spherical object about one micrometer in size. What's a micro? A micrometer is a millionth of a meter or a thousandth of a millimeter across. Now, I put my two fingers together. The closest you can see those two fingers apart is about a half of a millimeter. That's about the limit of the human eye to see. So, we can't see things that are smaller. Well, this agent is smaller than that, so you have to use a microscope to see it. If you take this agent and you prove that it causes pneumonia by Koch's experimental series, you can grow it in the laboratory if you supply it with sugars, and water, and things for it to grow. It will grow and reproduce very quickly. If you look at its chemistry, it's very complex. It's got thousands of different chemicals inside of it—water being the majority, but thousands of other chemicals as well. This is a bacterium. The name of the bacterium is *Pneumococcus*, and the bacterium will grow in a laboratory setting.

The second type of agent also causes pneumonia. Just like Koch's postulates, it goes through all of the experimental series—isolate, infect, symptoms, and then repeat. The second agent is much smaller than the other agent that causes pneumonia. It's about 1% the size. You can't even see that through a regular microscope. You've got to use a fancy microscope called an electron microscope that magnifies even more. This thing is very different from the bacteria. It's not only smaller, but it can't grow and reproduce on its own in a laboratory environment. It needs other tissues to grow. It's a parasite in its growth characteristics, and it's chemically simple. It's a virus. In this case the virus is called respiratory syncytial virus.

Bacteria—they're complex and exhibit all of the characteristics of living things—are cells. Viruses, much simpler, are not cells.

Cell theory tells us cells make up living things. In the case of bacteria, they are living things. Cells exhibit all of the characteristics of living things. For example, some of these characteristics are that they're complex. Viruses, of course, are very simple. Living things have many chemical reactions that go on in them. Living things have the ability to grow and reproduce. Living things can determine what comes in and out. They have a boundary between them and the environment that determines what things come in and out of the cells. Nonliving things can't do all of these things. Snowballs can grow. Snowballs can reproduce, right, but snowballs can't refashion things inside. They don't have these complex chemical reactions, and snowballs can't say, well, I'm going to let some snow in and not let snow in. They don't have this ability to determine what comes in and out. So, cells have all of these characteristics. There are two types of cells in nature. We recognize prokaryotic cells. The term *karyon* does not mean baggage. It means a body. It's a Greek term that means the body. *Prokaryon* means "before the body." It's a cell that is relatively simple. It doesn't have complex bodies inside of it. So, bacteria are examples of a prokaryotic cell. You'll know what I mean when I talk about the other type, which are the eukaryotic, the true cells of complex organisms, like cells in us. They all have complex internal substructures including the most obvious cell structure, which is the cell nucleus. When you look at a cell under the microscope, the cell nucleus is by far the most important and prominent part of the cell.

The cell nucleus is where the genes reside. Now, how do we know this? We know it through experiments, not by just saying that's where the genes are but by proving that's where the genes are by experiment. Let's do a couple of experiments on the cell nucleus. One of the cells that's a favorite of high school biology and grade school biology is the amoeba. It's this blob-shaped thing. It's pretty big, a couple of hundred micrometers in size, and it kind of flows around on a microscope slide. You see a nucleus inside the amoeba, and because it's so big, we can do the following experiment. We take a glorified straw—now in science we don't use the term "straw." We use the term "pipette." It's a glass straw. Okay, it's a straw. We suck out the nucleus. So, we puncture the boundary of the cell, and we suck out the nucleus. We're going to see what happens. Now, of course we have to compare that to a cell that is equally treated but you don't suck out the nucleus. So, we do what's called a sham, or fake, operation where we puncture the cell but we don't suck out the nucleus. So, we do exactly the same things, but we don't suck out the nucleus. Well, what happens? The cell with the nucleus survives. The cell without the nucleus dies. Conclusion—the nucleus is vital to the survival of the cell. Please send Nobel Prize to the following address …

That doesn't tell us much about genetics. Well, we can start looking at genetics when we look at cells that have a little bit more complexity. There's a plant called *Acetabularia* that lives in the intertidal zone, in the Pacific Northwest through western Canada, and this cell has specialized parts to it. The specialized part is on the top of the cell. It adheres to a rock with the bottom of the cell, has a nucleus, and the specialized part is on the top. One of the amazing things about this organism is you can cut it off, and if you cut off the top, it regenerates the specialized part. Now, there are different species. One of these species has a top that looks like an umbrella. Another has a top that looks like a flower—so they have different-shaped tops. A series of experiments has been done that shows that it's the nucleus part that determines what the top will be. If we cut off the top from the cell and the nucleus is still there, it will regenerate a top but it's always species specific. So, now we know that the cell nucleus determines genetically the inheritance of this particular organism—what type of top it will make.

What about complex organisms like a carrot? A carrot has a root, a stem, a leaf, a flower, and the root has different tissues, etc. The part of the carrot we eat is the carrot root, and it has different types of tissues inside of it just like your arm has different tissues. It's got muscle and bone, etc. The carrot root has different tissues. In 1958, Frederick Steward at Cornell University took a specialized cell from the root of a carrot and asked the following question: Does the nucleus of that specialized cell still have all of the genes for the rest of the cells of the organism? We know that the fertilized egg of the carrot is totipotent, meaning it has the potential to be everything, to be "toti." In other words, it has all of the genetic information to form the root, the stem, the leaf, and the flower. What about when the cell specializes? Does this nucleus still have that genetic information?

Steward did the following experiment, and it's a very historic experiment even though it's almost 50 years old. He took the root of a carrot plant, took some cells out of it, put them in a defined chemical medium, and lo and behold, the chemical medium that he defined, which was an embryo extract, told this root cell to stop being a root cell and start being an embryo. It reverted to where it was before, and it divided and formed a carrot embryo and formed an entire carrot plant that would reproduce. If he took ten cells from the carrot, he got ten identical plants. These cells are cloned—a clone is an identical group of cells or organisms that is genetically the same as the original progenitor of that group of cells or organisms. Here we could have ten carrot plants that came from a single carrot. Now, the cloning aspect is something we'll come back to later on in the course. The genetic aspect is what I want to emphasize here, and that is that the carrot root cell hasn't lost any of its genetic capabilities. It has all of the genes to give a whole carrot.

Now, the gene in the nucleus is carried on large, visible structures called chromosomes, and I want to turn to them now as our quest to further define the gene goes on and gets down to a finer physical level. Chromosomes provide an explanation for Mendel's laws of genetics. Remember what Mendel said? Mendel said that every organism has two copies of every gene, every element—one from mom and one from dad, one from the male and one from the female. By the same token, every organism has two copies of every chromosome. Genes are located on long strands of genetic material that are packaged into compact structures called chromosomes. We can see the chromosomes when cells reproduce. Now, when cells reproduce, all of the genes have to duplicate because if I have 10 genes, 5 from mom and 5 from dad, let's say, and I want to produce two new cells from one cell, if there are 10 genes in that cell, I have to have 10 genes in each of the new cells. So, that implies that before reproduction happens, before these genes are separated, I have to duplicate them. That's exactly what happens. There's this dance of the chromosomes in this beautiful process called cell division. It's really cell reproduction, in which the chromosomes first duplicate, and then one copy of each chromosome goes to the end of the cell. Then two nuclei form, and the important thing is these two nuclei in the new cell contain, each of them, a complete set of all of the chromosomes. So, the chromosomes have to duplicate before.

In humans, there are 23 pairs of chromosomes. For each pair, of course, we inherit one from mom and one from dad. Our gametes, or sex cells—eggs or sperm—contain one copy of each of these chromosomes. So, a gamete will have only 23 chromosomes and not 23 pairs. Specific genes have been linked to specific chromosomes, and since we have undertaken genome sequencing, we know with quite a degree of specificity where genes are on which chromosomes. As I mentioned, because humans have 24,000 genes and 23 pairs of chromosomes, we have about 1000 genes per chromosome. Think of the genome, the entire genetic complement, the sum total of all the genes, as a library, and the chromosomes as volumes, and the genes as paragraphs. That's a good way to look at it.

Now, in mammals, which include us, there's a special set of chromosomes, and this special set of chromosomes are the X and Y chromosomes. The X and Y are rather different from each other. The X is a large chromosome typical of most chromosomes, and it contains several thousand genes. The Y chromosome contains very few genes even though it's part of the pair with the X. People with Y chromosomes are males. People without Y chromosomes are females. Now, everyone has X chromosomes because X chromosomes contain many genes that are essential to the survival of a human or other mammal. It just happens to be one of those volumes in the encyclopedia, but it's the Y chromosome uniquely that contains the male-determining gene.

Now, first of all, how do we know that the Y chromosome is necessary for maleness? Well, that's not too hard. We know it from clinical cases. Some people inherit more chromosomes through some abnormalities in cell division when forming gametes from their parents. So, for example, there are people who have not an X and a Y but instead have an X, an X, and a Y: two Xs and a Y. So, these people have 23 pairs of chromosomes and one more: 47 chromosomes. The X, X, Y: The person is a male even though they have two Xs. There are people who have X, X, X, Y: male. There are other people who have 45 chromosomes and just an X. Now, you have to have at least one copy of every chromosome. You're not going to be missing 1000 genes and survive, and if they have one X chromosome with no other chromosome along with it, they have, of course, 45 chromosomes: 22 pairs plus the X. These people are female. So, it's the Y chromosome that determines maleness.

In fact, in the embryo, we all start out looking like a female in our anatomy very early on in the human embryo, and if the Y chromosome is present, the female plumbing kind of is degenerated and the male takes over. It's an interesting way to look at life to say we all start out in some ways looking like women. What are the genes on the X chromosome? We know the genes on the Y for maleness. The genes on the X chromosome include the gene involved in blood clotting that is defective in hemophilia, which I described earlier on in the opening story. Another gene on the X chromosome is a gene which, when defective, leads to red-green color blindness. Both of these are recessive, and they are both much more common in males than females. Why? Well, again, think of a male. A male has a Y chromosome that doesn't have the genes that are on the X. So, any gene in the X, dominant or recessive, will be expressed in males whereas if a female inherits, for example, the recessive allele that would lead to hemophilia, that woman will not express that recessive allele if she also has the dominant allele on her other X. So, that's why X-linked abnormalities are much more common in males than females.

Sex determination, male or female, forming sperm or eggs, is called "primary sex," and to show you how genetics works, scientists have recently been able to narrow down even on the X chromosome the location and identity of the sex-determining region. The sex-determining region on the Y chromosome is called not surprising, SRY. Listen—SRY, well "S," sex-determining; "R," region; "Y," on the Y chromosome. Now, we know it's there somewhere. How are we going to find out where it is? Well, take the case of a girl who had an X and a Y chromosome. The doctor went, "What? You have a Y chromosome. You must be a boy. How could you be a girl and have an X and a Y chromosome?" When they looked carefully, they found a very small piece of the Y chromosome was missing, and they figured, uh-oh, that's the region that causes maleness. It must be missing.

Take the case of a boy who is XX, 46 chromosomes, two Xs, no Y. When they looked carefully at his chromosomes, they found an additional piece of genetic material on one of his chromosomes. It turned out to be, you guessed it, that same piece that was missing in that girl—the sex-determining region on the Y chromosome. The lesson in this, and the reason I bring it up, is that these clinical cases tell us cause and effect in biology. By looking at what goes wrong, we can infer it in the normal situation and what is right. So, science can do experiments in this way, not actually manipulating themselves the chromosomes but by looking at people who are born with already defective chromosomes in some way.

Secondary sex, the outward appearance of us, the deep voice of men and the hair on the chest, or the higher voice on women and breast development, et cetera, is determined by hormones. It's not determined by the X and the Y chromosomes. The hormones will be familiar to you, estrogen in women and testosterone in men.

In this lecture, I've tried to describe the particulate nature of genes all the way down now to a specific region on a chromosome. Now, we turn to the chemical identification of the genetic material, and that is DNA, in the next lecture. Thank you.

Lecture Four
The Search for the Gene—DNA

Scope: The link between smoking and lung cancer, long proposed from clinical case histories and population studies, only became incontrovertibly strong after a substance from cigarette smoke was shown to cause genetic damage on DNA. To act as the genetic material, DNA must contain information, must duplicate (replicate) accurately and change (mutate) occasionally, and must be able to be expressed. There was early circumstantial evidence from its location in the nucleus and amount that DNA might be the genetic material. But this was only demonstrated conclusively by dynamic experiments. First, scientists isolated DNA from one genetic strain of bacteria, introduced it into a second, different strain, and showed that the second strain was genetically transformed into the first one. Later, this was repeated on many other kinds of cells from many different organisms. DNA was even shown to be the genetic material of viruses, being injected into host cells to convert them into virus manufacturers.

Outline

I. Opening story.
   A. The smoking gun is in DNA.
      1. In 1948, Ernst Wynder, a medical student at Washington University in St. Louis, attended an autopsy of a man who died of lung cancer. He noticed that the lungs were black, and when he saw the man's medical record he knew why: The man was a long-term cigarette smoker of two packs a day.
      2. Curious, Wynder looked at many more such cases over the next two years. Using a case-control approach, he found that comparing 649 cases (lung cancer) with 600 controls (no lung cancer), the rate of smoking was 40 times higher in the cases. This is the science of epidemiology.
      3. At the same time, British scientist Richard Doll was doing a cohort study. He followed doctors who smoked and those who did not over many years and found that far more smokers developed lung cancer.

4. However, these studies were controversial. For instance, people who had lung cancer might have been exposed to more air pollution or have a poor diet.

5. Finally, in the 1990s an incontrovertible link was found between smoking and lung cancer. As we will see later in the course, cancer is in part caused by genetic damage. A gene called p53 gets mutated (permanently changed). In cancerous lung tissues, these changes occur only at certain locations in the gene, called "hot spots."

6. When tobacco smoke was analyzed by sophisticated chemical machines to separate out its many products, one, called benzpyrene (BP) stood out. In the lung, BP is converted to a highly active form called BPDE, and it is this that binds to and damages genes. When scientists looked at the p53 gene in the lungs of smokers, they found BPDE binding to it and causing damage—right at the hot spots for genetic change. This closed the circle of evidence.

B. The p53 gene, like all other genes in most organisms, is made of DNA.

II. DNA fits several requirements for the genetic material.

A. It must be able to contain lots of information. Organisms have many genes (humans have 24,000), and these can be and are encoded by DNA. Few other molecules have the ability to carry so much information.

B. It must be able to replicate (a scientific word for duplicate) in an error-free fashion. A human has 60 trillion cells. These came from a single cell, the fertilized egg. Imagine the consequences if replication had a lot of errors that were then perpetuated. As we will see, DNA replication is impressively accurate.

C. It must be able to be expressed as the phenotype. As we have seen, genes encode the capability for phenotype: A gene in peas gives them the capacity to form spherical seeds, for example. It turns out that the substances ultimately responsible for phenotype, such as pea seed shape, are proteins. Cells have machinery to express DNA, usually as proteins in the phenotype. Of course, this expression can be modified by the environment.

D. It must be able to change. This might seem odd, since we have said that replication must be error free and that damage, as in lung cancer, is harmful. But variation is the spice of life and the raw material for evolution by natural selection. So some errors in genes are a good thing over the long term of generations. As we will see, DNA has ability to mutate.

III. There was circumstantial evidence for DNA as the genetic material.

- **A.** It is in the right place.
    1. A Swiss physician, Friedrich Miescher, had isolated DNA from nuclei of white blood cells in 1868, calling it "nuclein."
    2. Later evidence showed that the nucleus has the genes.
- **B.** It was there in the right amounts.
    1. A dye was developed that quantitatively stained DNA red. When cell nuclei were examined, each species had its own unique content, all somatic cells of that species had the same amounts, and the sex cells had half as much of the DNA as somatic cells. All of this would be expected if DNA was the gene. No other molecule in the nucleus (e.g., proteins) had these quantitative characteristics.
    2. But circumstantial evidence is not cause and effect in science. We need experiments to prove the hypothesis that DNA is the gene.

IV. Experiments proved that DNA is the genetic material.

- **A.** Frederick Griffith got sidetracked as he investigated a vaccine for bacterial pneumonia in 1928. There were no antibiotics yet.
    1. There were two genetic (pure breeding) strains of the bacteria: S, smooth coat (virulent, caused pneumonia in mice); and R, rough coat (not virulent).
    2. He wanted to see if heat-killed S could be used as vaccine to immunize against pneumonia. Heat-killed S did not cause pneumonia. But it did not work as a vaccine in mice.
    3. So he tried combining it with a booster of live R cells (these do not cause pneumonia). Once again, there was no vaccine effect. But to his surprise, the mice injected with heat-killed S and live R got pneumonia! And he found live S cells in their bodies. The dead S cells had genetically transformed the live R cells into live S cells!
    4. Now it became straightforward to find out what the chemical nature of this genetic transformation principle was. It took 15

years. In 1944, Oswald Avery and colleagues identified it as DNA.

5. DNA transformation in all cells has been possible since the 1970s and is now widely used in laboratories.

B. DNA is the genetic material of viruses as well.

1. Just like eukaryotic cells, prokaryotic bacterial cells get attacked by viruses. When a bacteriophage (virus) attaches to a bacterial cell, it injects something into the cell that takes over the cell's chemistry, directing it to be a virus manufacturer. Half an hour later, the cell bursts, releasing several hundred viruses that then go hunting for more cells to infect. Clearly, the genetic material is injected to take over the cell.

2. As noted earlier, viruses are very simple. Bacteriophage have only DNA and proteins. In 1952, Alfred Hershey and Martha Chase set out to show that it was the DNA, not the proteins, that got injected into the bacteria and must be the genetic material.

3. They looked for a way to label proteins and DNA differently. They used two different radioactive atoms, one that was specific for DNA and the other for proteins.

4. Bacteriophage with labeled DNA or protein were allowed to attach to the bacteria and inject genetic material into the cells. Then suspension of cells was agitated in a blender to shake the phage off the cells. The scientists looked inside the cells for some injected phage material. Only labeled DNA entered the cells; labeled protein did not. This showed that the DNA must be the genetic material of viruses as well as cells.

Essential Reading:

Michael Cain, Hans Damman, Robert Lue, and Carol Yoon, *Discover Biology*, 3rd ed. (New York: W. W. Norton, 2007), chap. 12.

David Sadava, Craig Heller, Gordon Orians, William Purves, and David Hillis, *Life: The Science of Biology*, 8th ed. (Sunderland, MA: Sinauer Associates; New York: W. H. Freeman and Co., 2008), chap. 11.

Supplemental Reading:

Anthony Griffiths, Susan Wessler, Richard Lewontin, William Gelbart, David Suzuki, and Jeffrey Miller, *An Introduction to Genetic Analysis*, 8th ed. (New York: W. H. Freeman and Co., 2007).

Benjamin Lewin, *Genes VIII* (Upper Saddle River, NJ: Pearson Prentice-Hall, 2005).

Questions to Consider:

1. There have been many claims of using DNA to transform complex organisms. Early on in the 1950s, scientists reported that injecting white ducks with DNA from black ducks gradually turned the latter ducks black. Others reported that feeding naive animals DNA from the same species of animal that had learned a task made the naive animals smarter. You can even find DNA tablets at stores in the vitamin section. These experiments have never been reliably repeated. Why don't they work?

2. Until 1970, it was very hard to reliably transform cells using DNA. This phenomenon was confined to just a few species, including bacteria that had been used by Griffith and Avery. Then, some scientists discovered that the reason that cells would not take up added DNA was that the surfaces of cells are negatively charged, and so is DNA. Things with the same charge repel one another, so DNA would be repelled from the cells' surface. To get around this, the scientists added a salt to the cells and DNA. This neutralized the charges, and cells readily took up any DNA they were given. This simple method revolutionized genetics, as it made possible all of modern biotechnology. The scientists did not patent this method, and so neither they nor their university have received royalties for their discovery. Jonas Salk, who made the first polio vaccine, likewise did not patent it, saying that he made his discovery for all people and not for himself. Today, scientists take out patents on many of their discoveries. Do you think they should?

Lecture Four—Transcript
The Search for the Gene—DNA

Welcome back. In the previous lecture, I described how scientists began looking for the gene in mechanistic terms. We found genes first in the cell, then in the nucleus—a part of the cell—and then in chromosomes, a part of the nucleus. And at the very end of the lecture, a gene was localized as positioned in a single chromosome, mainly the sex-determining region of the Y chromosome, SRY. In this lecture, we'll see how scientists hit pay dirt and found the gene and identified it as DNA. My opening story describes a smoking gun. In 1948, Ernst Wynder was a medical student at Washington University in St. Louis, and he attended, as medical students do, an autopsy, which is a dissection of a person who is deceased. This man had died of lung cancer, and when they opened him up, Wynder looked at the lungs of this man, and they were totally black.

Wynder noted that these lungs being black was correlated with the fact that the man was a long-term cigarette smoker. He smoked two packs a day for the last 35 years of his life. He was puzzled at this and came to the conclusion that it could be that smoking had something to do with the man's lung cancer. After all, the cigarette smoke got into the lung. Now, the link between smoking and lung cancer was not a new one in medical science in 1948. In fact, when cigarettes were imported to Europe 200 to 300 years before that, there was a link between smoking and cancer. There were publications in the 1600s in England that correlated snuff, which was essentially inhaling tobacco, with oral cancer and cancer of the pharynx and the mouth, so the smoking-cancer link was not a novelty.

Wynder decided to look at it in a more serious way, and he decided to do what is called a case-control study. He compared 649 cases at autopsy of people who died of lung cancer with 600 controls of people of similar age and similar gender who did not die of lung cancer. Then he looked back through their medical records for which ones were the smokers. Wynder found that the lung cancer people had a 40 times greater smoking rate than the people who had no lung cancer. This case-control approach is an example of a science called epidemiology. Now we all know what an epidemic is—it's the rapid spread of a disease in a population. In a more formal sense, epidemiology is the medical study of the states of disease—and no disease—in a population, not necessarily just the spread.

At the same time in the early 1950s that Wynder was doing his study, a British scientist by the name of Richard Doll followed doctors who smoked and doctors who didn't smoke over many years. Now Doll was doing kind of the flip side of what Wynder did. Doll was doing what is called a cohort approach. In the cohort approach, a scientist looks at people who are doing the bad causative thing and people who are not doing the bad causative thing—in this case, smokers versus nonsmokers—and then looks to see which ones are developing lung cancer. Not surprisingly, Doll found that there were far more smokers who developed lung cancer in his sample of doctors.

Now you'd say, doctors smoking? It doesn't make much sense, does it? Well, people at that time thought smoking was a fine and relaxing activity. I can recall buying a magazine for a friend's birthday. You can buy *Life* magazine for the week you were born. They sell these, and you can buy one. On the back cover is a picture of a kindly physician and a patient. The physician obviously is a male, and is smoking a cigarette, and at the bottom it says, you know, this brand of cigarettes is the one favored by most doctors. You won't see that anymore.

Now, there are severe limitations with these kinds of studies: The case-control study where you look at cases and controls and see who is the smoker, or the cohort study where you look at the smokers and nonsmokers and see who gets lung cancer. Here's some of the limitations in interpretation. What if smoking versus nonsmoking is something that relaxes people, and the people who are smokers are generally more stressed and have a bad diet? What if smoking is an activity that poor people do more than wealthy people? The poor people might have an inferior diet; they might be exposed to more air pollution. So equalizing the two groups is very, very difficult in epidemiology. When you open up a daily newspaper or watch TV, almost every day there are epidemiological results reported in populations of people. Always keep in mind the fact that the groups are never quite equal. They're not identical twins that we're comparing. They're usually people of large population groups, and we hope that they're equal in every respect except the variable—in this case, smoking—that we're studying.

So the notion that smoking causes lung cancer was one that still had some doubts for some time. In the 1990s, an incontrovertible link between smoking and lung cancer was found. Later on in this course, I'm going to describe how cancer is caused in large part by damage to genes. In lung cancer, there is a gene called p53. Remember that for later on, but for now just accept the fact that that's the name of the gene, called p53, that gets permanently changed. Permanent changes in genes are called mutations. I want to reiterate that definition because that's a very important term in genetics that I'm introducing for the first time. Mutations are permanent changes in genes, and those changes, therefore, are passed on to the next generation. Now, if the next generation is an offspring—that is, if these genetic changes happen in the cells that produce eggs and sperm—the offspring will inherit those mutations. If the mutation happens in any other cell of the body, it's called a somatic mutation. Somatic cells are the nonsex cells, so every cell in my body except my sperm are somatic cells.

In lung tissues that were cancerous, the p53 gene was mutated, and the mutations occurred along this gene. You can envision the gene as not being a single point, but a piece of information, and certain places where the p53 gene mutated were called "hot spots." In the 1990s, tobacco smoke was analyzed by sophisticated chemical machines to separate out its components, and one of these products stood out as being present in all types of tobacco smoke. There are hundreds of molecules in tobacco smoke; it's not just smoke. One of the molecules that stood out was called benzpyrene; I'll abbreviate it BP. In the lung, benzpyrene is converted to a highly active molecule; that is, a substance that will react with other substances very readily. This substance I will abbreviate BPDE; I'm not going to give you the chemical name. And what BPDE does is it binds to and damages genes.

So now we have BPDE, a derivative of something that's in cigarette smoke, binding to and damaging genes. When scientists in the 1990s looked at the p53 gene—remember, the one that becomes mutated in cancer—they found the smoking gun. They found BPDE actually binding to the p53 gene. They found it in the act of changing the p53 gene. And you'll never guess where they found it. They found it right at the hot spots where this gene is usually changed in lung cancer. This finding in the '90s closed the circle of evidence for smoking and lung cancer. We no longer relied on epidemiology of population studies with all of their possible caveats. This was solid evidence. Now this is not a course on lung cancer; we'll talk about cancer later on in the course. But the point I want to make now is that the p53 gene, like all other genes in humans, is made of DNA, deoxyribonucleic acid. DNA was found by Wynder in these lungs, and Wynder and later people found damaged DNA that was the p53 gene in the lungs of the lung cancer patients.

DNA fulfills the requirements for the genetic material. Now what are those requirements? There are four requirements for genetic material, and those four requirements are the following. First, information storage; second, accurate duplication. Now scientists don't talk about duplication of DNA, making two copies of DNA where there is one. We use the word replication. Don't ask me why we use the word replication. It sounds more scientific, so bear with me. I'll use the word DNA replication here rather than DNA duplication. Third, genetic material must be able to be expressed in some outward way as the phenotype. Just having a gene residing in the nucleus is very different than the outward expression of the gene: hair color, eye color, whatever. And fourth, DNA should be able to change, mutate. We just saw that in a somatic mutation in the lung in lung cancer. DNA has to be able to change because that's just the way the genetic material is; it does get changed sometimes.

Let's go back and describe each one of these. First, storage of information. Most organisms have a lot of genes. The tiniest bacteria have hundreds to a thousand genes. A human has 24,000 genes, a lot more; we're more complicated. These genes are all encoded for by DNA. There are few other substances in the body of an organism that have the ability to carry so much information. You know, we're made up of about 70% water. Could water be an informational molecule? No, it's just H_2O, H_2O, H_2O. There's no difference between one water molecule and the next water molecule. That's not going to carry variable information. It's like building a language from one letter, all Ts. I don't think that would work. DNA has a terrific ability to encode information, and we'll see this as we study it.

Second, DNA must be able to—I'm going to use the word now—replicate in an error-free fashion, or at least as error free as we can. Humans come from a single cell; we all accept that. The single cell is called the fertilized egg. It comes from the egg and sperm. And from that cell come all the cells of the body. Typically, at the last count, a human has 60 trillion cells. That's an estimate, please; no one has made an exact count, 60 trillion. I usually tell my students that professors have at least twice that number of cells because of our complex brains, and the students dutifully write this down and about one minute later put their pens down and look at me in a very strange way. Tenured professors, of course, have even more. Okay, imagine the consequences for duplicating a cell if the DNA, the genetic material, duplicated with a lot of errors. Those errors would accumulate over time, and I've already described how somatic cell errors can lead to cancer. It did in the lung cancer case. So DNA structure, as we'll study later on, is very important to study because it'll tell us that DNA can replicate, duplicate, very accurately.

My third requirement for genetic material is that it should be able to be expressed outwardly as the phenotype. For example, you remember Mendel's pea plants. There were the spherical seeds, coded for by a gene, and the wrinkled seeds, by its mutant—I'll use that word—allele. It turns out that the substances ultimately responsible for the phenotype, such as the spherical seed or the wrinkled seed, are proteins. We'll talk a lot more about proteins in the next lecture. Cells have a machinery to express DNA as proteins in the phenotype. However, and I always will say this, this expression can be modified by the environment. So just because the gene is there, it doesn't necessarily mean that that protein will have its normal function.

My fourth requirement for genetic material is the ability to change. Now that might seem odd, as I said a couple of minutes ago that DNA replication must be error free. You can't have any mistakes when DNA is replicating and cells are dividing; otherwise you'll get cancer or genetic damage. But you know, variation is the spice of life, and when you look around in humans, we don't all look the same. We all have mutations, and there are also environmental differences. Variety is the raw material of evolution by natural selection. You'll recall natural selection in evolution as one of the three major ideas that hold biology together. So some errors in genes might be a good thing because they might be beneficial ones later on. It's a paradox because most of these errors are harmful. So we put up with a lot of harmful errors in DNA duplication to put up with some ones that will be useful later on in terms of evolution. DNA has the ability to mutate. So DNA does fulfill these requirements, and I'll talk about them again when we look at the structure of DNA in more detail.

Now I'd like to describe the evidence for DNA as the gene. There are two types of evidence I'm going to describe. The first type is circumstantial, and the second type is experimental. First, the circumstantial evidence. DNA is in the right place. Where is the right place? It's in the nucleus. We know from evidence, experimental evidence I described previously, that the nucleus is the location of the genetic material. A Swiss physician that I'll describe later on, Friedrich Miescher, in the 1870s isolated DNA from nuclei of white blood cells, and he called it "nuclein." Later it was called nucleic acid, and later DNA. Since the nucleus has the genes, and the DNA is in the nucleus, well, it's in the right place—circumstantial evidence. Of course, nuclei have other things inside of them, notably a lot of different proteins, so we're not quite sure, just because the DNA is there, that the proteins aren't the genetic material.

Well, here's a little bit better piece of circumstantial evidence. It's there in the right amounts. About 70 or 80 years ago, a dye was developed that has the ability to bind to DNA and turn red. The more DNA that's there, the more red color there is there. Now scientists don't look under a microscope at nuclei and say that one's really red, that one's light red, that one's moderately red, that one's super red. That's not good enough. So scientists have instruments that will put numbers on this. And so looking at nuclei that are stained red by this special dye, we can determine how much DNA is in a nucleus. Here's what people found. They found each species—Homo sapiens, humans, pine trees, worms, ants, *E. coli* bacteria—had its own unique DNA content. Well, that's kind of pleasing. It says the amount of DNA is a species-specific thing.

Second, looking at DNA contents, they found, importantly, all somatic cells—remember, those are the cells that are not the sex cells—had the same DNA content. That makes sense. I showed you experiments from the carrot. You'll remember the cloning experiment that F. C. Stewart did that showed that all cells of an organism, somatic cells, have the entire genetic complement, have all genes present. Therefore, they should all have the same DNA content, and they do. That's nice evidence. Third, the sex cells, the gametes, the eggs and sperm, have half the DNA of the somatic cells. Remember Mendel? Mendel said for each—he called them "elementen"; we call them "genes"—a person inherits one from mom and one from dad. So we have two copies of each gene, and only one of those two copies is passed on in the gametes to the next generation. So you would expect half of the genetic material total, half of those two copies—one of those copies of every gene—to be in every gamete, and it is. The gametes have half the DNA of a somatic cell. No other molecule behaves this way—certainly not proteins—in the nucleus.

But this is circumstantial evidence. It's not necessarily cause and effect. Circumstantial evidence, as I've mentioned before, is for politicians who say the economy is terrible because person x happens to be president; whereas an economist might tell you those cycles happen whether we like it or not.

That's circumstantial evidence. Circumstantial evidence is you'll feel better if you ride in this car. That's just circumstantial; it's not necessarily cause and effect. You may feel better just because you're a happier person or because you're listening to The Teaching Company courses. We need experiments to prove the hypothesis that DNA is the gene. Several experiments were done to really prove that DNA is a genetic material, and I want to describe in a little bit of detail two of them.

The first experiment involves bacteria. Now bacteria are nice organisms to work on in the laboratory. They're easy to grow. They have genetic variations. They have true-breeding strains. They grow very rapidly. Bacteria will reproduce once every 30 minutes, so you can get a large number of bacteria very quickly. In 1928, Frederick Griffith, a public health microbiologist—that is, a biologist who studies bacteria but is studying bacteria involved with disease—was investigating making a vaccine for bacterial pneumonia. This is 1928, and there were no antibiotics yet available. Tens of thousands of people every day were dying of pneumonia worldwide, and even in this country the death rate was very, very high, so there was a desperate need for treatment.

Now Griffith had two, just like Mendel did, pure-breeding strains of bacteria. One strain would cause pneumonia if he injected it into mice. The other strain did not cause pneumonia. Now it turned out that the causing of pneumonia was related to a phenotype on the outer surface of the bacteria. The bacteria that caused pneumonia had a smooth coating. The bacteria that didn't cause pneumonia had a rough coating. This has to do with the ability of the bacteria to bind to tissues. Now here's what Griffith figured he would do. He would kill the smooth—that is, the bacteria that causes pneumonia—cells, and he'd kill them by heat. It was well known from Pasteur: Louis Pasteur showed that if you boil bacteria, you kill them. That led to pasteurization. So he decided he'll kill the smooth bacteria, the ones that normally cause pneumonia, and inject them into the animal, and hope that the animal will mount a response to them that will then protect it from a real infection of live bacteria.

Well, first he found that the heat-killed smooth bacteria did not cause pneumonia; that's a good thing. He destroyed them; they didn't cause pneumonia. Then he challenged these mice, who had received his possible vaccine of heat-killed cells, with live smooth bacteria. Unfortunately, it didn't work. The bacteria caused pneumonia, and the mice got the disease. So Griffith scratched his head, and he said well, why don't I try a booster of living cells? We can't use the smooth cells, so he took heat-killed smooth cells—the ones that normally will cause disease, but now they're not—and he gave them a booster of live rough cells, the ones that don't cause disease. His intent was: I'll challenge these in a couple of days. I will add to them; I will inject live smooth bacteria and see if they cause disease now, see if this booster worked.

Well, the upshot of his experiment was the booster didn't work. They still were susceptible to getting the disease. But something very strange happened as he watched the mice during those couple of days before the challenge with the smooth bacteria. Remember what they had in them: They had been injected with dead smooth bacteria and live rough bacteria. What happened was the mice got pneumonia. And Griffith said: Wait a minute. They can't get pneumonia; they have the rough strain that's live in them. The smooth strain is dead. How could they get pneumonia? He looked at the bacteria that were causing this pneumonia in the mice, and they weren't rough bacteria at all. They were smooth bacteria. He said, What have I done? Have I created life and caused these dead smooth bacteria to become live? No, he did some experiments to rule that out.

What he had done was to transform the live rough bacteria into live smooth bacteria. Something in the dead smooth bacteria extract had genetically transformed the rough bacteria into smooth ones. What was this genetic transforming principle, as they called it? It took 15 years to find out what it was. In 1944, Oswald Avery, at Rockefeller University, identified the substance—and it was DNA. So here we have a dynamic experiment. The DNA of a dead cell, of a smooth bacterium, alone could genetically transform a rough bacterium into a smooth one; pretty impressive results. Since the 1970s, it's been possible through chemical techniques to transform any cell we want with DNA from another cell. We could take human cells and add DNA from other sources. We'll talk about this technology later on in the course.

So this experiment that Griffith, and later Avery, reported was very strong evidence for DNA as genetic material of bacteria. A second experiment was concerning the DNA of viruses rather than bacteria. Now the life cycle of a virus is a very interesting thing. A virus is, as I mentioned before when I talked about pneumonia in the previous lecture, a small particle. This small particle is made up of two components. The two components are DNA and protein. There are viruses that actually attack *E. coli* bacteria, just like there are viruses that attack us. What happens is, in the biography of the virus, the virus attaches to the outside of the bacteria. Then something happens. The virus injects something into the bacteria cell and turns the bacteria cell from a bacteria cell into a virus factory. Come back half an hour later, and the bacteria cell is dead, and there's a couple hundred viruses that have been produced.

Now what could that be? It's got to be genetic material that does this. So Alfred Hershey and Martha Chase decided to find out what was injected. What they did was label, using radioactive isotopes, either the protein coat of a virus or the DNA. They were able to do this because there are different radioisotopes that will label proteins or DNA. So now they added a virus to these bacteria cells that was labeled with protein, for example. So now they had the protein labeled with radioactivity, and they let the virus sit in the bacteria, and then they did something rather cruel. They put the thing in a blender, and they shook it very violently. Now the virus, of course, fell off, but not the stuff that was injected; that's already in, right? They asked the question, what's inside? Is there any radioactive protein inside?

Then they did their second experiment where they shook the virus off after having the virus DNA labeled, and they asked, is there DNA labeled inside? Well, only the DNA got inside the cell; only the DNA was entering the cell. Therefore, it's the virus DNA that genetically transforms or changes the bacteria from a bacteria cell to a viral factory. The generality of this—DNA is the genetic material not just of cells like bacteria—but even of particles that sometimes are alive, like viruses. Attention now turned to the nature of DNA itself, and that's the subject of our next lecture. Thank you.

Lecture Five
DNA Structure and Replication

Scope: DNA is a remarkably stable molecule. It has been isolated from fossils and even from a man who was encased in ice for 5000 years. DNA was first purified from nuclei of white blood cells in 1868. When the nucleus was established as the location of the genetic material, attention focused on DNA, and this was intensified by finding DNAs with highly variable sequences of the four bases, A, T, G, and C. Watson and Crick evaluated two lines of evidence from chemistry (in DNA, the proportions of A=T and G=C) and physics (the crystal of DNA is in a helical form) and came up with a double-helical model with A fitting opposite T and G opposite C. This model fits the requirements for genetic material in terms of information content and mutability. DNA is replicated accurately by semiconservative replication where each parental strand serves as a template for a new strand.

Outline

I. Opening story.
   A. The Ice Man and his DNA.
      1. In 1991, hikers in the Alps between Austria and Italy spotted a corpse frozen in the ice, with some tools and a dagger nearby. Four days later, the body, now known as Ice Man, was removed and brought to the University of Innsbruck in Austria, where scientists found that it was 5000 years old. An arrow had killed him, and he froze into the ice.
      2. Remarkably, his DNA was preserved inside his bones. When its information was analyzed, it was similar in its information content to the DNAs of Europeans currently living in the European alpine regions. That DNA lasts so long is testimony to its durability. Its structure is testimony to something else.
   B. DNA as secular icon.
      1. An icon is an image or symbolic representation, often with sacred significance. The 20th century saw the emergence of two great icons that symbolized science in the public mind: the atom, with its whizzing electrons, and DNA— deoxyribonucleic acid—with its double helix.

2. People talk about DNA all the time, as a shorthand. An ad for a financial services company tells customers that it "understands the DNA of business." A perfume called DNA is the "essence of life." A media software system is the "DNA server." A clothing line called DNA Divewear advertises "genetic design-extreme behavior." And of course, a biotechnology company has the stock market symbol DNA.

3. DNA is a subject for artists as well. Salvador Dali used the double helix. A portrait of Nobel laureate Sir John Sulston has parts of his DNA inside bacteria cells. Brazilian artist Eduardo Kac used the chemical building blocks of DNA to translate verses from the Bible; viewers can change the DNA and the verses it represents at will. Playgrounds have DNA-shaped slides. And of course, many DNA-based sculptures adorn the lobbies of laboratories and pharmaceutical companies.

II. Early studies of DNA suggested its structure.

    A. Friedrich Miescher was the first to isolate DNA.

        1. The son of a doctor, Miescher graduated from medical school at the University of Basel. Because of partial deafness, he did not pursue clinical medicine but instead chose a career in research. He began working on the chemistry of the cell nucleus with the German biochemist Ernest Felix Hoppe-Seyler. Using pus from dressings at the nearby hospital, in 1868 Miescher isolated nuclei from white blood cells and then extracted a complex substance rich in phosphorus and nitrogen that he called "nuclein." A student later called it "nucleic acid." It turned out to be DNA. Hoppe-Seyler was so surprised by this novel substance that he personally repeated all Miescher's work before letting him publish it.

        2. Nucleic acid was a curiosity until it was realized that the genetic material resides in the nucleus. Now it became a candidate for the genetic material, along with protein, which is also abundant in the nucleus. In the 1890s, Albrecht Kossel found that nucleic acid was actually a polymer: a long chain of "beads" or monomer units of chemicals. In nucleic acid, these monomers are the nitrogenous bases adenine (A), thymine (T), guanine (G), and cytosine (C).

    B. Chemists analyzed the makeup of DNA.

1. In New York, Phoebus Levene spent the first 30 years of the 20th century studying DNA. He found that the four bases (A, T, G, and C) were not linked to each other in a direct chain. Rather, they were attached to a backbone of sugar and phosphate. The sugar is deoxyribose; hence the name *d*eoxyribo*n*ucleic *a*cid (DNA).

2. Levene proposed that DNA was a very, very, very, long chain consisting of repeating units of ATGC: something like ATGCATGCATGCATGC, etc. If he was correct, and he thought he was, this meant that DNA lacked the variable information content to be the genetic material. Levene was a towering intellectual figure, and so most people believed him. Attention focused on proteins as the gene.

3. During the late 1940s, another great biochemist took a stab at DNA. Erwin Chargaff, at Columbia University, found that DNA was not just a repeating four-unit structure but was highly variable: ATCGTTCAATACGATGACTT, etc. The information content was there. This came at the same time as the identification of DNA as the genetic material in experiments on bacteria and viruses.

4. Chargaff made another discovery whose significance came to be fully appreciated soon after: For each species he examined, there was a constant ratio of the proportions of bases, and that A=T and G=C. So for one species, it might have 20% A and 20% T, and 30% G and 30% C. Another species might have 18% A and 18% T, and 32% G and 32% C.

5. Now the problem was fitting the observations together.

III. The structure of DNA is a double helix.

    A. Physical chemists found that DNA was a helix.

        1. Physical chemists study the arrangement of atoms in three dimensions when atoms combine to make molecules. For example, water (H_2O), with three atoms, can form regularly shaped molecules in liquid and ice crystals. Larger molecules such as DNA have millions of atoms. Is there any regularity to their arrangement?

        2. When X rays are shone at a large molecule in solid form, the rays get bounced around before they pass through the molecule. By looking at the pattern that comes out the other side, chemists can figure out if there is a regular pattern to the

arrangement of atoms in the molecule. Rosalind Franklin and Maurice Wilkins at King's College, London did X-ray analyses of DNA and found a regularity in the shape of a helix.

B. Watson and Crick solved the structure of DNA.

    1. Nearby, in Cambridge, the young American geneticist James Watson and somewhat older British physicist Francis Crick looked at the X-ray evidence of a helix, and the notion that A=T and G=C, and came up with an inspiring idea: Maybe the structure of DNA was a double helix with two chains of bases opposite one another.

    2. They made chemical models of the four bases and found that A just fit into T and G just fit into C; no other fits worked. Crick's wife, an artist, drew the double helix, and they published their structure in the spring of 1953. It was immediately accepted for its elegance as well as its science.

IV. The DNA double helix fulfills the requirements for the genetic material.

    A. DNA has huge potential information content.

        1. The polymer of DNA is very long, ranging in size from 1 million base pairs in some bacteria to 100 million base pairs in humans.

        2. These large molecules containing genetic information are what biologists now call chromosomes.

    B. DNA can be accurately replicated.

        1. Watson and Crick said in their 1953 article that their model suggested a way that the genetic material could replicate. This was confirmed a few years later in living cells and involved several steps:

        2. The two parental DNA strands separate, exposing their bases.

            a. New bases come in a pair with the exposed bases. Thus an AT base pair on the parental strand gets exposed GA and CT. These then get paired up with appropriate bases GA-*CT* and *GA*-CT, and voila: There are two new strands with the same sequence as the parent.

            b. Because each new double-stranded DNA molecule has one strand from the parent and one newly built one, this is referred to as semiconservative DNA replication. Contrast this with conservative replication, which, like Xerox copying, has one brand new double-stranded molecule and the old double-stranded parent still intact.

C. DNA can be mutated. Errors do occur in replication (one in a million). They are mostly repaired by a proofreading mechanism, but sometimes are not. Errors change the base sequence in the new DNA, and so cause a change in information content of the new cell that is formed. This is mutation, the raw material for evolution.

D. DNA is expressed as the phenotype. This is the topic of the next lecture.

Essential Reading:

Francis Crick, *What Mad Pursuit* (New York: Basic Books, 1988).

Benjamin Pierce, *Genetics: A Conceptual Approach* (New York: W. H. Freeman, 2007), chap. 10.

James D. Watson, *The Double Helix* (New York: Athenaeum, 1968).

Supplemental Reading:

Anthony Griffiths, Susan Wessler, Richard Lewontin, William Gelbart, David Suzuki, and Jeffrey Miller, *An Introduction to Genetic Analysis*, 8th ed. (New York: W. H. Freeman and Co., 2007).

Benjamin Lewin, *Genes VIII* (Upper Saddle River, NJ: Pearson Prentice-Hall, 2005).

Questions to Consider:

1. Trace the changes in thinking about whether DNA was the genetic material from Miescher's time until Watson and Crick. This is an excellent example of the scientific process, where an idea is put out to the community and gets accepted, rejected, or modified with time.

2. It is important at this stage to understand base pairing and DNA replication. One strand of DNA has the sequence AGCTTCTGGATCTTTAGTCAGTGTAC. Write out the other strand that is paired with this one. Now, outline the steps by which this DNA is replicated: Draw the two separated strands and add new bases (in a different color, say red). Having one old and the new strand in the newly made DNAs is called semiconservative duplication. (Conservative duplication, which does not happen, would be like a copy machine, where there is an old piece and a new piece of paper.)

Lecture Five—Transcript
DNA Structure and Replication

Welcome back. My last two lectures have concerned the search for the genetic material, for the mechanism of heredity. First we found it in cells, then in the nucleus of the cell, then in chromosomes of the nucleus, then in a region of the chromosome. Remember that sex-determining region in the Y chromosome. In the last lecture, we found it inside the nucleus as DNA, and I described experimental evidence in several different systems for DNA as a gene. Now let's see what DNA really is and how its structure fulfills the requirements we have for the genetic material. My opening story concerns the Ice Man. In 1991, a group of hikers in the Alps between Austria and Italy spotted a corpse frozen in the ice. There were some tools and a dagger nearby. The body was carefully removed, and four days later the body now known as the Ice Man was at the University of Innsbruck in Austria. Scientists determined that this body was 5000 years old. It was a male, and it had been killed by an arrow; so he was a victim of homicide and then somehow froze into the ice.

There are many remarkable things about the Ice Man, but to me the most remarkable is his DNA was preserved in his bones, virtually intact. When scientists looked at the information content of his DNA, they found that this information content placed him smack in the genetic group of the current Europeans who live in the alpine regions of Europe. So this is one of the forefathers of the people who currently live there. That DNA can last so long is testimony to its durability. It's nice to have a genetic material that will be stable and not break down very readily. The structure of DNA is testimony to something else. I call DNA a secular icon in our society. Now what's an icon? An icon is an image or symbolic representation that is often used in sacred situations. In this case, it's secular. The 20th century had two great icons that symbolized science in the public mind. One is the atom, with the whizzing electrons going around a nucleus. The other is DNA, with the double helix.

People now talk about DNA all the time as a shorthand. An advertisement for a financial services company tells customers, We understand the DNA of business. A perfume that I actually tried—it didn't go over big—is called DNA. On the bottle, it says this is the "essence of life." It didn't liven me up very much at all. There's a media software system called the "DNA server." There's a clothing line called DNA Divewear, and it advertises that this is the "genetic design-extreme behavior." And of course there's the original biotechnology company whose stock market symbol is, you guessed it, DNA. DNA is the subject of artists as well. Salvador Dali used the DNA double helix in some of his art.

There is a portrait in England of a Nobel laureate, Sir John Sulston, who worked on cell cycling, cell division, in yeast cells. What it has is parts of his DNA inside of bacterial cells in the portrait. A Brazilian artist named Eduardo Kac used the chemical building blocks of DNA to translate verses of the Bible, and viewers looking at this work of art can change the DNA and change the verses that it represents at will. I've seen playgrounds with slides shaped in the helical form of DNA. And of course, it's hard to visit a pharmaceutical company or biotechnology laboratory that doesn't have a DNA sculpture somewhere. So DNA really is everywhere in our society these days.

I want to talk about DNA structure in terms of its function as genetic material in three ways. First I'll describe the early studies that suggested its structure, and I'll take you through how we determined what DNA was structurally. Then I'll describe some of the properties of DNA as a double helix, and finally I'll describe how this double-helix structure of DNA fulfills the requirements of genetic material that I talked about in the last lecture.

First, the early studies of DNA structure. I mentioned in the last lecture that Friedrich Miescher was the first person to isolate DNA from cell nuclei. Miescher is a very interesting man. He was the son of a doctor and graduated from medical school at the top of his class at the University of Basel. Unfortunately, Miescher was partially deaf, and decided for this reason not to pursue clinical medicine. Today, many physicians who have handicaps are in medicine. In those days, it was wise not to do so, so instead Miescher chose a career in research.

He began working on the chemistry of the cell nucleus, about which people knew nothing. His mentor was a world-famous, at that time, German biochemist named Ernst Felix Hoppe-Seyler. In fact, Hoppe-Seyler is so famous there's a journal called *Hoppe-Seyler's Journal of Biochemistry*, which until recently was called that name. Now it has a different name. For some reason, they wanted a shorter title, maybe for indexing purposes. Working in Hoppe-Seyler's laboratory, Miescher, in 1868, isolated nuclei from the cells of blood that was on dressings at a nearby military hospital.

From these dressings, he got white blood cells, isolated their nuclei, and then from the nuclei, he busted them open and extracted a substance that was rich in the usual things that you find in biological molecules: carbon, hydrogen, oxygen.

But two other elements were there, phosphorus and nitrogen. Because this substance was in the nucleus, he called it "nuclein." One of his students later called it nucleic acid, and later on when we found out what it was made of, of course, it turned out to be DNA. Now, Miescher's boss, Hoppe-Seyler, was so amazed at this new substance. It formed these long, long fibers. DNA is not that hard to isolate. I've done it with grade school students, it's so easy. These long fibers impressed the boss, Hoppe-Seyler, so much that before he let Miescher publish his work, he went into the lab personally and repeated all of Miescher's experiments. This was so novel, Hoppe-Seyler wanted to make darn sure that this stuff is for real. Well, he repeated all of Miescher's work and then allowed Miescher to publish the research.

Nucleic acid was a curiosity, even though Hoppe-Seyler had published it as something in the nucleus, until it was realized sometime in the next 30 years after this—remember this is the mid- to late 1800s—that the genetic material is in the nucleus. You'll remember those experiments I described of nuclear transplants and of regenerating cells, and the genetic material in the nucleus that's species-specific. So right away, when people found DNA in the nucleus, they said this is a candidate for the genetic material. But I mentioned previously that there's not just DNA inside the nucleus; there are proteins as well. So people wanted to find out, well, which one is it? Now we know the answer in advance, but I want to take you through some of the reasoning that led to that answer, especially the chemical reasoning, because it's important that we understand the chemistry of DNA. Not down to the last atom, but in terms of its information content and what it can do in terms of genetics.

In the 1890s, a chemist, Albrecht Kossel, found that DNA was a polymer. Now there's a new word for you. A polymer can be considered like beads on a chain. The long chain is the polymer. The individual beads that make up the chain are monomers. So, "monomer" and "polymer." The DNA fibers that Miescher had isolated were these long, long polymers of probably millions of units of monomers. The monomers were the things that had nitrogen in them, as well as carbon and hydrogen and oxygen. There were four of what are called nitrogen bases that make up DNA. These are bases, as the spelling in the "bases" on a baseball diamond, and they're called adenine, thymine, guanine, and cytosine. Now we abbreviate them A, T, G, and C.

Those are the different monomers that make up DNA. So if we're talking about a long chain, we only have four types of beads in it; red, orange, yellow, and green, let's say. And so our chain is made up of information that contains red, orange, yellow, and green. So the chain might be red, orange, yellow, green; red, green, orange, yellow; red—I'm not going to continue on that. There can be very many different orders of the beads on the chain in different amounts. Let me give you the names of the four of them again, and then I will not mention the names again in the course. I'll just call them A, adenine; T, thymine; G, guanine; and C, cytosine. Students often are so used to the shorthand of A, T, G, and C, they think they're part of the alphabet and they don't stand for substances, complex molecules in themselves, so I wanted you to give them a name.

Between 1900 and 1930, working at the Rockefeller Institute in New York, a nuclear chemist named Phoebus Levene spent 30 years studying DNA. Levene found that the four monomers—those bases A, T, G, and C—were not linked to each other in DNA. Instead, they were attached to a backbone, and the backbone was made up of a sugar and a phosphate group. Phosphate is phosphorus with oxygens attached, and the sugar is a multicarbon molecule that has ten hydrogens and five oxygens. The sugar is called deoxyribose, and so the name deoxyribonucleic acid. Deoxyribose is the sugar; nucleic acid is the name that Miescher's student gave to this stuff. "Deoxyribonucleic acid" was coined for this stuff by Levene, and it was called, from then on, "DNA."

Levene again showed that the bases A, T, G, and C are not directly hooked onto each other but are hooked onto this boring backbone of sugar and phosphate. So it's kind of like a chain that is a gold chain, that has little subchains hanging from it, and then the beads are on the subchains. The gold chain can be the sugar-phosphate backbone, and then the beads hanging off of those individual chains are the bases: A, T, G, and C. Now Levene proposed that DNA was indeed a very, very, very, very, very long polymer, and it consisted of repeating units. He said the repeating unit was ATGC. So we could define a DNA molecule as ATGCATGCATGCATGCATGC; and as I ask my students, can I stop now? Some of them say yes, and thank God, then I stop. If they don't say yes, I keep going for the hour. So it was just the repeating unit of ATGC, according to Levene.

If Levene was correct—remember this is about 1930—and Levene certainly thought he was correct, this meant that DNA lacked the variable information content to be the genetic material. Something as boring as that, the same unit repeating many times, that's not going to give 24,000 genes, or even 1000 genes. Levene was a towering intellect, a stupendous chemist, a strong personality—so people believed him. I like to think, in terms of nucleic acid, Levene is the Aristotle of the early 20th century. So everybody said, well, that's it for DNA. That's not going to be genetic material. Levene said it's just repeating units of ATGC. So people started looking at proteins for the genetic material. This is the 1930s, and remember DNA was not identified experimentally until the mid-'40s as the genetic material in the bacteria transformation experiment.

In the late 1940s, another great biochemist took a stab at DNA, by the name of Erwin Chargaff, working at Columbia University. Chargaff found that Levene was wrong about the polymer of DNA. It wasn't ATGCATGC at all; it was highly variable. So if our DNA starts with ATGC, Chargaff said, no, it's ATGCTTCAATACCA—did you get that exactly—GCTTA. It was highly variable, a very important finding because right away people said, whoa, there's a terrific information content here. Chargaff made other discoveries whose significance came to be fully appreciated shortly afterwards. First of all, for each species he examined when he chopped up the DNA into individual beads, monomers, he found a constant ratio of the proportion of bases. So for every human being, there was a certain percentage of A that was the same, a certain percentage of T, a certain percentage of G, and a certain percentage of C; they added up to 100%. For each eucalyptus plant, there was a different percentage of A, T, G, and C.

The second thing chemically that Chargaff found was that the ratios of A and T, and G and C, were the same. That is, if the species had 20% A, there would be about 20% T. Therefore, working out to 100%, 30% G and 30% C. So A was always equal to T in proportion, and G was always equal to C. Another species, another creature, might have 18% A and 18% T, and of course 32% G and 32% C. Now here's your homework assignment: 15% A; tell me the T, G, and C. Hand in the answer tomorrow; send it to The Teaching Company.

Now, the problem was fitting all of these observations together. Physical chemists came into the picture now; not biochemists who look at what things are, but physical chemists who look at the arrangement of atoms in three-dimensional space. Consider water. Water is H_2O; there's an O with a couple of Hs attached. It's very regularly shaped. All water molecules are the same. Now, consider DNA, millions of atoms. Was there a regular shape to DNA? Well, there's a physical way to examine DNA, and that's by shining

X-rays on the DNA molecule when it's in a solid form. Now, an X-ray is shone on a DNA molecule in a solid form. What happens is the rays go into DNA, and then they get bounced around by all the atoms that are there; then they come out the other end. Now if we put a photographic plate at the other end, we're going to get a pattern depending on how much bouncing around that ray has gone through. So the ray goes through the DNA molecule; then it bounces, and you get what are called X-ray patterns. The X-ray pattern of DNA was very regular.

Two scientists working at King's College, London, in the early 1950s, Rosalind Franklin and Maurice Wilkins, did X-ray analysis of DNA and found a regularity that they interpreted to be in the shape of a helix, a coil. So now we had a lot of evidence for the shape of DNA as a helix. We had a sugar-phosphate backbone that Levene had found. We had A = T and G = C that Chargaff had found. Working at Cambridge University, up the road from London, a young American geneticist, James Watson, and a somewhat older British physicist, Francis Crick, looked at all of this evidence and came up with an inspiring idea. Maybe, just maybe, DNA is a double helix; that there are two polymers here, and that the sugar and phosphate are on the outside—the regular sugar-phosphate—and the bases are on the inside.

To show that this might be true, Watson and Crick made ball-and-stick models of the bases of DNA, and the sugar and phosphate, and tried to fit them together tightly. The only way they would fit together as a double helix was by having the sugar and phosphate on the outside and the bases on the inside, and the As and Ts just fit together, and the Gs and Cs just fit together, like a ball into a baseball mitt. Now they fit; they didn't bond very tightly. They fit very weakly together, but they fit. No other type of structure worked than the double helix. Crick's wife was an artist, and she drew a double-helical shape, with the bases on the inside and the ribbon on the outside being the sugar and phosphate, for the article they published in the spring of 1953. It's a one-page brief article describing the evidence and their proposal for the double-helix model. This model was immediately accepted as the model for the genetic material; not only for its science, but for its elegance. It's a beautiful structure. And of course, this brief one-page paper won them the Nobel Prize. The Nobel Prize is given for people who think, not necessarily for people who do a lot of grunt work in the laboratory.

The DNA double helix fulfills the requirements for the genetic material. Now, what are those requirements? There are four of them. First, DNA should have a huge information content. Second, DNA can be accurately replicated. Third, DNA should be expressed as the phenotype. And fourth, you should be able to mutate DNA, to change it and get genetic mutation. I'm going to deal with three of the four now, and I will defer to the next lecture the aspect of expressing DNA as the phenotype. First, the information content of DNA. Well, this really came from Chargaff, as I mentioned. DNA has a huge information content. With just four bases in any amounts, we can make all types of words, right? It's a language that has a great number of possibilities. So, for example, there are 469 base pairs of DNA in insulin. Insulin is a hormone, and the gene that codes for insulin has 469 base pairs of DNA.

Now, when we draw in a structure of a DNA molecule, we go ATGC, and I'm going to read out the beginning of the insulin gene. I'm reading you a human gene, information content: AGCCCTCCAGGAC. We assume the other strand is there. Now how do I know what the other strand is? Everywhere there's an A, there's a T; A and T go together. Everywhere there's a G, there's a C, right? So we know one strand, we know the other strand. Everywhere there's an A, there's a T on the other strand; everywhere there's a G, there's a C on the other strand. Everywhere there's a C, there's a G on the other strand; everywhere there's a T, there's an A on the other strand. So if we know one strand, we know the other. Generally, when biologists look at DNA sequences, they look at only one of the two strands of DNA. There's a huge information content. Humans have over three billion base pairs of DNA, so there's a lot of information there. We can get lots of different sequences out of DNA, the four bases.

DNA replication. How is DNA duplicated? One of the great coy statements in the history of modern biology was the statement that Watson and Crick made in their paper where they unveiled the double-helix model. They said, it has not escaped our notice that the structure we propose will provide a mechanism for accurately replicating DNA, genetic material. What was not escaping their notice was that the double strands of DNA could unwind very easily. The base pairs of DNA—that is, the A and the T that are inside the double helix—are weakly attached to each other, and so we can envision the two strands of DNA unzipping. So the two strands separate, and each one of the old strands can act as a template for the new strands.

Let me give you an illustration of that. Let us say we have a DNA molecule—I'll make it really simple—that is AAAAA. The other strand of DNA, of course, will be TTTTT; five Ts to five As. The strands unzip. Now on one side we have the AAAAA; on the other side we have the TTTTT. And now there should be an enzyme or a mechanism coming in to duplicate this, and the AAAAA here gets bonded to TTTTT, so now we have an AT double helix. And the TTTTT here gets bonded to AAA, and so we have two new helices, just by unwinding and replicating in that way. This is called semiconservative replication; not because of the politics of the people who proposed the model, but because you are semiconservative. You are conserving both old strands of DNA, and you're adding the complementary, or the opposite, strand to the old strands of DNA.

It's not like doing a Xerox copy. In a Xerox copy, we put the old copy on the machine, and we get a brand new copy, right? So we have two copies, one old and one brand new. That would be conservative replication. It's not like that at all. It's semiconservative, where DNA is retaining the old strand for the new strand. And there's a very interesting question we can ask about this, and that is the following: I am the product of a single cell, the fertilized egg. It had DNA in it from my mother and father. When that cell reproduced, each new cell—semiconservative replication—had an old strand of DNA and a new strand of DNA.

So in the early embryo, the first cell had both original strands of DNA, parental strands from mom and dad; and when it divided, reproduced, each new cell had one old strand and one new strand. When those new cells replicated, each one of those cells ended up with an old strand and a new strand, one new cell, and the other cell has, of course, two new strands because its second strand of DNA is new. So is it possible that in my body still is my parents' DNA after all of those cell divisions? Answer? I guess it's possible. I haven't seen evidence that it's there; I haven't seen evidence that it isn't. But it would be nice to think that somewhere in my body might be a cell that contains the actual DNA from my parents in those 60 trillion cells.

My third requirement for DNA—the other two that I've talked about are information content and accurate replication—is DNA mutation or changes that are permanent and passed on to the next generation. So, we can envision a normal DNA sequence might be ATCGGTTA, and you change it. Instead of ATCG, it's ATCA or something. You change one base pair in DNA. It turns out that the duplication mechanism of DNA is error-prone; errors do happen. About one in a million times, an error is made. Now if you're replicating a billion building blocks, you're going to change one in a million. Most of these are repaired in DNA. So DNA is constantly being scanned by a system of DNA repair mechanisms that will remove the bad base and put in the good base.

Now how do we know a bad base? Well, if you put in a C opposite an A— normally you're supposed to put in a T opposite an A—that's bad. There is actually scanning going on all the time along your DNA to repair those errors. Any errors that are not caught, of course, are passed on to the next cell and the next generation. This is the raw material for evolution and for genetic diversity. The fourth requirement for DNA as genetic material is the expression as the phenotype. That's the topic of my next lecture. Thank you.

Lecture Six
DNA Expression in Proteins

Scope: Proteins are polymers (long chains of chemical "beads") composed of monomers called amino acids. With 20 amino acids, there are many possible orders of them in proteins up to 1000 units long. Because the amino acids vary in their chemical properties, proteins will also have these properties. Spider silk proteins are an example. One type of silk protein is in flat interlocking sheets that provide strength. Another type of silk is made up of a protein that stretches and is more flexible. Proteins can fold to expose surfaces not only for structure, but also for functioning as enzymes: catalysts essential to speeding up chemical transformations in living things. Protein is the major expression of a gene, called the phenotype. The relationship between DNA and its protein expression was worked out with mutant strains of simple organisms such as bacteria.

Outline

I. Opening story.
    A. Spider silk is an amazing protein.
        1. A spider web has three roles: It is home, it is where the spider mates, and it is where it captures food. The web must be strong and stretch, yet not break, nor wobble so much as to get out of control. Webs are thinner than hair, and indeed strong: stronger than steel and more elastic than nylon.
        2. Spider webs are made of a protein called silk. The silk proteins are giant molecules—macromolecules composed of millions of atoms of hydrogen, carbon, oxygen, nitrogen, sulfur, and phosphorus hooked together in a specific way. Silk is made in glands at the rear of the animal and spun out as fibers.
    B. Proteins are polymers made up of monomers—beads on a chain. Like the nucleotides that make up DNA, amino acids make up proteins. Only instead of four monomers, there are 20 different amino acids. Each protein has its own composition of these 20, and spider silk has a unique collection in a specific order that determines its structure and function.

      1. There are two kinds of silk.

          a. The strong fibers have strands of protein that fold into flat sheets, with ratchets that fit them together (like Lego blocks) so they won't slip apart.

          b. The flexible fibers have strands of protein that allow them to curl around and slip by one another.

      2. These structures are determined by spider genes in their cell nuclei.

II. What are proteins?

    A. Proteins are polymers composed of monomers.

      1. Twenty amino acids are linked together in a specific order for each protein. The amino acids are important in human nutrition. They contain amino groups (NH_2), which humans can only get from eating other creatures. Some organisms have the genetic capacity to get nitrogen from the air (79% N_2) and turn it into amino groups. Humans cannot breathe in steak!

      2. Humans lack the genetic capacity to make 8 of the 20 amino acids; these must be eaten as part of proteins in the diet. This has great implications in human nutrition, to which we will return in Lecture Twenty-Three.

    B. The specific order of the amino acids in a protein (they range from 10–1000 amino acids long) determines how the protein will fold in three dimensions.

      1. This is a chemically spontaneous process in the cell once the protein is made.

      2. Protein shape is very sensitive to the environment: Heat changes it, often irreversibly (boiling an egg).

      3. Protein shape presents specific surfaces to its surroundings (see spider silk, above). These can fit other substances like a lock and key (or baseball and glove).

III. Proteins have essential functions in the organism.

    A. Some proteins are structural.

      1. The shape of proteins allows for structural specificity. See spider silk for examples. Other structural proteins include: hair (keratin), muscle (actin and myosin), antibodies (immunoglobulin), and connective tissue (collagen).

2. These all have a unique composition of the 20 amino acids in a unique order.

3. They are only made by certain tissues at certain times (you don't have hair growing on your eyeball).

B. Some proteins act as enzymes.

1. The shape of proteins allows for a surface where chemical reactions can occur. Example: Consider DNA replication. In humans, a single DNA molecule (chromosome) has millions of base pairs. These must be replicated in just a few hours during cell division. If you put DNA into a text tube (or cell) and give it the building blocks for new DNA, the various steps of replication will eventually happen just because the building blocks will randomly bump into the DNA as it happens to unwind. But this will take thousands of years!

2. To speed things up, we might heat the cell to make the DNA unwind faster and the building blocks move faster. This might work, but we know that living tissues generally cannot tolerate heat. The reason is that their proteins will change shape (like the cooked egg).

3. Another way to speed things up is to provide a "workbench" to grab and line up the DNA and building blocks. This needs a specific surface, and proteins provide this. They are catalysts called enzymes.

4. The enzyme DNA polymerase binds to DNA and its building blocks in such a way as to speed up the polymerization many millionfold.

5. There is an enzyme for virtually every one of the thousands of chemical transformations in a cell (e.g., digestion of food).

6. Proteins are the phenotypic expression of genes.

IV. Mutations in model organisms relate genes to proteins.

A. The strategy of mutations proves cause and effect.

1. In biology, mere correlation does not prove causation. If we want to show that A causes B, we need to have a way of experimentally disrupting A and then seeing that B does not occur to prove our hypothesis.

2. Genetics is a way to do this. If there is an organism that has a genetic mutation that disrupts the gene for A, and B does not occur, then our hypothesis is correct.

B. Simple organisms can be genetically manipulated and tested in the laboratory.

   1. Bacteria such as the gut bacterium *Escherichia coli* and molds such as the bread mold have only one set of genes (all mutations show up), and it is easy to grow them in the lab. They are especially useful for showing nutritional mutations.

   2. Unlike humans, bacteria can make all 20 amino acids. Sometimes, a genetic mutation occurs so that the strain of bacteria no longer makes the amino acid. Now it's mutated, like us, and like us needs that amino acid to grow. Scientists can compare the chemistry of these mutant bacteria with those normal ones that can make the amino acid. And when they do, they find that an enzyme is missing: one of the enzymes that catalyzes the transformation of chemicals to that amino acid. So the normal gene must be expressed as that enzyme.

   3. A bacterium arose that genetically could not make DNA. (It just sat there and did not reproduce.) The missing enzyme in this case was DNA polymerase.

   4. These observations, repeated many times for many organisms, led to the one gene–one enzyme concept.

   5. And since almost all genes are proteins, it's "one gene–one protein." The mystery of genotype and phenotype is solved: The gene is DNA, and the phenotype is protein.

Essential Reading:

Anthony Griffiths, Susan Wessler, Richard Lewontin, William Gelbart, David Suzuki, and Jeffrey Miller, *An Introduction to Genetic Analysis*, 8th ed. (New York: W. H. Freeman, 2007).

David Sadava, Craig Heller, Gordon Orians, William Purves, and David Hillis, *Life: The Science of Biology*, 8th ed. (Sunderland, MA: Sinauer Associates; New York: W. H. Freeman and Co., 2008), chap. 12.

Supplemental Reading:

Horace Freeland Judson, *The Eighth Day of Creation: Makers of the Revolution in Biology* (Woodbury, NY: Cold Spring Harbor Laboratory Press, 1996).

Benjamin Lewin, *Genes VIII*, (Upper Saddle River, NJ: Pearson Prentice-Hall, 2005).

Questions to Consider:

1. Spider silk is as strong as Kevlar, the strongest synthetic material known. What uses can you suggest for the silk (for humans)?

2. With 20 amino acids and proteins up to 1000 amino acids long, the possibilities for different amino acid sequences and protein shapes seem virtually endless (20^{1000} is a very big number). Yet there are far fewer protein sequences—and hence, shapes—in the living world. Thinking about evolution by natural selection, why might this be so?

Lecture Six—Transcript
DNA Expression in Proteins

Welcome back. In the last lecture, I described four requirements for the genetic material. First, it needs to have a large information content. Second, it should be able to duplicate precisely. Third, it should be able to change raw material for evolution. And fourth, it should be able to be expressed in some outward way as the phenotype. In the last lecture, I showed you how DNA as a genetic material fulfills the first three criteria: information, replication, and mutation. Now I want to begin to talk about the fourth: expression. My opening story is about spider silk. A spider web is a phenomenal structure. When you look at a spider web next time, think of the three functions that the web has. First, it's home; it's where the spider lives. Second, it's where the spider mates, males and females, to have offspring; and third, it's obviously where the spider captures its food.

Spider webs have to be strong, and they have to be able to stretch, yet they can't break or wobble so much as to get out of control. Spider webs are thinner than hair, and indeed strong. In fact, spider web fibers are stronger than steel and more elastic than nylon. Spider webs are made of proteins called silk. And if we could figure out how to duplicate what the spider does, we could use spider silk for a number of functions, and there are biotechnology companies trying to do this. For example, some proposed uses are for surgical sutures, for the little strings that are involved with parachutes, and for bulletproof vests; they're that strong. This is different than the silk that's in clothing that's made by a silkworm. It's a different molecule. Silk proteins are giant molecules. They're macromolecules composed of millions of atoms of carbon, hydrogen, oxygen, nitrogen, sulfur, and phosphorus all hooked together in a highly specific way. The silk is made in glands at the rear of the spider, and it's spun out as fibers. We know a lot about silk, but we just don't know how the animal gets to spin it out and how the fibers are formed. We're getting there.

Silk, as I mentioned, is proteins. Proteins are polymers made of monomers. Remember what that was from DNA; they're chemical "beads" on a chain. And like the building blocks of DNA, the amino acids hook together to make proteins as building blocks. And instead of four monomers or building blocks of DNA, like A, T, G, and C in DNA—a DNA strand, remember it's double stranded, but one of the strands might read AGTTCTAGC, etc.— there are 20 different amino acid building blocks in proteins. Not 4, but 20.

So a protein might have a sequence amino acid 1, 2, 4, 6, 9, 11, 11, 9, 3, 4, 18, 20. They all have names; I'm just giving them numbers. Each protein has its own composition and order of these 20 amino acids, so the possibilities are very, very large. I wouldn't say they're endless—there's 20 amino acids—but it's pretty large. DNA, you'll recall, is a long, long molecule. Each DNA molecule in a human, for example, has 100 million base pairs. Proteins are not that long. Proteins have between 10 and about 1000 amino acid building blocks. Spider silk has a unique collection of these amino acids in a specific order that determines its structure and its function.

Now there are two kinds of spider silk. There are strong fibers, and there are flexible fibers. Strong fibers are composed of polymers—long strands of these building blocks put together—of protein that fold into flat sheets, and they've got ratchets on the end that fit them together like Lego blocks, so they won't slip apart. It's an amazing structure, and you can see that chemically in the building blocks as they fold. The flexible fibers have strands of protein that fold it into a different three-dimensional structure, and they allow them to curl around and slip by one another. You can see these at different locations in the web. These structures of the proteins and of the spider web itself are determined by spider genes in spider cell nuclei.

I want to talk about proteins in this lecture. First, I'll try to answer the question of what they are. I've intimated as to what they are, but we'll go into somewhat more detail on what proteins are. They're amazing. Second, what do they do? We'll see that they have two major functions in tissues. And third, I'll describe how mutations—changes in genes in model organisms—relate genes to proteins.

First, what are proteins? Proteins, as I've mentioned, are polymers of monomers put together, and the beads on the chain, the monomers, are called amino acids. One of my favorite bumper stickers sponsored by the Chemical Society says, "It's amino world without chemists." The 20 amino acids all have a basic similarity to them, just like the building blocks of DNA are somewhat similar, but there are slight variations. I want to discuss this in a little bit more detail.

The amino acids all have a central atom of carbon, and attached to that atom are four other chemical groupings. Grouping number one is a hydrogen atom. Well, that's not too interesting; cool, hydrogen atom. Grouping number two is the amino group, and the amino group has the formula H_2N;

water H_2O, amino group H_2N—where N is for nitrogen. Amino acids are important in human nutrition. We don't make amino groups. You know, we're in the air and breathing the air; the air is 79% nitrogen, so it stands to reason. Why don't we use that nitrogen, hook it together with some hydrogens, and we've got amino groups to hook to amino acids? Can't do it. The reaction of nitrogen and hydrogen is a reaction that very few biological organisms have the genetic capacity to do. The biological organisms include certain bacteria, and we'll talk about that later on in the course. They can take nitrogen from the air, nitrogen gas, which is N_2, just nitrogens, and add some hydrogen, H_2, to it to make the H_2N, the amino group.

Another way of saying this is we humans can't breathe in steak. You know, steak has a lot of proteins, a lot of amino acid. We can't breathe in steak, but these little bacteria can—clever. Humans lack the genetic capacity to make 8 of the 20 amino acids. Bacteria can do it; plants can do it. They can take carbon atoms, and as long as they've got amino groups, they can rearrange the carbons and the oxygens and the hydrogens and the phosphoruses and the sulfurs. They can rearrange them, jiggle them around, and make all 20 amino acids. We are mutant. We have genetic, inherited, defects in our structure such that we don't have the genes to be able to make 8 of them. We can make 12 of them; we have to get the other 8 in our diet, whole amino acids. We have to get those particular colored beads in our diet. This has great implications for human nutrition and agriculture, as I will describe later on in Lecture Twenty-Three.

Now, back to our amino acid. I described two of the four groups. I said there's a carbon atom in the middle, and there's a hydrogen attached to it, and there's this amino group. Now what about this acid? Acid is a carbon with some oxygens attached. It's actually essentially like a carbon dioxide molecule, CO_2. There's a little bit of a difference, but it's like a CO_2 attached to the carbon. The acid group is not that interesting. All amino acids have the amino group and the hydrogen group and the acid; three out of the four groups attach to the carbon. It's the fourth group I want to focus on now. The fourth group gives the amino acid its particular properties. This group, abbreviated in whatever way we want—it can be called alanine or valine; there are names for all the amino acids—contains atoms of carbon, hydrogen, oxygen, and sulfur arranged in certain ways. These atoms that are arranged in certain ways give the amino acid distinctive properties at that point in the chain.

You know, suppose you had a chain around your neck of beads, and at every red bead, you hung something on it—you hung a key or another piece of jewelry on it. Well, those red beads give the chain a certain property. And if a bunch of red beads are in the middle, you'd have the chains hanging on the middle. If the red beads were evenly spaced apart, you'd have chains hanging spaced apart. By the same analogy, in amino acids it's these variable groups that have distinctive properties and cause the chain of amino acids to fold or do something in a certain way; especially folding in three dimensions. These processes of folding are spontaneous in the watery environment of the cell. It's absolutely amazing. Once you make an amino acid out of certain chemical groups, and you put that amino acid in a certain location in the protein, that amino acid will cause the protein to fold in a certain way.

Let me give you an example. There are some amino acids that love to be near water. Remember, the environment of the cell is water; it's a watery environment. About 75% of the contents of the cell is a molecule that's otherwise pretty boring; it's water. The other 25% is what we're interested in, the DNA and the proteins and the fats and other things. Now there are some amino acids that like to be near water. We call them hydrophilic. A bibliophile loves books; a hydrophile loves to be near water. So this amino acid will want to be near water. There are other amino acids that are hydrophobic; they hate water. They want to be on the inside of the protein, away from water. So you can envision if we begin with a protein chain as just a flat chain with beads on it, it'll fold up so that the hydrophobic, the water-fearing, amino acids are away from the water, all huddled in the inside, and the hydrophilic ones are near water on the outside. Well, that's going to give the protein a three-dimensional shape, and that's where proteins have their structure, and therefore their function, the three-dimensional shape.

The shape of a protein is highly sensitive to the environment. For example, heat disrupts these interactions I've just described; the hydrophobic and other interactions that cause a protein that's a linear sequence to fold into three dimensions. It disrupts it permanently. You boil an egg; the egg changes its structure, doesn't it, from liquid to very hard? What's happening is the liquid is a protein called albumin, and you're changing the three-dimensional structure of it such that it no longer has its own entity, and they kind of glob together to make something that's solid. You can't unboil an egg; these changes are irreversible. As you'll see later in this lecture and in other lectures, folding of proteins is highly important in biology, and disrupting it is going to be a bad thing. Now if we've got a protein folded in three dimensions, it's going to present a shape that's specific to the environment around it, like the spider silk is going to be in a certain shape, and they'll ratchet together. In addition, these shapes can fit other substances in the cell like a lock and key or a baseball fitting into a baseball glove.

Well, what are the functions that these structures can perform in the cell? There are two general classifications of protein function. One of them is structural, and the other is as enzymes. First, structural proteins. Well, I've just described spider silk as a structural protein. It's a protein that has a three-dimensional shape that causes these fibers to form. Other structural proteins you'll be familiar with? Hair; it's made of a structural protein called keratin. Muscle has structural proteins called actin and myosin. Antibodies, things that fight disease in the immune system, are structural proteins called immunoglobulins; these have a three-dimensional shape for their function. Connective tissue has collagen; you may hear of collagen in skin. So there are structural proteins that have a unique composition of the 20 amino acids in a unique order, causing them to fold in a unique way, and they're only made by certain tissue at certain times. You don't have hair growing out of your eyeball, for example: structural proteins.

The other types of proteins are proteins that do something, they're called enzymes. Here we're dealing with the shape of a protein being presented as a surface for chemical reactions to occur. Consider something I talked about in the last lecture, namely DNA replication; the duplication of DNA. In humans, a single DNA molecule has about 100 million base pairs; it's a long, long double-stranded molecule. In a few hours during cell division, this thing has to be duplicated completely. Now let's see what's going to happen. The DNA has to unwind so that the two strands that are going to be templates for the new strands are available, and then the A, T, G, and C have to be brought in, and everywhere there's a T in DNA, an A will be in the new strand; everywhere there's a G, a C, etc. So we can make the two new strands off of the template.

If you put DNA into a cell or a test tube with the building blocks for new DNA—the A, T, G, and C—these steps will eventually happen just by random chance. By random chance, the DNA might open up a little bit; and by random chance, an A will come in and be right next to a T, and you'll start to build the DNA that way. It'll take thousands to millions of years for this to happen by random chance. It's a very, very unlikely and random event. So, you want to speed things up? Okay, let's speed things up in the cell for DNA replication. Let's do what the chemists would do; give the molecules more energy, heat them up. So we'll heat the cell. Yes, that'll make the DNA unwind real fast, and the building blocks will move fast, and they might replicate the DNA faster. Yes, it might work, but we know that living tissues cannot tolerate heat. Well, I've just told you why; their proteins get destroyed, so bad idea. We can't unboil an egg, right?

Another way to speed things up is to provide some sort of "workbench." We'll get a three-dimensional workbench that'll grab the DNA and grab the monomers—the A, T, G, and C—and line them up right beside one another. This workbench will also wedge its way into DNA so it'll unwind. That's going to need a specific surface. Well, proteins provide the specific surface for doing this. This function is called catalysis; the protein is called a catalyst. It speeds the reaction up but doesn't get used. All it is, is a workbench. It's not getting used up in any way; it's just the workbench. It brings the DNA in, and the A, T, G, and C, and lets it replicate and then goes on with its life and is unchanged after the reaction is done.

The enzyme involved in making DNA is called DNA polymerase. Enzyme names usually end in "ase." So if you look carefully in detergents, you might see "–ase" in there; that's a detergent enzyme. The DNA polymerase binds to DNA and its building blocks in such a way as to speed up the polymerization reaction millionsfold. There is an enzyme activity for virtually every one of the thousands of chemical transformations that go on in a cell—for instance, digestion of food. There's an enzyme for breaking down proteins; there's one for breaking down starch, etc. Proteins, as enzymes in this way, or as structural proteins, are the phenotypic expression of genes. We can't see it outwardly, but we can see its consequences.

Now how do we prove that proteins and enzymes are the products or the expression of genes? We can use what is called a genetic strategy to look at cause and effect. In biology, and in science as a whole, correlation—just two events happening at the same time—does not prove cause and effect. You know, just because there are genes and there are proteins and enzymes and structural proteins out there doesn't mean that genes determine proteins. I've said that they do, but don't take my word for it; prove it. Politicians try to prove this all the time; correlation is cause and effect. Because I'm in office, the economy is better. A scientist would say, well, prove it. Here's the way to prove it, of course; kick the person out of office, put someone else in, and do the same policies and see if the economy changes or not. Advertisers say if you'll just drive this car, you'll feel a lot better about yourself. That's correlation, right, driving the car and feeling better? Is that cause and effect?

Well, in science, we don't go for correlation; we want cause and effect. So if we want to show that phenotype A causes phenotype B—that's our hypothesis—what we need to do is experimentally disrupt A in some way and prove that B no longer happens. One way to disrupt A is by genetics. If an organism has a genetic mutation that disrupts the gene for A, and B now doesn't happen, then our hypothesis is correct. We can do this in the laboratory using simple organisms, model organisms that are easy to manipulate in the lab. A good example is bacteria such as the gut bacterium that lives in the human gut, *Escherichia coli*. Most biologists call this *E. coli*, and that's what I'm going to call it from now on, but I'll say it once more, it does have a name, *Escherichia*. It's named after a scientist named Escherich; *Escherichia coli, E. coli*.

Now the gut bacterium has only one set of genes. It doesn't have two copies of every gene as Mendel would say. It's only got a single set, so it's easy to grow and to see mutations in the laboratory. So if I take one bacterium, and I put it onto a solid medium like Jell-O, with some goodies for bacteria to grow, that one will divide every half hour, so you have two, four, eight, sixteen, thirty-two that kind of stick together. And come the next morning, we'll have millions of bacteria in a single colony. If we come two days from now, the colony will take up the entire plate or the entire dish that we're growing in the lab. You could grow these bacteria also, of course, in a liquid medium, and it'll make the whole medium cloudy and full of bacteria.

Bacteria can make all 20 amino acids. They're good at this. As I said, we're not; we can only make 12 of them. Sometimes, however, there's a genetic mutation in a bacterium—bacterium, singular—such that this particular genetic strain of bacteria no longer makes an amino acid. It requires an amino acid in order to grow. So if we try to grow these bacteria in a growth medium that has vitamins and minerals and sugars, and say, go, grow, it'll say, I'm not going to grow. I'm on strike. I can't grow. I can't make proteins. The cell just sits there and eventually dies because it doesn't have all 20 amino acids. It's missing one of them. I mentioned all proteins, virtually all proteins, have all 20 amino acids in various amounts.

So if you're missing an amino acid, you can't make most proteins. You can't substitute either. So that's going to be pretty bad for the bacterium; it'll just sit there and eventually die. You're not going to get much of a colony or growth of bacteria. Now, of course, we can then ask the question; okay, what is the phenotype here? Which amino acid does it need? So one by one, we can add the amino acids, all 20 of them, to this bacterium, this mutant, and say, this is one that requires amino acid number six to survive and grow. It will not grow unless I add amino acid number six. If I add amino acid number three, the bacterium says, I've got that already; that's not what I need.

What can scientists do at this point? At this point, scientists can zero in on the chemistry inside the bacteria cell; look inside the mutant bacteria cells that can't make the amino acid and compare them, the chemistry, to the normal ones that can make the amino acid. And when they do this, they find, lo and behold, there's an enzyme missing in the mutant. The enzyme activity isn't there. The protein might be there; it just might have a mutant that causes an amino acid or other changes, so the protein doesn't fold right, so it doesn't hasten the reaction. Well, now we're in pretty bad shape, right? This enzyme is missing, so you must supply the amino acid. But the important conclusion we can draw from this particular analysis is that enzymes relate to genes because the mutant enzyme is related to a mutant gene. It's using a genetic argument to prove something in biology.

In the cell, simple transformations don't occur in one step. In my next lecture, I'm going to talk about a phenomenon called metabolism, where stepwise conversions of substances take place inside the cell. This can be quite complicated, but the chemistry is fairly straightforward for a chemist, anyway. In a biochemical pathway, A, for example, gets converted to B, and B gets converted to C, and C gets converted to D, and D gets converted to E, and E gets converted to F, for example. F might be our amino acid, and A might start off by being sugar; just plain old sugar that the bacterium gets from growing in the intestine or in a growth medium in the laboratory. So this bacterium is converting this sugar and rearranging its carbon, hydrogen, and oxygen atoms, then adding the amino group, the H_2N, at some point to it, to make the amino acid F.

Now it's doing it A to B, to C, to D, to E, to F, in five steps. I can define those steps. A is converted to B, B is converted to C, C is converted to D, D is converted to E, and E is converted to F. You can't do it in one step. It's like doing a double play in baseball in one step—no, you have to go from one man to another—or a football analogy where the center passes the ball to the quarterback, who gives the ball to the halfback, who runs to the side and is doing a tricky play where the halfback passes the ball to the tight end. Several steps, and the end product, of course, is, they hope, a touchdown. Okay, our end product is an amino acid, and there are five steps. What biochemistry shows us is each of those steps is catalyzed, or hastened, by its own enzyme. It's very important to understand that. Each of the steps is catalyzed by its own enzyme. So the organism I've just described that has all five enzymes makes this amino acid.

What happens if the organism has a genetic mutation in one of the genes coding for one of these enzymes? Well, what will happen will be, for example, if there is a genetic mutation in the last step—the conversion of E to F—two things happen. Number one, A gets converted to B—the sugar gets converted to B—which goes to C, which goes to D, which goes to E, which stops because the enzyme is not there to speed up the reaction. Enzymes speed up reactions millionfold by having a workbench on which the reaction can occur. So E starts piling up and just sits there, and you don't make the amino acid. The phenotypic consequence is this bacterium, as I described earlier on, requires this particular amino acid to grow, so we'll have to supply the amino acid. The second consequence, of course, of the missing enzyme is we're missing F; we're missing the amino acid. So the molecule that was going to be converted doesn't get converted, and it piles up.

This genetic reasoning of one gene coding for one enzyme has been used to elucidate, or fully describe, all of the biochemical pathways that exist in the cell. A number of Nobel Prizes were given out for people using model organisms to do this, and this genetic reasoning was very important in doing it. These observations that I've just described, which have been repeated many times for many organisms—we began with bacteria, then we went to bread molds, then we went to fruit flies, then we went to model plants; you can do this as well, as you'll see in the next lecture, in humans—have led to the concept of one gene–one enzyme. But you know from the earlier part of the lecture, I described that most enzymes are proteins. So really, the idea here is one gene–one protein. The mystery of genotype and phenotype is therefore solved. The gene is DNA; the phenotype, the gene's expression, is protein. We'll see in the next lecture how this phenotype plays out in the chemistry of the cell. Thank you.

Lecture Seven
Genes, Enzymes, and Metabolism

Scope: Genetically inherited diseases such as phenylketonuria and alkaptonuria led to the one gene–one enzyme hypothesis in humans. Biochemistry is the expression of the phenotype, and enzymes are the actors that determine conversions in biochemical pathways. Metabolism is the sum total of the biochemical conversions in a cell, tissue, or organism. Cells obey the same physical laws of thermodynamics as the rest of the inanimate universe. Anabolism is using energy in chemical conversions to make energy-rich substances, and catabolism is releasing energy for use in other conversions. In both cases, energy is not created or destroyed, only changed. In biology, where each step in a biochemical pathway is determined by the presence of an enzyme encoded by a gene, the biochemical capabilities of an organism are genetically determined.

Outline

I. Opening story: Phenylketonuria is a human genetic disease.
    A. Dr. Asbjorn Folling solved a medical mystery.
        1. A Norwegian mother had watched her children, a 6-year-old daughter and a 4-year-old son, get progressively sicker over time. By mid-1934, both were profoundly mentally retarded. Her family physician told her that he could do nothing to help the children and advised her to see Dr. Asbjorn Folling, a medical specialist in both chemistry and mental retardation.
        2. Folling thought that the children's symptoms might be related to blood sugar, so he tested their urine by adding a solution of ferric chloride, which turns from brown to purple when there are a lot of ketones from sugar. To his surprise, the solution turned green!
        3. Folling first had to rule out that whatever was causing this color change came not from the children's own body chemistry but from something they consumed. So he asked the mother to stop giving them any of the special medicines they were taking for a week and retested. Once again, the green color appeared.

4. Folling now used his chemistry knowledge to extract the mystery substance from the kids' urine and identified it as phenylpyruvic acid. He named the disorder with the rather cumbersome Latin "imbecillitas phenylpyruvica." Later, it was called phenylketonuria (PKU).

5. Over the next decade, Folling saw other mentally retarded people who excreted (put into urine) phenylpyruvic acid and had PKU. Over half of them were siblings, like the original pair. In all four families, both parents were mentally normal and did not excrete phenylpyruvic acid. Knowing Mendelian genetics, he realized that PKU must be inherited as a recessive.

B. Other human genetic diseases were known.

1. In 1896, English physician Archibald Garrod saw patients with a rare disorder known as alkaptonuria, where the urine turns black when exposed to air. Because the disease seemed to occur most often in children of first-cousin marriages, he concluded that alkaptonuria is a genetic disease caused by a recessive allele.

2. Garrod took this one important step further. Enzymes had just been discovered as essential biological catalysts, and he proposed that the error in alkaptonuria was due to a lack of an enzyme that converts a molecular product of protein breakdown. Now knowing about the identity of genes and proteins, he came up with the one gene–one protein hypothesis. He called alkaptonuria an "inborn error" of biochemistry.

3. "I believe that no two individuals," wrote Garrod, "are exactly alike chemically any more than structurally." This was an amazing and true prediction.

II. Protein is the phenotype, and biochemistry is the expression of the phenotype.

A. A biochemical pathway describes the sequential conversions of substances in the body.

1. Each step in a pathway is catalyzed by a specific enzyme, encoded by a gene.

2. A single pathway involves the enzymes that are deficient in PKU and alkaptonuria. That pathway involves the conversions of an amino acid, phenylalanine.

3. Because phenylalanine is an amino acid and part of proteins, and because phenylalanine cannot be made by humans, we need to take it in our food. Proteins containing phenylalanine (e.g., in corn) are digested to amino acids. These are absorbed into the blood and transported to the liver.

4. In the liver, some of the phenylalanine is converted to other substances. Each step in this pathway is catalyzed by an enzyme. The enzyme step in converting phenylalanine to tyrosine is called phenylalanine hydroxylase. The product of the conversion is tyrosine, which is phenylalanine with a hydroxyl group.

5. To summarize: The substrate is phenylalanine, the product is tyrosine, and the enzyme is phenylalanine hydroxylase.

6. Other genetic disorders along the pathway include, besides alkaptonuria, the more familiar albinism.

B. Each enzyme is coded for by a gene. A gene can be mutated such that the expressed enzyme is not functional. When people are heterozygous (one normal and one mutant allele), the normal allele determines the good enzyme, and enough of it is made to provide normal function. So the parents who saw Dr. Folling were not mentally retarded and did not excrete phenylpyruvic acid into their urine.

III. Metabolism is the totality of biochemistry.

A. Metabolism is the sum total of all of the chemical transformations that occur in a biological entity: a cell, tissue, or organism. It is the expression of the phenotype.

1. Much of metabolism involves energy. Thermodynamics is the study of energy in physics and chemistry. There are two laws of thermodynamics.

a. The first law states that energy is not created or destroyed, only changed. This means that in any metabolic conversion, energy gets changed. For example, we eat sugar. The sugar gets converted to carbon dioxide (CO_2), which we breathe out. Sugar has a lot of energy stored in its chemical bonds. CO_2 has much less energy. So where does the energy go in this conversion? It gets released as heat and gets transferred to a conversion in the body that needs energy, like making fat!

     b.   The second law states that in any conversion, disorder increases and usable energy is lost (recall the old Woody Allen film in which the child gets depressed because the sun is "running down" and will be out of usable energy … in billions of years). What this means in biology is that it takes an input of energy to make complex substances from simple ones (or for a teenager to clean his or her room).

    2.   Biology is part of the physical universe. Life obeys these laws, just as the sun does. Scientists do not believe that there is a vital force that is different in life than elsewhere in the universe. This unity of nature is called "mechanism."

  B. Anabolism is the term for building up, and catabolism is the term for breaking down in biochemistry.

IV. There are several rules for metabolism.

  A. Metabolism occurs in small steps to release energy in small, usable packets. For example, consider sugar being converted to CO_2. This releases a lot of energy, about 50 times more than is needed for any single anabolic conversion in the cell. So if it happened in one step, most of the energy released would be lost as heat. Instead, it happens in over 40 steps, and energy is released in about a dozen of them.

  B. Because each metabolic conversion is determined by a gene, the pathways present in an organism are genetically determined. For example, bacteria have genes that code for enzymes that can take the carbon, hydrogen, and oxygen atoms in simple sugar and rearrange them to make ascorbic acid, vitamin C. We can't do this because we lack the enzymes. Other bacteria have the ability to take cellulose from wood or paper and convert it to sugar so they can use that for energy. Again, we lack the gene (and enzyme) to do this. Of course, there are many things we can do that bacteria can't. The point is, metabolism means phenotype, and this is determined by genes.

Essential Reading:
Jeremy M. Berg, John Tymoczko, and Lubert Stryer, *Biochemistry*, 6th ed. (New York: W. H. Freeman, 2006).

Michael Cain, Hans Damman, Robert Lue, and Carol Yoon, *Discover Biology*, 3rd ed. (New York: W. W. Norton, 2007), chap. 7.

Supplemental Reading:

Katherine Denniston and Joseph Topping, *Introduction to General, Organic and Biochemistry*, 4th ed. (New York: McGraw-Hill, 2003).

Thomas Devlin, *Textbook of Biochemistry with Clinical Correlations*, 6th ed. (Hoboken, NJ: Wiley-Liss, 2006).

Questions to Consider:

1. Think about your daily activities. Which are catabolic and which are anabolic? If you could get the genes for it, what biochemical pathway that some other organism has would you want?

2. PKU and alkaptonuria both occur because of enzyme deficiencies that result in accumulation of certain toxic substances. Both diseases are in the same pathway, which metabolizes the amino acid phenylalanine. Can you suggest a nutritional treatment to prevent the symptoms of these diseases? What would be the problems with nutritional treatment?

Lecture Seven—Transcript
Genes, Enzymes, and Metabolism

Welcome back. In the last lecture, I described how DNA is the gene and protein is the phenotype, and genetic arguments were used to establish this relationship. I want to continue that line of reasoning in this lecture and also describe how the phenotype plays itself out in the overall chemistry of tissues. My opening story concerns a human genetic disease. A Norwegian mother watched her six-year-old daughter and four-year-old son get progressively sicker over time. It was mid-1934, and both children were now profoundly, severely mentally retarded. Her family physician told her he couldn't help anymore and advised her to see a doctor Asbjorn Folling, who was a medical specialist in both chemistry and mental retardation. Folling saw the children with the mother and figured that the children's symptoms—this mental retardation and some other symptoms—might be related to blood sugar.

Sugar contains a chemical grouping called a ketone; it's carbon with some oxygens present. We don't have to know the chemistry as such, but I just want you to know that sugar does contain ketones. So Folling decided to test for excess ketones and an abnormality in sugars by testing the urine and adding to it a solution of a chemical called ferric chloride. Ferric chloride happens to be brown in color; I've used it myself in the lab. And when you add it to ketones, the solution turns purple. That's a diagnostic test of the presence of ketones derived from sugar. Folling did this; he added some ferric chloride to the urine of these two children, and lo and behold, the urine turned green; not purple, green. He said, I have never seen this before. What's going on? There's a ketone there, but it's doing something different to the ferric chloride and turning it green. What is this stuff?

Well, he first had to rule out that whatever was causing this color change came from the children's own body chemistry and not something they ate on the outside, so he did an experiment. His hypothesis was that this green color-changing stuff came from something the kids were taking; maybe one of their special medicines. They were on a whole bunch of medications that the mother gave them, which the other doctors had prescribed. So his hypothesis was, well, those medicines have something in them that is causing this green color change—that those ketones have nothing to do with the inherent biochemistry of these two children. To test the hypothesis, he asked the mother to stop giving these kids any of the special medications they were taking for the next week—this would clear them out of their system—and then he retested.

The result was the green color was still there. That means he could reject his hypothesis that the green-colored substance, the substance that turned ferric chloride green, came from the outside, because when you eliminated the outside stuff, the green color was still there, so it must be from the body chemistry. I mentioned that Folling was a medical specialist in chemistry, as well as mental retardation, so now he used his knowledge of chemistry. If you talk to your physician, you might ask them how was premedical education, and very often they will say well, the toughest course was chemistry—organic chemistry, they call it, the chemistry of carbons. That always has the reputation of being a tough course for students who are headed for a medical career. Folling actually did pretty well in chemistry, and did doctoral-level work in it.

What he did was extract this mystery substance, whatever it was causing the green color. Over a period of many, many long hours in the lab, he extracted this substance from the urine of these two children, and he identified it. The identity was something no one had ever seen before in urine, and it was called phenylpyruvic acid. That's the name—I'm going to give it to you for a reason—phenylpyruvic acid. It has a ketone in it, and so that's what caused the color change in ferric chloride from brown—but not to purple, to green. Folling now named this disorder in these two children. He looked in the literature, in scientific journals. He'd never seen anything like this described, with this strange chemical imbalance. He gave it the rather cumbersome Latin name "imbecillitas phenylpyruvica." It sounds descriptive. "Imbecile" was an old name—we no longer use it—to describe a severely retarded person; "phenylpyruvica" is, of course, phenylpyruvic acid. Later on, it was called "phenylketonuria," the ketones from the phenyl. Phenyl is a chemical grouping, so phenylketonuria, in the urine. So I will abbreviate phenylketonuria as PKU.

Over the next decade, Folling saw other mentally retarded people who put into their urine this phenylpyruvic acid, this combination, and he made the diagnosis of PKU. Over half of his PKU patients were siblings—brother/sister, brother/brother—just like the original pair of patients. In all of the families he saw when he had siblings, both parents were mentally normal, and they did not put this unusual chemical, phenylpyruvic acid, into their urine. Now this is the 1930s to 1940s. Folling knew Mendelian genetics, and he realized that PKU must be inherited as a recessively inherited allele because both parents were carriers. They had a normal allele taking care of their phenyl ketones, not allowing them to be put into the urine—whatever the chemical error was—and they also had the bad allele that would cause PKU.

The chances of having a child with PKU, therefore, are one half of the gametes the mother is going to make will have this bad allele; one half of the gametes of the sperm, that the father makes, will have the bad allele. So the combined probability is one in four. When he had large families, typically it was one in four children who had PKU. Now you might say well, how did it happen that this woman was bringing in two children who had PKU? She must have had eight kids, right, and the other six were normal? That's a lesson in statistics. In the average, it's going to be one in four, but it's certainly possible to have two consecutive children who have this one-in-four chance of inheriting the recessive allele.

Other human genetic diseases were known by Folling's time. In 1886, and into the 20th century, an English physician named Archibald Garrod began to see patients with a rare disorder. The rare disorder was called alkaptonuria. Again, it's something in the urine, but in this case the urine turned black when it was exposed to air. Garrod noted that this disease occurred most often in children of first-cousin marriages. First cousins have a grandparent in common, and he concluded that this must be a genetic disease—because in the first-cousin marriages, it seems to be more common, and it's caused by a recessive allele. Garrod took this one important step further in studying this particular disease. Enzymes had just been discovered. In fact, the idea of enzymes was first discovered literally at the turn of the 20th century, in the first couple of years of the 20th century, and Garrod, I told you, was working at the end of the 19th and the early 20th centuries. There was huge publicity about what enzymes were, their catalysts, and their proteins.

Garrod went out on a limb, and he proposed that the error in alkaptonuria was expressed as a lack of an enzyme activity—the lack of a functional enzyme—and that the normal function of this enzyme was to convert some product of protein breakdown. He didn't know what it was. Knowing about genes and proteins, he came up with the one gene–one protein idea long before the people who worked on bacteria did, as I described in the previous lecture. Garrod called alkaptonuria an "inborn error" of biochemistry, and to this day there are journals of inborn errors, and there's a Society of Inborn Errors. People still use that term. Inborn, of course, means genetic. Garrod made the following statement: "I believe that no two individuals are exactly alike chemically any more than structurally." Let me repeat. "I believe that no two individuals are exactly alike chemically any more than structurally"—an amazing and true prediction. We are all unique in our genetic makeup and in our phenotype, as it turns out, and Garrod said this 100 years ago.

I want to talk about protein as the phenotype now, and biochemistry as the expression of the phenotype. A biochemical pathway, as I described in the last lecture, describes a sequential conversion of substances in the body. Each step in a biochemical pathway, as I said in the last lecture, is catalyzed by its own specific protein, its enzyme, that is encoded for by a gene. So we can envision a gene, DNA, encoding, or having the information that will determine, an enzyme. The enzyme folds into a three-dimensional structure because it is a protein that can do that. You'll recall proteins do this in a spontaneous fashion depending on the order and chemistry of the amino acids in that order. These enzymes then bind substances, line them up, to allow products to form. The substances that bind to enzymes are called substrates—a substrate is a substance that is acted upon by an enzyme to form a product—and the products, well, they're called products.

Now back to a biochemical pathway. A single biochemical pathway involves the enzymes that are deficient or that have inherited errors in their genes, in a wide variety of diseases, including the two that we have described—in phenylketonuria, PKU, in alkaptonuria, in a couple of other diseases. For example, in albinism, albinos lack a product that comes from the product of phenylalanine metabolism. So phenylalanine is converted by an enzyme into its product, and that ends up being converted into pigment. If the enzyme that converts the product into pigment isn't there or isn't active, you get albinism. So several genetic disorders exist in this, and every, biochemical pathway.

Some pathways are more important than others, and so there are some genetic disorders we never see because the people just don't get born. Imagine the genetic disorder in the ability to have cells have energy in some way. If you have that, you couldn't have any energy. The cell couldn't do anything, and so it's not going to survive much in the embryo. Phenylalanine, which is the substrate involved with PKU, gets converted into this phenylpyruvic acid because phenylalanine—it's a side-shunt pathway that normally doesn't happen—normally gets converted into another amino acid in the liver called tyrosine. Phenylalanine is an amino acid, and it's one of the essential amino acids we cannot make, and so we take it in in our food. When proteins containing phenylalanine are taken in—like, for example, corn protein—they are digested in the intestine to their individual building blocks, the amino acids. One of those amino acids happens to be phenylalanine.

Now here's what happens in the body after digestion. The amino acids, or any digestion products, end up in the blood. The blood goes from the intestine, and the first stop before it goes to the heart, or anywhere else in the body, is the liver. The liver is an amazing organ. It is what I call a chemostat. You know, a thermostat is a piece of machinery that detects the temperature in the atmosphere surrounding it and then sends an instruction—turn on the heat or turn on the air conditioning—depending on the temperature. That's a thermostat; it keeps the temperature at the level that you want. The liver is like that; it's a chemostat. It looks at the chemical composition of blood that arrives in it, and then says well, should we convert some of the chemicals that arrive into other things? There might not be enough blood sugar, so we'll convert some of the protein into sugars, etc. All those conversions go on in the liver.

Now in the liver, typically some of the phenylalanine that is part of protein is converted to other substances, and each of these conversions is catalyzed by an enzyme present in the liver. The enzyme that is responsible for catalyzing the conversion of phenylalanine into its product, which is another amino acid called tyrosine, has a name: It's called phenylalanine hydroxylase. That's the name of the enzyme that can do this. The product, as I mentioned, is tyrosine, which is phenylalanine with a hydroxyl group; that's why it's called hydroxylase. To summarize, what are we dealing with in biochemistry here? The substrate of this reaction is phenylalanine. The product of this reaction is tyrosine. The enzyme that speeds it up is called phenylalanine hydroxylase. It's the enzyme whose structure and function are determined by DNA, the gene. I mentioned, of course, the other genetic disorders along this pathway.

Now each enzyme in a pathway is encoded for by its own gene, and genes can be changed in some way. That is, the information content of DNA can be changed—we will specify this later on in the course—and by changing the information content in DNA, you can change the expression of that information content as protein. If you change the order of amino acids in protein, the expression, the protein will fold differently. If it doesn't fold in the right way, it will not present the surface for the substrate, for phenylalanine, to bind and do its thing and get converted into tyrosine. The parents of the children who had PKU that Folling originally saw were not mentally retarded, as I mentioned. They didn't put phenylpyruvic acid in their urine. Why? Because they had one of their two copies of DNA coding for this enzyme as being the good copy; the DNA that had not been changed, the DNA that had not been mutated. They were essentially carriers of the mutant gene, the mutant allele.

I want now to turn to the overall aspects of biochemistry and how that reflects the genetics of an organism. Metabolism is a term that you often hear, and it is essentially the sum total of all of the chemical transformations that occur in some sort of biological entity. It could be the metabolism of a cell, a single cell's metabolism. It could be the metabolism of a tissue, a muscle. So we can talk about muscle metabolism—that means all the chemical reactions and changes going on in a muscle—or it could be the metabolism of a whole person, a whole organism. So we talk about the metabolic rate of a human's metabolism. Some people are high metabolizers; others are lower metabolizers. That's a general term for saying they just do a lot of chemistry in a high level or low level, especially in regards to energy metabolism. Metabolism is the expression of the phenotype, and much of metabolism involves energy, transferring energy.

I mentioned earlier on in the course that there are three major ideas that tie biology together: mechanism, cell theory, evolution. Mechanism of metabolism is reflected by the study called thermodynamics. Thermodynamics is the physical study of energy—thermo, heat; dynamic, change—changing heat. It's not really heat; it's energy. There are lots of forms of energy. There's heat energy, there's chemical energy, there's light energy—you know those three—and there's electrical energy, there's nuclear energy. There are two laws of thermodynamics that physicists, chemists, and biologists agree apply in biological systems as well as the rest of the universe. The two laws are appropriately called the first law of thermodynamics and the second law of thermodynamics; really good names.

The first law says that energy is neither created nor destroyed. If you look in the whole universe, the sum total of the energy is constant. All we're doing is changing energy into one form or another. We can't create energy. This means that in living tissues, in any metabolic conversion, we're just changing energy from one form to another.

Let me give you an example. We eat some sugar—good food energy in sugar—and the sugar gets converted, ultimately, into carbon dioxide, which we breathe out. So our reaction is sugar, lots of bonds, and sugar and carbon dioxide. Sugar has a lot of energy stored in its chemical bonds. I'll give you the formula for sugar—$C_6H_{12}O_6$. Lots of carbons and oxygens and hydrogens all tied together. The tying together requires and stores energy. CO_2, carbon dioxide, not much energy at all. Well, where does the energy go? We're converting this complex thing that has a lot of stored energy into a simple molecule that has very little energy. Energy is neither created nor destroyed. Some of the energy goes off as heat—and that heats up our body, by the way—and other aspects of this energy are used immediately by reactions in the body that need energy; like, for instance, making fat. So if you eat excess food, of carbohydrate, you can use that excess energy, but you don't really take it off as so much heat. The body doesn't want a lot of heat coming off, so instead you use that energy chemically to store it as fat. That's the first law.

The second law of thermodynamics says that in any conversion involving energy, disorder increases, and usable energy is lost. I said some energy comes off as heat. Well, if we trapped all that heat, and we trapped all that chemical energy, we're still missing some energy. Chemists and physicists recognize that the universe is kind of running down, that the tendency of the universe is to have energy in a form that is disordered. We call that entropy. There's an old Woody Allen film that I recall in which Woody has a kind of daydream in which he recalls his youth. He's a young kid in the 1940s, and his mother has taken him to a doctor because Woody is very depressed. He just read in a magazine that the sun, all the chemical reactions going on in the sun, are converting one energy into another, and some of it's going off as heat, and some of it's going off as light. But some of it is being converted to this unusable form, entropy, and gradually—astronomers have said in the article Woody has read—the sun is running down and will be out of usable energy, and the earth will no longer have life on it at that point because there won't be any more sun.

The doctor, who was smoking a cigarette, as I recall, in this scene, says to Woody in a kindly way, "But that's not going to happen for billions of years." And the mother, of course, screams at Woody, saying, "Hear that? Billions of years. Go do your homework. Stop worrying about it." Now what this idea of unusable energy in biology means is that it requires an input of energy to make complex substances from simple ones. If you want to build a complex protein, you're going to need energy for that building, and you'll see how this happens later on in the course. It's just like a teenager and cleaning up his or her room, you know, it requires an input of energy to do so. So "mechanism" tells us biology is part of the physical universe, and life obeys these laws of thermodynamics, just like the sun does.

We recognize, in terms of energy, two types of chemical pathways in cells and tissues, in living tissues. These two pathways are called catabolism and anabolism. Catabolism means breaking down complex substances like sugar to simple ones like carbon dioxide, and releasing energy for use in the cell. So that's what catabolism is, breaking down the complex to the simple and releasing energy; an example, of course, being the breakdown of sugar. Anabolism—you know, anabolic things—build up, so anabolism builds up complex substances, and therefore requires energy. So anabolic steroids are drugs or hormones that cause a buildup of muscle tissues, and you can get all buff, etc. I always tell my students that I'm doing that in the gym every day, and they laugh because I'm a rather thin person.

There are several rules for metabolism that biological tissues obey, and they are genetically determined. These two rules are, first, metabolism occurs in small steps to release energy in small usable amounts; and second, that metabolism and conversions and pathways are genetically determined. First, the small steps. Consider sugar, as I mentioned before in catabolism, the breakdown, being converted into carbon dioxide, this simple molecule. I mentioned it releases a lot of energy. Those stored bonds in the $C_6H_{12}O_6$— all these bonds between the carbons and the hydrogens and oxygens—store a lot of energy. The amount of energy if you did this in one fell swoop, one single reaction, is 50 times more than a cell would ever need for a single anabolic reaction in the cell, a single building-up chemical reaction. So you lose a lot of the energy; you lose 98% of it because you don't need that much energy. It's like using an atomic bomb for a firecracker, right?

So this is not really good. You're going to lose most of the energy as heat. Instead, in biochemistry, in the cell, this conversion of $C_6H_{12}O_6$, of this complicated sugar, into simple CO_2, carbon dioxide, happens in 40 steps, and the energy is released bit by bit. Each bit then can be used efficiently for anabolism. There's about a dozen steps in this conversion, and 40 steps that actually release some energy, because we have to rearrange the molecules. It's a fascinating series of events that biochemistry students have to learn. Because each of these conversions is catalyzed by an enzyme and therefore determined by a gene, the overall pathway I've just described—these 40 events that happen, going on to CO_2—is genetically determined because there's a gene for an enzyme for each one of the steps in this particular pathway. Just as I could say A to B to C to D, there are 40 steps involved.

Let me give you an example of genes determining biochemical pathways because there's a great diversity in nature. Just getting energy out of sugar; well, a lot of organisms can do that. Let's look at some that are particular. I'll talk about the lowly bacteria. They're not necessarily lowly; they're just complicated in their own way. For instance, bacteria have genes that determine the enzymes that can take carbon, hydrogen, and oxygen, and mix them up and put them together in a simple sugar to rearrange them to make ascorbic acid, also known as vitamin C. We can't do that. We can't rearrange atoms to make vitamin C. We don't have that gene and that enzyme. Another example: There's some other bacteria that can take cellulose, which is paper or indigestible things that we can't digest from wood or paper or grass, and convert this cellulose, which is a polymer of glucose—glucoses hooked together—and convert it into glucose sugar. Glucose is one of the sugars. And so they can use this sugar for energy. We can't do it. We lack the gene, and therefore the enzyme, for this biochemical pathway.

Well, of course, there are many things that we can do and that bacteria can't, so I mean we can get back at them in our own way. My point is metabolism—sum total of chemical reactions—means phenotype, and this is determined ultimately by genes and the enzymes that they determine. We now turn in the next lecture to the way that DNA as the gene actually determines protein as the phenotype. Thank you.

Lecture Eight
From DNA to Protein

Scope: The gene (DNA) resides in the cell nucleus, but its expression (protein) occurs outside the nucleus at a molecular "workbench" called the ribosome. A gene is transcribed into messenger RNA (mRNA), which is a copy of the gene that is sent to the ribosome. A specific sequence of DNA bases near the gene called the promoter determines whether a gene will be transcribed and therefore expressed in the phenotype. Substances such as hormones that cause cells to specialize may act as promoters to enhance transcription of certain genes. The gene and its mRNA contain a sequence of nucleotide bases. This sequence is translated at the ribosome into a sequence of amino acids to make a protein. The intermediary between the mRNA and amino acids is transfer RNA (tRNA), which carries the amino acid to the ribosome and binds to the appropriate sequence on mRNA. This sequence is determined by the genetic code. So the order of amino acids in a protein is determined by the order of codons in mRNA, which is determined by the order of nucleotides in DNA. A mutation is a change in the base sequence of DNA. A single base-pair change can lead to an amino acid change, which leads to a change in the function of a protein in the phenotype.

Outline

I. Opening story: toxic revenge on gene expression.

    A. Journalist Georgi Markov was waiting for a bus in London.

        1. A man carrying an umbrella (not an unusual sight) brushed up against him, and Markov felt a pinprick in the leg as the man's umbrella poked him. Within a few hours he felt weak, and two days later he was dead.

        2. The police found a tiny pellet where the umbrella had poked him, and chemical analysis revealed it was coated with ricin, a poison extracted from the seeds of the castor bean plant. I remember taking castor oil as a child, with my mother telling me it would clean out my stomach. Fortunately, ricin is a protein that does not dissolve in the oil; otherwise, I might have had an excuse to avoid the oil's awful taste.

3. Since the Markov assassination in 1978, ricin has been in the news. It was probably used by Iraq in its war with Iran in the 1980s and was the partial basis of possible weapons of mass destruction that the government of Iraq allegedly stockpiled prior to 2003. In 2002, ricin was found in caves in Afghanistan abandoned by Al-Qaeda. In 2004, traces of it were found in a mailroom at the U.S. Senate building, prompting evacuation. Less than 1/10,000 of an ounce can kill a person.

B. Ricin inhibits gene expression.
   1. As Markov found out the hard way, ricin is very toxic to people. The plant makes it as a storage protein in its seeds. As they germinate, the ricin is broken down (catabolized) to amino acids for the growing plant embryo to use.
   2. Unfortunately, the ricin protein has enzyme activity. It catalyzes the modification and breakage of an essential molecule in the ribosome, the part of the cell that is used to make proteins. Inactivation of the ribosome essentially inactivates gene expression, and the cell dies.

II. Translating the information in the gene (DNA) to its expression (protein).
   A. We have seen that a gene is expressed as a protein. This poses a chemical problem: These are very different molecules.
      1. Gene: DNA with a sequence of nucleotide bases (A, T, G, C).
      2. Expression: protein with a sequence of amino acids (20).
   B. The locations of the gene and its expression are different.
      1. Gene: in the nucleus.
      2. Protein: made in the cytoplasm (outside the nucleus).

III. Information signals for protein synthesis.
   A. DNA sends a copy of its instructions to the ribosome.
      1. There are many genes on a chromosome: For example, a human chromosome has thousands of genes.
      2. A cell only expresses certain genes as proteins (you don't make hemoglobin in your hair, and don't make hair in your red blood cells).
      3. Determining which genes to express is the central issue of cell differentiation.
      4. A copy of the gene is sent to the ribosome (similar to a copy of architectural plans sent to the job site). That copy is mRNA

(m = messenger). It is made by an enzyme, RNA polymerase, and is a base-paired copy:

If a region of DNA is: AAGTATGTTAGCCGT
                         TTCATACAATCGGCA,

then if the bottom strand is copied to RNA, it will be (RNA has U, not T):   AAGUAUGUUAGCCGU.

This is called gene transcription.

B. A signaling sequence on DNA attracts the RNA polymerase for copying.

    1. The signal is called a promoter sequence.

    2. The RNA polymerase is guided to the promoter by a host of other substances that bind to it: These are the factors that cause a cell to specialize.

    3. Example: Hemoglobin is made by developing red blood cells. A hormone is made to stimulate this. The hormone enters the cells and goes to the nucleus, where it acts at the promoter for hemoglobin, directing RNA polymerase to copy that gene (transcribe it).

C. The mRNA goes to the ribosome, where it sits and waits for the appropriate amino acid.

    1. Amino acids are each brought to the ribosome by a different RNA called tRNA (t = transfer).

    2. The tRNA can bind by base pairing to the mRNA. This is done by triplets of bases. For example, for the amino acid lysine, where there is AAA in mRNA, the appropriate lysine-carrying tRNA has UUU (U bonds with A in base pairing).

D. The genetic code is the key to translating the DNA information to amino acid information.

    1. The code is in three base letters: AAA in mRNA means lysine tRNA will bind and be put at that spot in the growing protein chain.

    2. It is very important to relate this to the gene (DNA). If the mRNA has AAA, then it must have come from a DNA that is:

        AAA
        TTT

    3. So the order of bases in the gene determines the order of amino acids in the protein.

    4. There are 64 codons of 3 bases each ($4 \times 4 \times 4$), and almost all code for amino acids.

5. The "meaning" of each codon was determined by clever test tube experiments using synthetic mRNAs.

6. The code is virtually universal for all of life on Earth: This is vital for understanding genetics, evolution, and biotechnology. We have a common language.

E. It takes a minute for a cell to make a protein with 500 amino acids. There are hundreds of ribosomes in a cell. Ricin blocks the ribosome in eukaryotic cells. Antibiotics such as tetracycline and neomycin block the ribosome in prokaryotic cells (bacteria) by binding to proteins. Genetically determined antibiotic resistance is a phenotype often caused by a gene mutation resulting in an altered ribosomal protein.

IV. The genetic code explains mutation.

A. Consider phenylketonuria, a genetically inherited disease caused by a defective enzyme, phenylalanine hydroxylase.

1. In its common genetic variant:

Normal:	Mutant:
Protein is 451 amino acids	Protein is 451 amino acids (but not functional)
Amino acid 408 is arginine	Amino acid 408 is tryptophan
Codon in DNA at 408 is	Codon in DNA at 408 is
CGG	TGG
GCC	ACC
mRNA from bottom	mRNA from bottom
CGG	UGG
Amino acid is arg	Amino acid is trp

2. Note that this is one base-pair change in a gene that is thousands of base pairs long. The human genome has 2 billion base pairs, and this one change leads to a protein with the incorrect shape to do its job.

B. There is a new way to define a gene and a mutation.

1. Genetic mutation can now be defined chemically as a change in DNA base.

2. Genetic capacity can now be defined as the presence of a DNA sequence that codes for a protein with a specific function.

Essential Reading:

Horace Freeland Judson, *The Eighth Day of Creation: Makers of the Revolution in Biology* (Woodbury, NY: Cold Spring Harbor Laboratory Press, 1996).

Harvey Lodish, Arnold Berk, Paul Matsudaira, Chris Kaiser, Monty Krieger, Matthew P. Scott, Lawrence Zipursky, and James Darnell, *Molecular Cell Biology*, 5th ed. (New York: W. H. Freeman, 2005), chaps. 4 and 11.

Supplemental Reading:

Benjamin Lewin, *Genes VIII* (Upper Saddle River, NJ: Pearson Prentice-Hall, 2005).

David Sadava, Craig Heller, Gordon Orians, William Purves, and David Hillis, *Life: The Science of Biology,* 8th ed. (Sunderland, MA: Sinauer Associates; New York: W. H. Freeman and Co., 2008).

Questions to Consider:

1. The ribosome is the workbench for protein synthesis. The molecules that make up the ribosome in bacteria differ from those in eukaryotes, although their roles are the same in making a protein. This is an example of convergent evolution. Antibiotics such as streptomycin, neomycin, and tetracycline block protein synthesis at only the prokaryotic ribosome (Otherwise they would kill the patient, like ricin!). Can you explain how these antibiotics might work and why they are specific?

2. What are the implications of a common genetic code for all organisms for the origin and evolution of life?

Lecture Eight—Transcript
From DNA to Protein

Welcome back. In the last two lectures, I've described how genes, composed of DNA, are expressed outwardly as the phenotype, which I defined as proteins. DNA has an information content in nucleotide bases. Protein has amino acids that allow a protein to fold and have a function. In this lecture, I'd like to describe how this happens; how information gets translated from DNA to protein. My opening story is about toxic revenge on gene expression. In 1978, Georgi Markov was a journalist waiting for a bus in London. Markov, a Bulgarian, was an expatriate who had written several articles critical of the government in his home country. A man carrying an umbrella, not an unusual sight in London, brushed up against Markov. Markov felt a pinprick as the man brushed by, and a few hours later, Markov felt rather weak. Two days later, he was dead.

Police found a tiny pellet where the umbrella had poked Markov, and chemical analysis of this pellet revealed a poison called ricin, which is extracted from seeds of the castor bean plant. Now, I remember when I was a kid, I was given castor oil once a month by my mother, and she told me it would clean out my stomach. I hated the stuff. It was the vilest-tasting thing I can recall. In fact, one of the great puzzles of my youth was listening to an ad on the radio saying children cry for this product—I won't give you the name of the product. I couldn't figure that out. I guess they were crying because of the anticipation of having to swallow that stuff. Well, fortunately, ricin as a protein doesn't dissolve well in castor oil; otherwise, I would have had a really good excuse to avoid the awful taste of that stuff.

Since the Markov assassination in 1978, ricin has continued to be in the news. It was used by the Iraqis in their war with Iran in the 1980s. It's the partial basis of weapons of mass destruction that the government of Iraq was allegedly stockpiling prior to 2003. In 2002, some ricin was found in caves in Afghanistan that had been abandoned by Al-Qaeda. In 2004, traces of ricin were found in the mailroom of the U.S. Senate building in Washington, DC, and the entire building had to be evacuated. This stuff is really poisonous: 1/10,000 of an ounce can kill a person. How does ricin work? It works by inhibiting gene expression. The castor bean plant makes ricin as a storage protein in its seeds. The seed of a plant, as I will describe when we talk about agriculture in Lecture Twenty-Three, is a lunchbox. It's got stored proteins and starch to provide, respectively, amino acids, which are the building blocks of proteins, and sugars, which are the building blocks of starch, for the developing embryo.

So, as the castor bean plant seed germinates, it sends out chemicals that will degrade or catabolize—now we have a word I talked about in the last lecture. It breaks down ricin to its amino acids, and those amino acids can be refashioned by the embryo of the plant for their own use. Now unfortunately, ricin has an enzymatic activity that affects animal ribosomes. Ribosomes are the place where proteins are made in the cell. This enzyme catalyzes the modification and breakage of an essential substance in this ribosome workbench for making proteins. So, when the substance is no longer present, the ribosome is no longer able to catalyze the formation of proteins. No making of proteins means no phenotype, expression of genes; cells die, and people die too.

This lecture is about translating information that is in the gene, as DNA, as its expression, phenotype, protein. I want to talk about that in a couple of ways. First of all, I'll try to set up the problem of translation. We've got two different languages here. Secondly, I'll try to talk about information signals for making proteins, and then get to something called the genetic code, which is an amazing translating device. We have seen how genes are expressed as proteins, and this poses a big chemical problem because genes, DNA, are really different from proteins. The building blocks of DNA are chemicals that are totally different than their expression as proteins. It's kind of like saying English is a totally different language from Hebrew. The letters look different, the meaning is different; they even do it from a different direction, right? English is read from left to right, Hebrew from right to left.

Proteins are composed of amino acids—carbons, hydrogens, oxygens—and they're pretty regular in their linear structure. DNA is a double helix composed of these nucleotides that have nitrogen and sugar and phosphate, a sugar-phosphate backbone with these DNA bases. You remember what they're called; A, T, G, and C. I'll give you the names again—adenine, thymine, guanine, and cytosine—and I promise not to give you those names ever again in the course. From now on, we'll call them A, T, G, and C. There's 20 amino acids in protein, not just four, as there are bases. There are 20 amino acids in protein.

These molecules' structures look totally different. DNA is a linear double helix. It can bend slightly, but it is largely a long fiber. Protein is in three dimensions, and I described when I described protein structure in a previous lecture how this thing folds spontaneously when it's put into water because of the properties of its constituent beads on the chain. These things are even different in their location in the cell. DNA—I think I've made this point abundantly in the course—is located overwhelmingly in the nucleus of the cell. The vast proportion of DNA is in the chromosomes residing in the nucleus, these huge molecules. Proteins, well, they're all over the cell, actually. There are proteins in the nucleus, as I mentioned before. There are proteins everywhere because of their vital functions as structural elements and as enzymes. This is the phenotypic expression of genes.

DNA has a linear sequence, and protein has a three-dimensional sequence. Protein is made in a location that's quite distant in cellular terms from DNA. Protein is made at the ribosome, and the ribosome is a small particle outside of the nucleus, out there in the soup of the cell. How do we know this? We know this because we can take a cell and feed it amino acids that are labeled in some way. The label I will choose will be a radioactive label, but you can think of it as amino acids labeled with red dye. And then you ask the question, where do we get proteins being hooked together? Where does that red dye get hooked together to form proteins? You look for the red proteins that are just being made. And if you catch a protein just in the stage of being made, that protein will be made at the ribosome, which is far away from the DNA. So right away, we have a geographical problem as well as a chemical problem.

Information signals are very important in protein synthesis. The first thing that has to happen is that DNA has to send some information and signals for protein synthesis out to the ribosome. Now there's two ways to look at this. The DNA itself could go out to the ribosome; that is, the gene or chromosome that we want to express could leave the nucleus and go out to the ribosome and say, I have the information to make this particular protein. Do it now. That's one way to look at it. The other way to look at it is the DNA would say well, I've got 1000 genes per chromosome and 23 chromosomes. It would not make sense for 1000 genes to be made at once, to be translated into protein at once. So if we're only going to translate or express a couple of those genes, why not just send a copy of the DNA out to the ribosome, and the DNA can stay in the nucleus?

Think of an architectural firm. Supposing you are building a house; well, you're supervising the building of a house. You're paying for the building of a house. A contractor is assigned to build the house for you, and the contractor has architectural plans from an architectural firm. The architectural firm might be downtown in your community, and you may live in the suburbs. Does the architectural firm take the original plans, the only copy, and drive out to your worksite and have those plans there as you build the house? No. That architectural firm might be supervising the building of 50 houses at that time. They all might be different, and so what they do is, of course, they make a copy. They go down to the local copy shop, and they make a copy of those plans, and they send it out. The original copy remains at the architectural firm. Think of gene expression, DNA expression, in the same way. DNA is expressed as proteins, and the copy of the DNA is being sent out to the ribosome.

The exact chemical nature of this copy is not as DNA. It's a different molecule called RNA. RNA is obviously a cousin of DNA because it's got an "R" instead of a "D." The D stands for deoxyribonucleic acid, DNA; R stands for ribonucleic acid. The sugar is the big difference. There are two differences. The biggest difference is the sugar, and the sugar in RNA is ribose sugar, whereas the sugar in DNA is deoxyribose. So they're slightly different. RNA is single-stranded; it's not a double-stranded molecule. That's very important because if RNA is single-stranded, its sugar-phosphate backbone exposes those beads to the outer world, doesn't it, because the beads are hanging down from the chain. If DNA is a double-stranded molecule, the beads are internal, right? It's two chains with the beads hanging down, and those beads are internal, inside the molecule. They're not exposed to the outside environment of the cell. So DNA and RNA are different in that way. RNA, being single-stranded, has its nucleotide bases exposed to the outside. That's going to be very important because RNA is going to act as a message from DNA. That's why, of course, it's called messenger RNA. It's a message from DNA that says, make this protein. But the language is still in nucleotides; it's still in bases.

The enzyme that catalyzes the production of RNA from DNA has a name, and like DNA polymerase, this is called RNA polymerase, and it makes a base-paired copy from DNA. Now what do I mean by that? Let's consider the base pairs in DNA. You'll recall A always pairs with T; G always pairs with C. Okay, T always pairs with A; C always pairs with G. I think I've got it across both ways. These bases fit into one another and recognize one another. So if we have a region of DNA that, for my hypothetical purposes, has the following sequence, AAAAAA, the other strand of DNA will be what is called "complementary"—will have the bases that fit into this—will be TTTTTT. So we've got two strands of DNA: AAAAAA and TTTTTT. Now let us say that the information content is in that first strand, AAAAAA. If we make an RNA copy from the opposite strand of DNA, TTTTTT, the opposite bases in RNA will be As, correct? In DNA, the opposite; the A goes with T, and now the bases opposite in RNA will be As again, so we're making a copy of that original gene, AAAAAA, and that's the molecule that goes out to the ribosome.

Let's step back a minute and think of the fact that DNA is double-stranded, and now think of why DNA might be double-stranded. What a marvelous molecule this is because the double-stranded DNA allows for its duplication. Each of the new strands of double strands of the DNA has a complement from the old strand of DNA, and so is semiconservative in its replication. That's really nice. If DNA was single-stranded, it wouldn't work that way because an AAAAAA, if it was just single-stranded, would make a TTTTTT. That's not AAAAAA. You can't make As off of As. You have to make it by the complementary, the bases that fit each other. So it's nice that DNA is double-stranded. It's nice that DNA is double-stranded for gene expression because we can have AAAAAA and then TTTTTT in the other strand, and now off of those Ts you can peel off a bunch of As and mimic the original strand.

So we have our AAAAAA going out of the nucleus, out to the ribosome. How's it get there? Well, there's a lot of mechanics going on here in the cell, and people have looked at all of the minor minutiae of how things leave the nucleus. The nucleus has little holes in it, through which the molecules of RNA can move, etc. I don't want to talk about that. That's just all complex machinery. But there's a really important aspect here we have to address, and that's the following. Each chromosome, piece of DNA, of the 23 chromosome pairs in a human genome has over 100 million base pairs of DNA. This is a long molecule. We only express at a given time in a cell certain genes. We don't express all genes at all times. I'll give you an example. You don't make hemoglobin in your hair. You don't make hair in your bone marrow. A profound and important conclusion; please send Nobel Prize to the following address.

Not trivial, though, because we have the genes for making them. So if we consider a long chromosome that might have the genes both for making hair and hemoglobin—the protein component of hemoglobin—the question now is what's going to cause, in an immature red blood cell in your bone marrow, the hemoglobin gene to be making its RNA copy, to make hemoglobin at the ribosome, and in the hair follicle to make the hair protein and not the hemoglobin protein? There has to be an information signal, and the information signal has to reside in the DNA itself. So a gene is not just a sequence of information that determines which protein is going to be made and the order of amino acids in that protein. The gene also has to have a sequence adjacent to it that says, turn me on here in the red blood cell and not in the hair.

That sequence is a group of nucleotides that's different, obviously, for the hair gene than it is for the hemoglobin gene. That sequence of nucleotides is called a promoter. This is a signaling sequence for gene expression. A promoter is a sequence of nucleotides that is recognized by proteins. Now what do I mean by that? I've given you the impression that in terms of information content, DNA is pretty important because the AGTCCCC has a language. But now I'm telling you that the AGT and certain sequence of nucleotides also have information of a three-dimensional nature that can be recognized by proteins that fold in a three-dimensional nature. So if we have a protein called RNA polymerase, RNA polymerase will land on DNA only at that promoter region. That's not helping us at all because RNA polymerase will land at the promoter for hair in my bone marrow, and my bone marrow will start making hair. If RNA polymerase just lands there, it'll start making the RNA copy of every particular gene because every gene has a promoter.

Promoters also attract other proteins, and it's called a "complex." It may be due to the people who study this thing psychologically, but it's a complex of proteins that land there. Let me give you an example. Hemoglobin, as I've mentioned, is made in red blood cells. There's a hormone that stimulates this. That's going to be the big difference. The hormone enters the red blood cell in the bone marrow, and the hormone binds to molecules of protein in the bone marrow, and they together go into the nucleus and bind to the promoter. And then they gather the RNA polymerase and say, okay, please make the copy here. That's really important because it says that the promoter is the place that stimulates and differentiates one cell and one gene from another.

This process of making an RNA copy of a gene, due to the promoter and the specific nature of the promoter—this will be important when we talk about biotechnology—is called gene transcription. The next stage is gene translation. So now we have an RNA copy at the ribosome, and we're going to translate that into amino acids and proteins. This is done by bringing the amino acids to the ribosome. How is this going to be accomplished? It's going to be accomplished by another type of RNA called "transfer RNA." Transfer RNA grabs the amino acid out there in the cell and brings it to the ribosome, and transfer RNA—it's made up of nucleotides—and the nucleotides in transfer RNA are opposite to those in messenger RNA. So when it sees AAA in messenger RNA, the transfer RNA will have the opposite nucleotides to that and bind to it.

What is the language? The language is called the genetic code, and the code words are three bases each. Let us say the language was only one base. Let us say in messenger RNA, every time there was an A, you would bring in amino acid number one; makes sense. So there'd be four different nucleotides, four different amino acids. That's not going to work because you have 20 different amino acids. You need 20 different words in the messenger RNA to bring 20 different amino acids. Okay, there are four bases; let's make two letters, right? AA, AG, GA, GC, right? There's 16 possibilities. That's not going to work either, right? We need at least 20 different words, and we have 20 different words if we have 64. So if there are $4 \times 4 \times 4$, or three nucleotides in the codeword in messenger RNA, we can essentially get the language that we need.

The code was actually deciphered first by a scientist named Marshall Nirenberg in 1961. Nirenberg did a very famous experiment where he took a test tube, and he added everything you need to make proteins except messenger RNA. And when he put in a messenger RNA that just contained U—it's the equivalent of T in messenger RNA, it's a different nucleotide called uracil—he put in a bunch of UUUUUs, and he asked which amino acid is going to be put into protein. So he had this in the test tube. He had all the amino acids there, and he said which amino acid will be put into protein if we have the signal UUU in messenger RNA? It turned out to be an amino acid called phenylalanine. Next he made a messenger RNA that had AAAAA, and it got lysine. Then he tried CCCC, and he got another amino acid called proline. So that's the way you decipher the code, with these artificial test tube experiments with messenger RNA.

The sociology was very interesting. Nirenberg was a very young, not famous scientist, and he was not a self-promoting kind of person. He presented a talk at the International Congress of Biochemistry in 1961 in Moscow to an audience of less than 10 people. Everyone was going after what the genetic code was. What's the messenger RNA that primes the synthesis of amino acid? And this guy that no one ever heard of had done it. It turned out that

Crick, of Watson and Crick, was in the audience because he had seen the title of this thing, and he said wow, this guy may have cracked the genetic code. Crick walked up to Nirenberg afterwards, and he said would you like to give your talk again tomorrow morning on the last day of the conference? And the guy said okay, I was going to leave, but I guess I'll give a talk again tomorrow. There were 2000 people in the audience, and they gave him a standing ovation. A couple of years later, he won the Nobel Prize.

The genetic code is a very fascinating thing. There are code words for all 20 amino acids, and these are determined, again, in the messenger RNA that comes from the DNA. That's the most important thing genetically that I want you to know. The DNA makes a messenger RNA that has the code word that determines the order of the amino acids, and the code is in the messenger RNA. The code is virtually universal for all life on earth; amazing. We use the same genetic code as coconuts, as bacteria. We have a common language. This implies that we're all related in some way, and evolutionarily we'd call that descent with modification. It takes about a minute for a cell to make a protein with 500 amino acids. Things are happening pretty fast down there.

Antibiotics such as tetracycline, for example, block the ribosome in prokaryotic cells like bacteria that infect us only because the ribosome has slightly different components in prokaryotes as it does in eukaryotes such as plants and animals. So these antibiotics can take advantage of that by binding to that particular ribosome. You might ask, well, how do I become resistant to an antibiotic? Obviously the gene coding for that particular protein that's in the ribosome, to which the antibiotic binds, might mutate. The protein in the ribosome will fold differently. The antibiotic can't bind anymore, and now you have antibiotic resistance. We'll talk about that later on in the course.

Genetic coding explains the phenomenon of mutation. Consider phenylketonuria, a disease I've talked about several times in the course. It's genetically inherited. A gene codes for a defective enzyme, when it's in mutant form, called phenylalanine hydroxylase. Remember phenylalanine is converted to tyrosine, and when this doesn't happen, mental retardation can be the result.

Let's now define this in the precise terms that we're able to do at this point in the course. In the normal situation, in the dominant gene that codes for the protein, the protein phenylalanine hydroxylase has 451 amino acids. In the most common mutant form, in phenylketonuria, the protein has 451 amino acids; same length. At position number 408 of the 451, the coding information in DNA is CGG in the normal situation. At position number 408 in the mutant situation, the coding information is TGG. A single base; a C in the normal, a T in the mutant. Now we're beginning to define what a mutation really is. It's a change in DNA; a single letter has changed. The amino acid that is primed from this, in the chain at position 408 of 451, is called arginine in the normal and tryptophan in the mutant.

Now the arginine at position 408 causes the protein to fold in a certain way, and it catalyzes the reaction of phenylalanine converted to tyrosine; all is well. That single amino acid changes to tryptophan, 1 out of 451 amino acids—causes the protein to fold abnormally. So now it doesn't catalyze the reaction going from phenylalanine to tyrosine, and all of the clinical results happen. A single base-pair change, a C to a T, out of three billion in the genome causes all of the clinical characteristics of this disease. So now we can define a mutation. A genetic mutation is defined chemically as a change in a single base, or multiple bases, in DNA; a C going to a T, for example. Then we can start talking about mutagens and what they do. We can define genetic capacity, the ability to produce a phenotype, now as the presence of DNA sequences that code for proteins with specific functions. Now we know what coding information is. We turn in the next lecture to the genome, where we look at the total genetic sequence and the capacity of an organism. Thank you.

Lecture Nine
Genomes

Scope: The Human Genome Project grew out of a desire to understand radiation damage to Japanese survivors of atom bomb explosions. DNA sequencing methods can determine the complete base sequence of 800 base-pair fragments. However, most chromosomes are much larger, so a way to order the fragments was needed. One way was to pinpoint specific short DNA marker sequences at intervals throughout the genome, then sequence the fragments and order them; this was developed by the publicly funded Human Genome Project. The other method was to sequence first, and then use computers to order the fragments. Both sequences were completed in 2003. Only 2% of the entire human genome is its 24,000 genes that get expressed as the phenotype. Over half of it is noncoding repeated sequences, and most of the other half appears to be noninformational. There are several ways that these relatively few genes can end up making a greater diversity of proteins. Many other genomes have been sequenced. A minimal genome of about 400 genes has been described for a prokaryote, and synthetic biologists are trying to make this genome in the lab, possibly creating life.

Outline

I. Opening story: Genome sequencing uses new technologies.

   A. The impetus for genome sequencing arose from radiation damage.

   1. From the early 1900s, when genetic mutations were first studied in fruit flies, scientists found that various chemicals could increase the mutation rate—they were mutagens. Recall that DNA can also spontaneously mutate due to errors when it is replicated. Among the mutagens was ionizing radiation. This was found the hard way by people working in uranium mines, and radium "painters" for dials on luminous watches developed mutations that caused cancer. By the 1930s, this type of mutagenesis was studied under controlled conditions in the lab, with a clear dose-mutation relationship.

   2. At the end of World War II, the U.S. exploded atomic bombs on the Japanese cities of Hiroshima and Nagasaki. Hundreds

of thousands were killed and many more exposed to radiation as fallout. These people and their descendants have been intensively studied for any increases in mutations, both in somatic cells (leading to cancer) and in sex cells (leading to genetic diseases in the next generation).

3. This has been a paradigm for studies of environmental mutagens.

B. By 1980, methods were developed to sequence DNA, about 800 base pairs at a time.

1. Up to then, the scientists studying genetic damage in the Japanese survivor group looked at genetic damage by its effects on the phenotype (e.g., cancer, inherited abnormalities). Now they realized that the best way to analyze genetic damage was to actually determine the DNA sequence and look for differences between people exposed to radiation and those not exposed.

2. In 1984, Nobel laureate Renato Dulbecco suggested that the entire human genome be sequenced. The U.S. Department of Energy, which oversaw the radiation damage project, was the first sponsor.

II. The human genome was sequenced in two ways.

A. The initial challenge was to get DNA signposts.

1. The problem: We can sequence DNA fragments that are 800 base pairs long. But each chromosome in humans is about 100 million base pairs long. So we cut the chromosome into 800 base-pair pieces (Can you figure out how many pieces that makes?), sequence each one, and then line them up. This seems straightforward.

2. But the problem is, how do we line up the sequenced fragments? If every word in this printed Guidebook was cut out and all the words put on the floor, could you line them up to make the sentences I have written?

B. Two methods revealed the signposts.

1. The first way was sponsored by the government. It set out to identify short sequences of one to several base pairs that would "mark" each segment of DNA. This would create a "marker map" along the chromosome. So if a sequenced fragment had that marker, it must be at a known location on the chromosome. It turns out that human DNA has short, often

repeated sequences at intervals along each chromosome. It took over 10 years to find them and another 2 years to sequence the fragments. It was painstaking work by thousands of scientists led by Francis Collins.

2. The second way was to break up the chromosome into fragments, sequence them, and then have a computer look for markers and arrange the fragments. A key was to do staggered breaks. For example, consider the sentence:

THIS COURSE IS GOOD.
It can be broken into four-letter fragments:
THIS COUR SEIS GOOD.
Or, if the break is internal:
TH ISCO URSE ISGOI OD, etc.

3. This approach was undertaken by a scientist-entrepreneur, Craig Venter, and relied on the development of bioinformatics, the use of very sophisticated computer programs to analyze a mountain of DNA sequence data. These programs were developed in the 1990s. It took less than a year to sequence the genome in this way.

III. There are several types of information from DNA sequences.

A. Open reading frames are regions of genes that code for proteins.

B. Amino acid sequences of proteins can be deduced from sequences by the genetic code.

C. Gene control sequences such as promoters can give information on regulation of gene expression.

IV. Nonhuman genomes have been sequenced.

A. Comparative genomics provides important information.

1. This information relates to gene functions: If a gene is also present in nonhuman genome and its function is known there, this may point to its function in humans or other organisms.

2. A gene sequence may have a new function in a different organism. This allows for evolution by natural selection and is an important argument for it.

B. The nonhuman genomes sequences have a wide range.

1. The first genome sequenced (in 1995) was the bacterium that causes meningitis: *Haemophilus influenzae*, which has 1,830,137 base pairs and 1743 genes.

2. Many new genes have been discovered in prokaryotic genomes, for example, genes for virulence in bacteria that cause typhus (*Rickettsia*); genes for cell surface attachment in the bacterium that causes TB (*Mycobacterium*); and genes for attachment to plants in nitrogen-fixing bacteria that colonize plants (*Rhizobium*) and are important in ecology and agriculture.

   a. The yeast genome was the first simple eukaryote: 12 million base pairs, 6000 genes. It is a model organism for eukaryotes. It has the basic bacteria set for metabolism but also genes for building cell compartments and targeting proteins to them.

   b. The nematode worm genome (1000-celled organism) has 97 million base pairs and 19,000 genes. It is a model for complex eukaryotes, with different tissues. It has genes for cell differentiation and signaling between cells.

   c. The rice genome has 430 million base pairs and 35,000 genes. Note that a lot of the genome is repeated sequences.

V. The human genome has been sequenced.

   A. The two groups finished a draft at the same time in the spring of 2000 and the final draft in the winter of 2003.

   B. The human genome has several characteristics.

      1. Of the 3.2 billion base pairs, less than 2% are coding, with about 24,000 genes.

      2. The average gene size is 27,000 base pairs, including control regions.

      3. Over half of the genome has short, repeated sequences that do not code for proteins.

      4. About 99% of the genome is the same in all people. There are 2 million single nucleotide polymorphisms (single base-pair changes) that differ in at least 1% of people.

      5. The functions of some protein-coding genes are not yet known.

      6. Other organisms have sequences very similar to human genes: The worm has hundreds of these, as do fruit flies.

      7. The first genomes sequenced from identifiable people were those of James Watson, codiscoverer of the DNA double helix, and Craig Venter, pioneer in shotgun sequencing.

VI. The problem of so few human genes can be explained in three ways.

    A. How can humans have 20% more genes than a 1000-celled worm or fewer genes than rice?

        1. Genes are interrupted by noncoding sequences called introns. These are removed after the initial mRNA transcription. So a gene is really:

        coding 1——intron 1——coding 2——intron 2——coding 3

        Many genes have dozens of introns that must be removed as the initial RNA is cut and spliced.

        2. This can be done in alternate ways: Remove intron 1 and intron 2: Product is coding 123. Remove intron 1, coding 2, and intron 2: Product is coding 13. These get translated to different products. In this way, the average human gene gets translated to about five proteins.

    B. After a protein is made, it is modified, and this gives it new functions. For example, sugars put on a protein that sticks out of the cell surface allow for cell-cell recognition and adhesion. These modifications occur far more often in human cells. So there is great variety there.

    C. Micro-RNAs are short transcripts from the genome that remain in the nucleus but are not translated. They appear to be involved in gene regulation, and there are more of them in humans than other genomes.

VII. The next frontiers of biology are the minimal genome and synthetic biology.

    A. The prokaryote *Mycoplasma genitalium* has only 482 genes.

    B. Scientists have inactivated these genes one by one and asked whether the cell still survives: 100 genes are dispensable. So the minimal genome for a cell is 382 genes.

    C. These genes code for proteins involved in basic cell structures (e.g., cell membrane, ribosome) and functions (e.g., enzymes for energy, tRNAs).

    D. Craig Venter and colleagues are trying to make each gene in the lab and put them together, creating life. This is called "synthetic biology."

    E. There are many potential uses of this technology, for example, custom-made bacteria that can perform any role we assign them:

ethanol for fuel, environmental cleanup, making plastics, biological warfare agents, etc.

Essential Reading:

Kevin Davies, *Cracking the Genome: Inside the Race to Unlock Human DNA* (New York: The Free Press, 2001).

David Sadava, Craig Heller, Gordon Orians, William Purves, and David Hillis, *Life: The Science of Biology*, 8th ed. (Sunderland, MA: Sinauer Associates; New York: W. H. Freeman and Co., 2008), chaps. 13, 14, and 18.

Supplemental Reading:

Benjamin Lewin, *Genes VIII* (Upper Saddle River, NJ: Pearson Prentice-Hall, 2005).

James D. Watson, Jan Witkowski, Richard Myers, and Amy Caudy, *Recombinant DNA: Genes and Genomics*, 3rd ed. (New York: W. H. Freeman, 2007).

Questions to Consider:

1. The Human Genome Project included a component studying the ethical and social implications of its findings. If you were in charge of this taxpayer-supported effort, what questions would you ask?

2. If the average human gene can code for five different proteins by alternate splicing out of introns when mRNA is made, and each protein can be modified at least five ways, with 24,000 genes, how many different proteins can be made? Does this ease your mind at the prospect of having far fewer genes than a rice plant?

Lecture Nine—Transcript
Genomes

Welcome back. In the last lecture, I talked about genetic capacity in terms of protein-coding genes, and these protein-coding genes then determine the phenotype of an organism. Now I want to extend this by looking at the whole genetic capacity of an organism in terms of the entire sequence of the nucleotides that are there in the genome. The genome is the entire complement of genes that make up an organism. My story is the history of genome sequencing, and it begins in the early 1900s when genetic mutations were first studied in the model organism of the fruit fly. That's the supermodel of genetics. Scientists found there were a number of things that would increase the rate of mutations. You'll recall that mutations can happen spontaneously when DNA replication makes errors. Mutations can be increased if something damages DNA. You'll recall in our last lecture that I defined DNA damage as mutation, basically a change.

One of these mutagens, things that cause mutations, was ionizing radiation, and we really found this out the hard way. Miners working in uranium mines got cancer because the uranium caused genetic damage, radiation leaking from it, and the genetic damage led to cancer. People making luminous watches in the early decades of the 20th century—to glow in the dark, you need some energy source, and the energy source they used was radium. These people would use very fine brushes, camel's hair brushes, to paint the dials, and they'd dab them with their tongue to get the brush together to paint the dial, and of course they got oral cancers. By the 1930s, this type of mutagenesis due to radiation had been studied enough that we could draw a graph, and the graph would have radiation on one axis and damage of genes on the other axis. The more radiation you got, the more damage of genes you got.

In the closing days of World War II, the United States exploded atomic bombs on the Japanese cities of Hiroshima and Nagasaki. Hundreds of thousands of people were killed. Many more were exposed to radiation in what is called fallout; particles of radioactivity that then gently came down to the ground. These survivors and their descendants have been intensively studied ever since that time for increases in mutations of somatic cells. Remember the vast majority of cells in our body are somatic cells, they are not sex cells—here genetic damage can lead to cancer—and germ line cells, so that we're looking at the offspring of people who were exposed, and now their great-great-grandchildren in some cases have been born. You're looking for genetic abnormalities in the next generation.

By the late 1970s, methods had been developed to get the sequence of DNA molecules, but you know, DNA molecules are very large, and the only way we can sequence them now with current technology is 800 base pairs or so at a time. So we can sequence fragments of DNA, 800 base pairs at a time, and you can do that even by machine. Until that time, the scientists who were studying genetic damage in the Japanese survivors and their descendants looked at genetic damage by inferring genetic damage from phenotype. People got more cancers—for example, thyroid cancers and leukemia—who were survivors of atomic bomb radiation. So you surmise, then, that there's genetic damage in DNA. Some of their offspring had some genetic damage as well, and you looked at it through the phenotype.

Well, now that we could sequence DNA, we could look at the genes directly. We could look at the base pairs that had changed due to the damage. In 1984, a Nobel laureate, Renato Dulbecco, who had won the Nobel Prize for studying cancer viruses, made the daring suggesting that we should sequence the entire human genome, because if we did that, we could compare the entire human genome: all the DNA, all 23 chromosome pairs of a human, and all the nucleotides. We could compare the people who were not exposed to those who were exposed, and we could get a very good handle on genetic damage. It's not surprising, then, that the first sponsor of what came to be known as the Human Genome Project was the U.S. Department of Energy. The U.S. Department of Energy oversaw the radiation damage project. Since then, it's been farmed out to other organizations.

The human genome sequence was determined in two ways. There was a huge challenge here in genome sequencing. The problem was the following: Chromosomes are extremely long. A typical human chromosome, on the average: 100 million base pairs of DNA. These machines can sequence—get the nucleotide sequence from start to finish—800 base pairs at a time. So what are we going to do? We'll cut the 100 million base pairs into 800-base-pair fragments. How many is that? That's your assignment. Please e-mail me or The Teaching Company with the number of fragments. It's a lot. Now we determine the sequence of each one of those fragments, and then, of course, you just fit them together.

Oh, yeah? How are you going to fit them together? How do you know which fragment is which? Because we're not cutting it end-on; we're cutting it randomly, so we're just taking the DNA, and we're hitting it with a restriction enzyme—with some sort of enzyme like you'll see later on in the course—that will cut DNA at certain places. Or we can just physically cut it. It doesn't matter. We're not cutting it end-on; we're just cutting a whole piece into 800-base-pair fragments. It's kind of like taking the printed guide for this Teaching Company course, cutting out each word, throwing them all up in the air, getting down on the floor, and then lining them up to make the sentences I have written. Good luck, because it would be very hard to do.

There were two methods to get some sort of signposts by which we could say this particular 800-base-pair fragment's on the left end, this one's in the middle, this is on the right end. That's the simplest way to look at it. The first method was called hierarchical sequencing, and the second method was called shotgun sequencing. The hierarchical sequencing was done by the government-sponsored Human Genome Project. This was not only sponsored by the U.S. government; it was sponsored by a consortium of governments from around the world. Thousands of scientists worked on this effort. It was led by a physician-scientist, Francis Collins, and is still is led by him.

What they decided to do was identify short sequences of DNA, a couple of base pairs long, that were at certain landmarks all the way down the chromosome. So if that short sequence is on the left end of the chromosome in the first 800-base-pair fragment, and then you randomly sequence fragments, and you see that short sequence, you'll say, oh, that's the one on the left end. These were the signposts they used. It's kind of like saying, well, supposing we were doing the word problem that I just had. You've got all the words for this manual, and they're all on the floor, and we need a signpost to say how about Lecture Two? Where is Lecture Two? Well, that's going to be about the middle of Lecture Two. The word Mendel appears in Lecture Two. So you look on the floor and say Mendel, oh, that's over here on the left near the start of his lecture series. That's going to be near the start of the manual because, indeed, that's where Mendel appears, and we don't use Mendel's name anywhere else. Well, I just used it, so now we're in trouble because Mendel appears several places.

So we had these short sequences. It took 10 years for scientists to look at all the human chromosomes and get these landmark sequences all along the chromosome. There were thousands of them all along the chromosome.

Then what they did was cut the chromosome into 800-base-pair fragments, sequence all the fragments, the 800 base pairs, look for the landmarks, those little sequences, and then arrange them along the chromosome, each chromosome. It took about 12–15 years, depending on how you define it, to do this human genome sequence.

The other way of doing it is called shotgun sequencing. Shotgun sequencing was done by private industry, led by a scientist named Craig Venter. What they did was the same thing using landmarks, only they had a computer find them, find the landmarks. What they did was take the chromosome, bust it into 800-base-pair fragments, sequence them all, feed the sequences into a computer, and have the computer line it up for you. This took amazingly sophisticated computer analysis. A whole new field was invented for this shotgun sequencing effort, and that field is called bioinformatics. It's a major field of computation, then. The computer would analyze a sequence, saying oh, that's on the left-hand end; Mendel is there, for example. That's going to be on the left-hand end of the chromosome, and this is on the right-hand end of the chromosome.

This was much more rapid. It took only a year to sequence the human genome using shotgun sequencing, as opposed to 15 years doing it the painstaking way. Having the computer do it was a lot faster. But when the people started the hierarchical sequencing, the Francis Collins–led Human Genome Project, originally the computational power wasn't there. The computer programs just weren't there to analyze DNA at that level. Now the computer programs are there, and so shotgun sequencing is much more common.

What information can we get from genome sequencing, from getting all this ATGCCCC, etc.? There are several types of information we can get. The first type are called coding sequences, open reading frames. A computer can scan along a chromosome sequence, along this long chromosome sequence, and the computer scans along and says, oh, look, that's a promoter. I've seen that before. Oh, look, that's the codons coding for amino acid. Codons are those three base code words in messenger RNA. So those are the code words of codons along the DNA that code for proteins, and those are different than random DNA sequences because they've got the promoter there. The promoter is kind of a signpost saying "The gene starts here." It's kind of like a capital letter starting a sentence or indentations starting a paragraph. We have that language.

The second thing, of course, you can see. Once you've got the code words there, and the DNA, you can look up the genetic code and say, well, here's the protein that that thing makes, so you can have that information. Related to that is something technically called annotation, where you can find the function of that protein. So now we have a genome sequence. We have the gene sequence; now we have the protein function that that gene codes for. And, of course, you can get gene control information from the promoter. In context of the Human Genome Project, a number of nonhuman genomes have been sequenced, and most of these are on the model organisms scientists study to represent other organisms in its class in nature. First the model organism was sequenced, and then other organisms afterwards.

There is a huge amount of information we can get from this. We can do what is called comparative genomics. When a gene is sequenced, or an entire genome is sequenced, the information, of course, is done on computer, and it goes to a big database. There are a number of these in the sky. It's not really in the sky; it's in computers, usually in Washington or some other place like Europe or a number of places that have repository computers for storing genetic information. And the amount of information is awesome. We have way more information than we have analysis. Analysis is behind the information. It's easy to get a sequence—much easier than it is to get the information from it.

So suppose we have the sequence of a human gene. We don't know what that protein does. We have the sequence of the protein, and it's hard to predict in some cases, just from the amino acid sequence of a protein, how it's going to fold and what it does. Well, we dial up the database, and we say, is there a similar protein to this somewhere else in nature? And they might say, well, there is a protein; it's a receptor for a hormone or something in the fruit fly. If that's true, then maybe it's the same hormone receptor in the human. Or it might have a different function, and we're looking at evolutionary change. Nonhuman genome sequences began with a bacterium. The first genome to be sequenced is, in the context of molecular biology, a long time ago—1995. This was a bacterium that causes meningitis. The bacterium is called *Haemophilus influenzae*. Just let me give you the data because you'll see how complex things got.

It had 1,830,137 base pairs, 1,743 protein-coding genes. Half the genes until that time were unknown, so we immediately doubled the amount of knowledge about this thing. This thing causes meningitis, so it was very interesting. When that was published, it was a sensation in biological thinking. It opened up a whole door of genome sequencing. I had never thought, in my career as a scientist, I would ever see this done. Many new genes have been discovered in these prokaryotic genomes. For example, genes for virulence or disease causing, like the typhus-causing bacteria. A gene for attaching to human tissues in the bacterium that causes tuberculosis. So if we have that gene, and we know its protein, we could make a vaccine. Genes for attaching to plants and bacteria that fix nitrogen. Remember I told you that nitrogen gas in the air cannot be converted into amino groups except by some organisms, most notably bacteria. Now we know how they do it, and we know the genes involved through the genome sequence there.

Well, one step up from bacterium—and many bacterial genomes have been sequenced now—is the model eukaryotic cell yeast. The yeast genome has 12 million base pairs. We only had a million and a half in bacteria; 12 million base pairs, 6000 genes. It's got all the genes for bacteria for basic metabolism, for building up and breaking down substances, but it's also got genes for being a eukaryote, such as building compartments in the cell, like the nucleus, and targeting proteins for those compartments. The model complex organism is a worm; I've mentioned this before. This particular worm has only 1000 cells, but it's an amazing worm. It's transparent. It's very small, a couple of millimeters in size. It only has 1000 cells, but in those 1000 cells is a reproductive system, a basic nervous system, a little bit of a digestive system. It's got organ systems; it's complex. All those 1000 cells formed from a single cell. You can watch it happen over three days. There is an amazing amount of information we can get from this particular organism. This organism has 97 million base pairs in its genome—now we're getting a little bigger—and 19,000 protein-coding genes. And a lot of these genes are doing similar things to making a complex body with organ systems like we have.

There is a model organism which led to genome sequencing of rice, a very important plant genome. The rice genome, well, we're making a real step up now—430 million base pairs—all these sequences have come out in the last five or six years—and 35,000 genes. So we've learned a lot about the genes of rice plants, and we'll talk about that when I talk about agricultural genetics in Lectures Twenty-Three and Twenty-Four. The human genome, of course, has been sequenced. The two groups—the publicly funded Human Genome Project and the privately funded group—announced their drafts of the genome at the same time, in the year 2000, to great fanfare.

There was a White House press conference with the president, etc. Craig Venter and Francis Collins were there with President Clinton. The final draft came out in the winter of 2003.

The human genome has several characteristics. One, of the 3.2 billion base pairs in the human genome, less than 2% for proteins; 98% of the genome is not coding for proteins. You're saying, what's going on here? We'll talk about that in a minute. There are 24,000 genes in a human. I just told you rice has 35,000 genes. Humans have 24,000 genes. I consider that a major affront. I think I'm more complicated than a rice plant. How come I have so few genes? We'll talk about that problem in a moment. The average gene size in protein coding is 27,000 base pairs, including the promoter. Over half of the human genome has short repeated sequences that don't code for proteins. Ninety-nine percent, give or take, of the human genome is identical in all people; 1% is different. Look around the room where you are; look in your car at the other people driving. Yes, you are different in your genes as well as the environment that influences them. Well, 1% of the human genome is a lot of base pairs that are different.

The functions of many—well, some, a good chunk—of these 24,000 genes coding for proteins in humans are not yet known, so we're trying to find out what they do. Other organisms have sequences very similar to us. The worm I just talked about—remember the worm has 19,000 genes; we have 24,000 genes. There are a bunch of genes in the worm that are very similar to genes in us. Humbling, again. Genome sequencing is getting faster and cheaper. In 2007, the genomes of James Watson, the discoverer of the DNA structure, and Craig Venter, the guy who sequenced the human genome by the private method, were made public. It took those genomes two months each to get sequenced—just two months, not a year now—and it cost about $2 million. The price is going down and down and down. Within a year or two as I speak, it may be about $10,000 to sequence a genome, and the objective is by 2010 to 2015 there may be a $1,000 gene sequence. It's possible.

Why do it? Screening for possible diseases: We'll talk a lot about this. Research: finding out what humans are, what they're made of. Origins: Where did we come from? We'll talk a lot about that when I talk about evolution. There's a problem; too few human genes. I am insulted that I have fewer genes than a rice plant. Of course, as I tell my students, of course tenured professors have many more genes because of our complex brains. And once again, they put down their pens and say, he's got to be kidding. No, we've all got the 24,000. There are three explanations, possible explanations, for this anomaly of so few genes in humans yet such a great amount of complexity.

First, something called alternate RNA splicing. Genes are interrupted in their information sequence by noncoding sequences. These intervening sequences, called introns, are kind of nonsense. You might say, what are they doing there? There are explanations, but I don't want to get into that right now, just to tell you that they're there in the gene. So, for example, I could say, this course is good. That's information, correct? But if this was the analogy of messenger RNA at the ribosome, it would say, this course is good. That's a meaningful statement. In the DNA that codes for "this course is good" might be all these intervening words. So, this Teaching Company (hair follicle, left toe) course (vice president, secretary of the Senate) is (dirt, air, water) good. Now we have to get rid of all those nonsense words to make sense out of this, and that is done in the nucleus.

But it has this cutting and splicing to get the words "this course is good," to get them together; it happens in the nucleus, it happens at signals. We could theoretically put those words together differently, couldn't we? We could just put "this course is" and leave out the word "good." Or we could put "this is good." That's called alternate splicing, and it happens to make proteins. In fact, every protein-coding gene has so many of these internal introns, or intervening sequences, that the coding regions can be mixed and matched together. Each human gene gets translated into about five proteins. So we don't just have 24,000 protein-coding genes. Those 24,000 can make about 120,000 different proteins.

The second way that we can deal with this problem of 24,000 is called post-translational modification. After a protein is made and completed, it folds into its three-dimensional shape, but other things happen too. Sugar-coating can happen, so it can't just be a plain donut; it could be a sugar-coated donut, which tastes quite different than a plain donut. Sugars can be put onto proteins and make them have different functions. We can have a whole set of genes that add sugars to various proteins. So a protein can add three sugars in one place and five sugars in another place and have a different function. Proteins with sugars on them very often act as flags on the outside of the cell that cause the cell to bind to and recognize the other cells. It's important in cancer. So these post-translational modifications add to the diversity of proteins that can be made. Just making a protein is not enough. You can add things to it to change its structure and function.

Third, there is a chunk of the 98% of the human genome that actually makes RNAs that don't get out of the nucleus, that don't end up getting translated into proteins, but that stay in the nucleus. These are very small RNAs called micro-RNAs, and they're very recently discovered. In fact, they're not even in most textbooks. In the eukaryotic, in the human genome, there are many of these small RNAs that seem to be made by the genome, and humans make a lot of these. These RNAs may be involved in gene regulation, in turning a gene on or off and having that gene make a protein or not make a protein; make a messenger RNA or not make a messenger RNA.

We're not quite sure what the micro-RNAs are doing, but humans have a lot of them, and they are obviously an informational part of the genome. You know, scientists used to say that the 98% of the human genome that doesn't code for proteins is junk. Well, it looks like this junk has a valuable function. The junkyard does have some gems there, and the gems are these micro-RNAs hanging around the nucleus, doing something we think is pretty important in controlling genes. So that's an added complexity. So we may get away with 24,000 genes because we do so much with them, and we can do many, many more things than we thought.

The Human Genome Project has led to a new frontier, and that frontier became realized when the most simple prokaryote was sequenced; the genome of *Mycoplasma genitalium*. This is a small prokaryote that, as its name implies (genitalium), lives in the genital tract. This genome is the smallest in nature. It has 482 genes; not 24,000, but 482 genes. Using technologies of manipulating DNA, some of which I will describe in future lectures, scientists have been able to inactivate these genes one by one and ask the following question: Does the cell survive? So you've got this cell with 482 genes, and you take gene one, and you knock it out. You ask the question: Okay, are you still alive? If the cell is alive, you say, you know, it really doesn't need that gene to survive. If the cell dies, it says it's essential for survival. In that way, scientists have knocked out 100 genes, and the cells still survive. So there are 100 genes that are dispensable and 382 genes that are indispensable for life. Wow, we are now down to a genome of 382 genes which are essential for life. You need all 382 of them, and you don't need much more to be alive as a very small bacterium living in the genital tract, but still alive.

What are these genes? These are genes that code for proteins involved in basic cell structures like the nucleus, the eukaryote, or the ribosome. And they're involved in functions of cells like enzymes for energy or making

RNAs and making proteins, etc., obviously things that all cells have to do: Make the structures and functions of every cell. Craig Venter and his colleagues in a private company are trying to make each gene of these 382 in the chemistry lab. As I'll describe in a later lecture, it's possible to do that. You can go in the chem lab and make genes. You can do that by just taking it—say the gene has the following sequence: ATGC. You go in the lab, and you say to the machine, take an A, add it to a T, add it to a G, add it to a C; that's just chemistry. It's tinker-toy stuff, but it's chemistry. So you can make each one of these genes. Then they want to put all these genes together, 382 of them, in a genome, artificial genome; put them in an empty cell and create life.

Is this just a stunt? No, because if you can do that, you could take any gene you want and put it into this prokaryotic cell. For example, you could have the prokaryotic cell make ethanol for you if you put the genes for the biochemical pathway there. You could have it degrade oil in what is called bioremediation for oil slicks. You could have it make plastics for you. There are many things you could do. You could also, of course, have it make ricin, which is a toxin. So there are very scary biological warfare aspects of this brand-new field, which is called synthetic biology: making artificial chromosomes by artificially making DNA because we know the genome sequences, and then putting it into an empty cell and having that cell do the things that you want.

Knowledge of DNA sequencing, as I just described—a knowledge of DNA in general—has allowed scientists to manipulate it, and I've just described one of those manipulations. In the next lecture, I'll step back and talk about one of the major manipulations of DNA, which is called recombinant DNA. Thank you.

Lecture Ten
Manipulating Genes—Recombinant DNA

Scope: The discovery of how bacteria protect themselves from a virus invasion led to a revolution in gene manipulation. Bacteria make an enzyme that recognizes a specific DNA sequence on the invader and cuts it at that sequence. There are many such restriction endonucleases in nature. They can be taken from cells that are brought into the lab, where they are used to cut any DNA in the test tube. The resulting DNA fragment can be spliced to another DNA molecule, creating recombinant DNA. If the DNA recipient is a chromosome, it can be introduced into its host cell, and now that cell has a new gene. Genes from any source can thereby be put into any cell. This circumvents the need for conventional reproductive processes to genetically modify a cell organism.

Outline

I. Opening story: A basic research study leads to a revolution.

    A. Werner Arber studied bacterial viruses (phage).

        1. Born in Switzerland in 1929, Arber graduated from one of the world's great universities, the Federal Institute of Technology, in Zurich. As a graduate student at the University of Geneva in the 1950s, he studied with a physics professor who had been converted from a pure physicist to a biophysicist and was interested in genetics. Arber, too, caught the "biology bug." The structure of DNA had just been described, and looking at genes was all the rage in science.

        2. Arber's thesis was on the phenomenon of bacteriophage restriction. He was trying to find out why a specific genetic type of bacterial virus successfully infects only one strain of host bacteria. Other bacteria were inhospitable.

        3. Recall from our earlier lecture how such viruses infect: They actually inject their DNA into the host cell, and the virus DNA takes over the cell, turning it into a virus factory. The cell soon dies, releasing hundreds of viruses.

        4. Arber's professors must have been impressed with him, for they hired him as a junior professor at the university in 1960. By 1962, he and his graduate student, Daisy Dussoix, had found that bacteria evade viral infection by chopping up the invading virus DNA into fragments. Successfully infective viruses don't get their DNA chopped.

  5. Arber now proposed a hypothesis for what he called virus restriction.

    a. The host bacteria make an enzyme that recognizes specific DNA sequences on viral DNA and chops it up at these sequences.

    b. The bacteria also have an enzyme that modifies their own DNA to make it resistant to chopping.

    c. Virus strains that are successful in infection must have mutations in their DNA that make them resistant to the chopping enzyme.

B. Arber's hypothesis was soon confirmed by the isolation of its components.

  1. Arber and a colleague found that successful virus strains had genetic mutations that made them resistant to getting their DNA cut.

  2. In the U.S., at Johns Hopkins University, Hamilton Smith and his team isolated and described the chopping enzyme from bacteria. Because it cut DNA only at a certain sequence, it was called a restriction endonuclease (or restriction enzyme).

  3. Arber also characterized the system that modifies the host bacteria's DNA to make it resistant to the restriction enzyme.

C. The revolution begins.

  1. Scientists soon described several other restriction enzymes for other invading viruses. Each recognized a specific DNA sequence on the virus and cut there.

  2. They realized that these enzymes could be removed from cells, and if they put them in a test tube along with a large DNA, scientists could cut that DNA at the specific locations. This essentially led to a way to "map" large DNAs. At Johns Hopkins, Daniel Nathans and his team used Smith's enzyme to cut up DNA of a tumor virus and map it in this way.

  3. Meanwhile, on the West Coast, Stanley Cohen at Stanford and Herbert Boyer at the University of California San Francisco saw Nathans's work and wondered whether they could take it one step further and put the DNA fragments back together after they were cut.

4. A colleague of theirs had described a joining enzyme that can do this. If their proposal worked, Cohen and Boyer realized that any two pieces of DNA could be cut and joined in this way. They tried their experiment with DNA from two different strains of bacteria. One bacterium had a chromosome with a gene for resistance to antibiotic A, and the other to antibiotic B. Cohen and Boyer cut them both with the restriction enzyme, got fragments containing the two genes, and glued them together. Indeed, testing showed that the new chromosome carried genes for both A and B resistance. When they put the DNA into a bacterium that was not resistant to the antibiotics, the bacteria were genetically transformed to be doubly resistant. Since these antibiotic resistant cells were genetically identical, they were clones. It was 1973. They had created genetically functional recombinant DNA (recDNA).

5. This was a revolutionary discovery. It meant that genes from any sources could be swapped and spliced. We were no longer limited by the normal processes, such as fertilization, to mix genes in a single cell. This new method was far broader than fertilization: Soon, human genes were put into bacterial chromosomes, something that could never happen in nature (we don't mate with bacteria).

D. Arber, Smith, and Nathans won Nobel Prizes. The two California universities patented the method to make recombinant DNA and have reaped millions of dollars in royalties. Boyer soon founded Genentech, the first major biotechnology company.

II. There was initially great concern about recombinant DNA.

A. Concerns were raised in several aspects:
1. The bacteria used were *Escherichia coli*, which commonly occur in the human intestine. What if the recDNA got out and into human DNA?
2. Since any gene could be out into the cells, what if a disease-causing (e.g., cancer) gene was under study and it got out?
3. What about just putting any DNA that was unidentified into bacteria (called shotgun cloning)?

B. In February 1975, a conference was held at Asilomar, California, that brought together scientists, ethicists, physicians, and lawyers. The meeting urged a moratorium on certain experiments and safety precautions on others. Oversight by government agencies and institutional boards that continues to this day was set up. It was an important event in government regulation of research. In retrospect the concerns were overblown, and untoward events have not occurred. Experiments that required severe precautions in 1975 are done in high school science labs today.

III. The methods of recombinant DNA are widely applicable.

    A. There are two goals for making recombinant DNA.

        1. The first goal is to study a particular DNA sequence, for example, to find out about promoter sequences within a gene. In this case, the recDNA is inserted into a cell, and when that cell divides, the recDNA is amplified along with it.

        2. The second goal is to take the recDNA and insert it into a cell and have the cell express the gene(s) carried by the recDNA. This can be done for two reasons.

            a. As an experiment to see what happens. Adding a new gene to a cell can be used to investigate cause-and-effect relationships. For example, suppose we think that a certain hormone (like adrenalin) must bind to a recognition protein on the surface of a muscle cell before acting on the cell. We can get the gene for that protein, insert it into any cell that normally does not respond to the hormone (e.g., a skin cell), set it up so that the gene is expressed in the new cell, and see if the skin cell now binds the hormone.

            b. To have the recipient cell make a product. For example, a hormone such as insulin is needed by many diabetics. The only way to get the hormone used to be by extracting it from the pancreases of animals. Now, bacteria can be used to make the protein.

    B. Many organisms are used as a host for recDNA. In theory any cell can be used, but in practice we use cells that we can manipulate in the lab and that are well characterized.

        1. Bacteria were the first cells used. But they are prokaryotic, and may not do all of the added things (e.g., add sugars) that make a protein active in eukaryotic cells.

        2. Yeast is a simple, single-celled eukaryote. Its genome is sequenced.

        3. Mammalian cells, even human cells, can grow and reproduce in the laboratory.

4. RecDNA can be added to the egg of an animal, and then the animal reproduces. This makes a transgenic organism.

5. Plant cells are easily grown in the lab. If plant cells are grown in an appropriate environment, they make a new, transgenic plant.

C. There are many restriction enzymes that cut DNA at specific sequences. For example, one cuts at

xxxxGAATTCxxxx

xxxxCTTAAGxxxx.

Whenever this sequence is in DNA, that DNA will be cut by that enzyme. This specificity is useful, as the scientist may know the sequence of a target DNA and can choose where to cut it.

D. There are two typical ways to get DNA into host cells.

1. DNA can enter cells naked if salts are used to neutralize the charges in the DNA and the cell.

a. The problem with this is that the recDNA often stays outside the nucleus and is not part of a chromosome.

b. So when the cell gets ready to divide and replicates its DNA, the recDNA will not be replicated and will not get to the new cell. Soon, it gets diluted out, and few cells have it. This is like buying a stock so that you have 10% of the company, and then the company issues more and more shares to other investors, so your actual ownership ends up at 1%.

2. A chromosome from the host organism can be isolated and put into the test tube. Then the chromosome is cut with the restriction enzyme and the new DNA spliced into it. This recDNA is then put into the host cell, and since it is part of normal chromosome, the host cell thinks that it "belongs," and the recDNA stays there and is replicated.

a. The carrier chromosome is called a vector.

b. Vectors are usually very small chromosomes so that they are easily manipulated in the lab and also contain, preferably, only one restriction enzyme recognition sequence, so they are cut only once for insertion.

c. Because vectors are chromosomes, they have genes, and these genes can be useful. Once they are expressed in the host cell, the vector genes may be "markers" for the presence of the vector and its new gene hitchhiker.

  d. Vector marker genes include antibiotic resistance, so any cell carrying the vector has that property and can be selected in a mixture of cells.

  e. In addition to small chromosomes, vectors include viruses that normally infect the host cells. These viruses are disabled by lab manipulations so that they inject their DNA into the cells but do not reproduce and kill the host.

IV. To summarize:

  A. A new gene is isolated for cloning. The gene is spliced into a vector chromosome or virus that also has a "flag" that makes its presence detectable.

  B. The recDNA is inserted into a host cell that lacks the "flag" gene (and the new gene). Those cells with the "flag" (and therefore the vector) are selected by the experimenter with appropriate environmental conditions.

  C. When the cells grow, the new gene is cloned.

Essential Reading:

Susan Barnum, *Biotechnology: An Introduction* (Belmont, CA: Thomson Brooks-Cole, 2005), chap. 3.

William Thieman and Michael Palladino, *Introduction to Biotechnology* (San Francisco: Benjamin-Cummings, 2004), chap. 3.

Supplemental Reading:

George Acquah, *Understanding Biotechnology* (Upper Saddle River, NJ: Pearson Prentice-Hall, 2004).

John Smith, *Biotechnology*, 4th ed. (Cambridge: Cambridge University Press, 2004).

Questions to Consider:

1. The initial reaction to the creation of recombinant DNA in the 1970s ranged from positive excitement to panic. This led to the Asilomar conference. In retrospect, the concerns about the dangers of this new technology were largely groundless. Can you think of any recent advances in science and technology that provoke similar concerns? Is it a good idea for society to be cautious, or are the concerns usually exaggerated?

2. The creation of genetically new organisms by recDNA manipulation led to a new industry. To protect their inventions, scientists can patent their discoveries. This led to the patenting of living organisms. Is this a good idea?

Lecture Ten—Transcript
Manipulating Genes—Recombinant DNA

Welcome back. In our last lecture, I described genomes as entire sequences of DNA, all the chromosomes, and the protein-coding regions being the most important in terms of the phenotype. At the end of the lecture, I gave you a preview of some coming attractions when I talked about manipulating genomes; remember, knocking out genes and getting the minimal genome of a bacterium, and then custom-making bacteria. This is a transition from basic science to technology. In this lecture, I'm going to continue that transition by talking about manipulating genes and creating recombinant DNA. The history of this whole field is my opening story because it's a real case lesson in learning about how basic research gets translated into applied research and industry.

A scientist named Werner Arber studied bacterial viruses. Bacterial viruses are also called bacteriophages. They eat—"phage" comes from eat— bacteria. Arber was born in Switzerland in 1929 and graduated from one of the world's great universities, the Swiss Federal Institute of Technology, in Zurich. As a graduate student at the University of Geneva in the 1950s, he studied with a physics professor, and he watched this physics professor get converted from doing pure physics to doing biophysics, being interested in genetics. This was the 1950s. The DNA structure and the double helix had just been announced, and looking at genes in science was all the rage. So, even physicists were catching the biology bug.

Arber's Ph.D. thesis was on the phenomenon of bacteriophage, or bacterial virus, restriction. Now what this is, is a phenomenon in which a specific type of bacterial virus can only infect a specific genetic strain of bacteria, host bacteria. Now recall from Lecture Four how such viruses do their infection. Remember, the virus particle with its protein and DNA lands on the outside of the bacterial cell, its host. It injects its DNA into the cell, and this DNA of the bacterial virus then takes over the cell, and half an hour later, that cell, which was converted from a bacterial cell into a virus factory, is dead. The cell is dead, and hundreds of virus particles are released. Arber was specifically interested in the fact that only certain host cells seemed to work for a particular virus. Other host cells didn't; it was restricted.

Now Arber's professors must have been really impressed with him because they hired him in 1960 as a junior professor at the university. In 1962, he and his graduate student, Daisy Dussoix, found that bacteria seemed to evade infection by viruses—that is, when the viral infection is not successful—by chopping up the invading virus DNA into fragments. So the virus DNA gets in, and all of a sudden it gets chopped up into fragments, so it's not going to be successful at all. Arber proposed a hypothesis to explain this phenomenon, and he called this "virus restriction." First, host bacteria, Arber proposed, make an enzyme that recognizes a specific DNA sequence on viral DNA. It's kind of like the viral DNA is wearing a red hat, and we're going to kill the guys with the red hats. This enzyme catalyzes the chopping-up of that invading DNA, the red hat.

Second, the bacteria have an enzyme that modifies their own DNA to make it resistant. So if their own DNA has a red hat as well, has a sequence identical to the virus DNA, they have some method of modifying their own DNA to make it resistant to the chopping enzyme. So they might put a brown beret on top of the red hat. Third—this is still his hypothesis—virus strains that are successful in infection must have mutations in DNA that make them resistant to the chopping enzyme. So they turn the red hat into a blue hat, and they say, well, I'm not a virus DNA; I'm just a regular old bacterial DNA. They fool the bacteria, and they take over. Arber's hypothesis, all three aspects, was soon confirmed in the 1960s.

In the U.S., at Johns Hopkins University—remember, Arber, of course, published his hypothesis so all scientists could read it—Hamilton Smith and a team isolated and described the chopping enzyme from bacteria. Because it only cut DNA at certain sequences—namely a sequence that was present in the bacteriophage—they called it a restriction endonuclease; we call it a restriction enzyme. I don't want to call it an endonuclease; that's too specific. Nuclease means it cuts DNA. I'll just call it a restriction enzyme. A restriction enzyme cuts DNA where there is a certain sequence present. You can imagine—it's that red hat—the bacteria make a restriction enzyme against the invading virus: clever.

The second aspect of Arber's hypothesis was that the host cell modifies itself to make itself resistant. And indeed, Arber, in his own laboratory in Switzerland, characterized this system that modifies its own DNA. There's an enzyme. There's a gene that codes for this enzyme in the bacterium that modifies its own DNA bases. It adds some chemical groups, and they're no longer recognized by the restriction enzyme, so it doesn't chop its own

DNA. That's very fortunate because if it did, it would be a former bacterium. The third aspect of his hypothesis was that successful virus strains must be mutated so they're no longer recognized. And indeed, these viruses had mutations in their DNA that altered the DNA base sequence so that it no longer had the site that the restriction enzyme recognized, and so it didn't cut anymore. So, all three aspects were confirmed.

Now so far, I'm describing basic research. If Arber's mother, in a hypothetical situation, had come around to him saying, what do you do for a living, he would say, I'm looking at viruses invading bacteria and why certain strains invade bacteria and others don't. Mom might ask, what's the use of that? He'd say, well, you never know in science. The scientific budget in this country is huge, and a lot of it goes into basic research because you never know. Well, now I'm going to show you how "you never know" turned into a revolution.

Scientists soon described other restriction enzymes that would cut DNA at other DNA sequence sites. Each of them was highly specific for a certain site that happened to be on a virus. Now early in the 20th century, it was recognized that if you take a protein out of the cell, the protein will fold in the same way it does inside the cell if you put the protein in water. The cell is mostly water, so you take a protein, and you put it in water; it'll fold the same way. It's a spontaneous process. It's a genetically determined sequence of amino acids that causes the protein to fold in its own specific way. So you can study proteins outside of the cell. You can study enzymes in a test tube. In the same way, you can study restriction enzymes in a test tube. You could take them outside the bacteria, give them some DNA, and they chop it up if the DNA had that particular site.

This led to the first way of mapping DNA. Suppose we had a sentence, "The quick, brown fox jumped over the lazy dog," and the map we're going to do is we're going to put red lettering everywhere there's the word "the." We've created a map, haven't we? So we look far away at that sentence. We have: The (quick brown fox jumped over) the (lazy dog.) Two "the"s at certain locations. Restriction enzymes could do this. If a restriction enzyme cut DNA wherever there was a sequence AATT, if you have a big piece of DNA, wherever there's an AATT, it'll cut. That was the first physical map of DNA in the 1970s. This was done at Johns Hopkins by a colleague of Hamilton Smith—who had done this restriction insight—named Daniel Nathans, and his graduate student, Kathleen Danna.

Meanwhile, on the West Coast, two scientists named Stanley Cohen at Stanford University and Herbert Boyer at the University of California at San Francisco saw, of course, the publication of Nathans's work of cutting DNA and mapping it that way in the test tube, and of course, of the restriction enzyme that had been discovered as a basis of Arber's work, by Hamilton Smith, and wanted to follow it up. Their idea was, look, if we can take a DNA, and we can cut it, maybe we can put it back together again. Well, at Stanford University, another scientist had discovered that there is an enzyme that would catalyze that; that an enzyme will put cut DNAs together. So then Cohen and Boyer apparently, by an anecdotal story, were sitting at a deli in Waikiki where they were at a conference. And ever the scientists, they weren't out there on the beach surfing; they were at this deli doodling on a napkin, and doodled two different DNAs, and cut them with a restriction enzyme, and put them together in the test tube. And they said, gee, if we can do this with two different DNAs, we can do this with any chromosome, and we can swap chromosome pieces in the test tube.

Well, they tried the experiment; they went back to the lab on the West Coast, and they tried the experiment using bacterial chromosomes, chromosomes from *E. coli*. They had two different strains of bacteria. One bacterium had resistance to one antibiotic; I'll call it antibiotic A. It had a gene that made the bacterium resistant to this antibiotic. Another bacterial strain had resistance to antibiotic B. It had a gene that made it resistant to antibiotic B. They isolated chromosomes from both of these, put them in a test tube; and just as they had planned on the beach there in the restaurant, they cut the chromosomes open with restriction enzymes and glued the two chromosomes together using this third enzyme that would glue the chromosomes together.

They had to prove that these chromosomes had been glued together, and so they took some naive bacteria that didn't have any bacterial resistance to antibiotics, and they put this new chromosome in with them. Lo and behold, these bacteria that never resisted anything now were resistant, in some cases, to both A and B. What had they done? It was 1973. These scientists had taken two chromosomes, cut them open, put them back together, and showed that they were functional in a cell. They had created genetically functional recombinant DNA, the recombination of the two different genomes. It was a revolutionary discovery. It meant that genes from any sources in nature could be taken out of a cell in a laboratory setting and swapped and spliced beside one another.

We were no longer limited in genetics by normal processes such as fertilization to mix genes in a single cell. This was way broader than fertilization. Soon, within a couple of months of their first announcement in 1973, they had taken human genes in a test tube and spliced them and put them into bacterial chromosomes, and had them function in bacteria cells. The bacteria did not turn into humans. It was a single gene that made RNA. It was a demonstration project. This could never happen in nature. We don't mate with bacteria; at least not in regular life. Arber—who made the original basic discoveries that led to this revolution—Smith, and Nathans all won Nobel Prizes. The two California universities, one of which turned out to be Stanford University of California where Cohen and Boyer worked, patented the method of making recombinant DNA and reaped millions of dollars in royalties. Boyer, one of the two people who made recombinant DNA, soon cofounded Genentech, the first major biotechnology company. So the revolution in recombinant DNA was profound. It had now begun, in the mid-1970s.

There was initially great concern about recombinant DNA. The concerns centered on several aspects of this work. First, the bacteria used in these experiments were our friend *Escherichia coli*, nicknamed *E. coli*. There's actually a cartoon that says the *E.* stands for Edward; no, it's *Escherichia*. It's *E. coli*, the bacteria that commonly occur in our intestines. So people were worried about, well, what if this laboratory recombinant DNA got out into a human and got into our gut bacteria? What would happen there? What if we're studying a disease-causing gene, and we're putting it into bacteria to do experiments with it, and this disease-causing gene somehow gets out of the bacteria in our laboratory dish and into us, and into our bacteria that are in us? What would happen? Could the bacteria lead to cancer in us? There were these kinds of fears.

It led to almost a hysteria. Municipalities passed laws banning all recombinant DNA work. A very famous scientist arrived at his laboratory one day to find it padlocked and police out front, saying, you have broken our municipal ordinance against doing any gene swapping. Doomsday scenarios were all over the place. People were very worried. And in 1975, in February, a conference was held at Asilomar, the Monterey area of California, on the coast, which brought together scientists, ethicists, physicians, and lawyers to deal with this situation. This was a unique event in the history of science and government relations. The meeting was really called by the scientists who were doing the work because they just wanted some sort of feedback on what they were doing, because they were worried about the dangers.

At this meeting, there were several days of very heated discussions among the senior scientists and ethicists, physicians, and lawyers present, and they decided to have a moratorium on certain types of experiments. For example, until they knew what they were doing, they weren't going to put cancer-causing genes into bacteria to study them. They just passed this moratorium. They had extreme safety precautions on all other types of recombinant DNA experiments. Government agencies and institutional boards at universities and research institutes were set up, and in fact, the mechanism that was set up then exists today. The scientists really asked for this oversight, which was very unusual because we are usually, as scientists, characterized as people who just want to do our work, and leave us alone. We would never harm you at all. Well, the scientists were quite worried because this was so profound a change in biological manipulation, to take genes from different organisms and swap them together. We were in a really unknown area.

In retrospect, these concerns were overblown, and no untoward or dangerous events have really occurred with recombinant DNA work. In fact, experiments that required severe precautions—you'd see people doing the experiments with white suits and masks, and sterile environments and hoods and things like this, in 1975 because of these rules—are now done in high school science labs with no problem. It doesn't mean that we don't need to constantly monitor this research. In fact, it still is monitored, and if you are dealing with harmful genes, you must take extreme precautions. But still, some of the precautions have been relaxed.

The methods of recombinant DNA, and the way that recombinant DNA is used, are very widely applicable. Why does recombinant DNA work? Is it a stunt? What's the purpose of putting a human gene into bacteria? Just to swap genes because we feel like it? There are two purposes. The first is if we want to study a particular DNA sequence. You know, I mentioned yesterday that there are machines that will sequence DNA, 800 base pairs at a time. Well, you can't take a single, small cell of DNA and put that DNA into the machine and have it sequenced; it's too small an amount. So we have to amplify genes. We have to amplify genes to get an amount that will make it available for sequencing and study. If we want to find out the promoter sequence of a gene, for example, we can put it into bacteria. And the nice thing about bacteria as a model organism is that if you take one bacteria with recombinant DNA in it that has a human gene, then you've got a vat of it the next day—because in half an hour, the time it takes to listen to this lecture, that bacteria will double its numbers. And in an hour, time for two lectures, the bacteria will quadruple; and if you do the whole course, you'll have a lot of bacteria. That's the first reason for doing recombinant DNA; amplifying DNA so we can determine its sequence and study it.

The second reason is to have that DNA express itself as a phenotype, as a protein, in the new cell that's the host. Why would you want to do that? Well, there are two reasons: First, to do an experiment, to do cause and effect in science. Let me give you an example. Supposing we think that for a hormone like adrenaline to act, the adrenaline binds to a recognition protein, which is made on a muscle cell to get that muscle cell to contract so I can run. Adrenaline is the fight-or-flight hormone. So you make the hormone; it goes to the muscle cell, and it binds to what is called a receptor protein. That's our hypothesis. But how do we prove that that's the case? We have circumstantial evidence. We see the protein; adrenaline binds to it.

Can we prove that's why the muscle responds? Well, if we isolate the gene and then, by recombinant DNA methods for this particular protein that's a receptor, put that gene in a cell that doesn't respond to adrenaline—a skin cell or any other cell, or even a bacterium—and then we have that skin cell make this protein for us, then we add adrenaline. All of a sudden, that cell will respond. That's cause and effect, right? These gene-swapping experiments allow us to do those cause and effect things, and so it's been very, very powerful—in fact, almost routine now—in biological science to do these kinds of experiments, the "what if," and to prove experiments using recombinant DNA. At the time it was done—I can't tell you how astounding it was for us in the field to be able to do this. It opened up incredible vistas, to do this.

A second way of expressing DNA is to make the protein in large amounts. So if we need insulin in human diabetics—a topic I will describe in a later lecture—one way to get a large amount of human insulin might be to extract it from the pancreas glands of dead humans. We don't have many pancreas glands, and insulin is in very small amounts. Another way might be to take the insulin gene and put it into bacteria and make a vat of bacteria, and have that gene express itself, and now we have a vat of insulin protein. So the two reasons for doing it are to study DNA and sequence it, and secondly to express it in the recombinant situation in a new cell.

Recombinant DNA can be put into any organism. In theory, any organism, any cell, can be used in this work. In practice, we use only the cells we can manipulate in the laboratory; the model organisms like bacteria, right? They're real easy to use. We can put DNA into them. We can control them. We have them in a nice controlled situation. The problem is, of course, if we're taking a gene that makes a protein in eukaryotes—for example, bacteria don't do gene splicing at the messenger RNA level, so they don't take that messenger RNA and take the introns out, as I described in the last lecture. Bacteria don't add sugar coatings to most of their proteins, so it really might not make a functional protein of a human type if it's in bacteria. You've got to be careful about that. So, instead, people use yeast as a model organism. So they'll take a recombinant DNA of a eukaryote and put it into yeast. We know a lot about its genome, as I've described in the last lecture. We know lots of things about yeast. It's easy to grow. We can get a large amount of yeast making the protein that we want.

Cells of mammals, even humans, can grow and reproduce in the laboratory, and we can add recombinant DNA to those cells. For example, we can even add recombinant DNA to the egg cell of an animal, or even a human, but it's not done on humans. It's been done on animals, and the animal will go ahead and grow up. So if we have a fertilized egg cell, and we add recombinant DNA to it—take a chromosome, add a recombinant DNA to it—that animal will now have a new gene. It's called a transgenic animal. Plant cells can be grown in the lab, so we can add those things to plant cells. And because they're totipotent, we can grow a whole plant from any plant cell. I've described that in an earlier lecture. So suffice it to say, there are many ways we can add recombinant DNA to different types of cells.

Because there are many restriction enzymes, we can cut DNA at will. We can cut it in whatever way that we want, and we know with specificity where we're cutting the DNA; and so where the cuts are determines where the DNAs will splice together. To get DNA into host cells, we have two ways. The first way is "naked DNA," and the second way is called a vector. First, naked DNA. No, that's not the scientist, and that's not what we have under our lab coats. Naked DNA just means DNA by itself with nothing there. It's just a gene, and maybe its promoter attached. Recall the experiment I described when people were proving—in Griffith's experiment, for example—that DNA was the gene. Remember in bacteria, Griffith added DNA from one strain of bacteria into another. Well, you can add just naked, regular DNA. The problem with doing it this way is that the recombinant DNA is just by itself. It's a piece of DNA; it's a single gene.

When the cell gets ready to divide and replicate its DNA, that single lonesome piece of DNA out there will not bind the enzyme DNA polymerase. You've got to be part of a chromosome for this DNA polymerase to unzip and add the new DNAs to make daughter DNA double helices. So if you're not in a chromosome—you're just a single gene—it doesn't work. The DNA polymerase doesn't replicate it. And so when you form two cells, one of the cells will still have the recombinant DNA, but the second one won't. And when those cells divide again, three of the cells will not have the recombinant DNA—they'll have the regular genome—and the one piece will still be in one cell. You're going to dilute it out. You'll really have very few cells with the recombinant DNA as the cell population continues to grow and double. It's kind of like buying stock. You buy stock, and you own 10% of the company: You get 10% of the profits. Then all of a sudden, the company issues more and more shares. Well, you're diluting your investment, right? Your investment goes down to 1%. Same thing with recombinant DNA.

We want the recombinant DNA to duplicate when the cell duplicates. The best way to do that is to put the recombinant DNA into a chromosome. That's what they did originally with the bacteria. They used whole chromosomes. Well, it turns out there are small chromosomes that exist, and we use them as vectors. A vector is a piece of DNA that can carry a gene from a test tube into an organism, and it's a regular chromosome that the DNA polymerase will recognize. So a piece of DNA that we want—I'll call it your favorite gene—can be added to a vector, which is a normal chromosome, and that piece of DNA that's now in the normal chromosome together, are put into the host cell, the bacteria cell. And the hapless bacteria cell—or human cell if it was a human vector and a human chromosome—would go ahead and duplicate that recombinant DNA along with all of its other chromosomes.

Now we need a way, because this process is not 100% efficient, to tell that a cell has a vector or not. So usually we use a vector chromosome—that is, a chromosome that's normally present in the organism—that has a flag on it that says, hello, I'm present. And the "hello, I'm present" flag may be antibiotic resistance, for example. Bacteria are usually not antibiotic resistant, so our vector might have a gene on it, on its chromosome—it's a regular chromosome—that codes for a protein that makes it resistant to an antibiotic like tetracycline. So we take this chromosome that is tetracycline resistant. We splice in our human gene. We infect it into a bunch of bacteria cells, and we can select those bacteria that have this chromosome because they are antibiotic resistant. They're carrying that new chromosome that we've put in.

To summarize, a gene is isolated for cloning, step one. Step two, the gene is spliced into a vector chromosome that also has some sort of gene that acts as a flag to make its presence detectable in the host cell. Third, the recombinant DNA is inserted into the host cell that doesn't have this "flag" gene; it's not antibiotic resistant, for example. Fourth, those cells with the "flag," with this antibiotic resistance, can be selected by the experimenter. What would you do? You'd just add antibiotic to a whole bunch of bacteria, right? The ones that don't have resistance; they're all going to be dead. The ones that survive have this chromosome that unwittingly carries our gene of interest. When those cells grow, the new gene has been cloned. In the next lecture, we'll turn to some of the properties of the genes that are isolated by recombinant DNA, and how that process occurred. Thank you.

Lecture Eleven
Isolating Genes and DNA

Scope: Finding the protein that is defective in muscular dystrophy presented a challenge because the protein is present in muscle in tiny amounts. So scientists first isolated the mutant gene responsible for the disease and then used the gene's DNA sequence to identify the protein. An important technique in finding genes is nucleic acid hybridization, in which single strands of DNA (or RNA) from different sources are incubated together to see if they will bind by base pairing (A to T and G to C). If that occurs, the sequences must be closely related. An entire genome can be chopped into fragments, and these displayed by cloning into bacteria (a gene library) or directly on a microarray (a DNA chip). In both cases, the fragment containing a certain DNA sequence can be "fished out" by using that sequence as a hybridization probe into the library or array. This has been useful not only in isolating genes but also in finding out patterns of gene expression. The latter may be important in new ways for medical diagnosis and prognosis. The ability to actually make DNA in the laboratory has freed scientists from looking for useful mutations in nature and opens up the possibility of making genes whose protein have customized properties.

Outline

I. Opening story: Muscular dystrophy was a genetic challenge.

    A. In traditional genetics, scientists went from phenotype to gene.

        1. As we have seen, genes were first identified as phenotypes, the genes were inferred, and then the genes were isolated.

        2. For example, PKU was described in terms of genetics (phenotype), and then the missing phenylalanine hydroxylase enzyme was isolated, and this led to the isolation of the actual DNA sequence coding for it.

    B. Muscular dystrophy was a challenge to this paradigm.

        1. The most common form of muscular dystrophy was first described by French neurologist Guillaume Amand Duchenne in 1861. He noted a progressive muscle wasting in boys, first with the pelvic and calf muscles before age 5, and then losing the ability to walk by age 12. The weakness spreads to all the so-called voluntary muscles and the breathing muscles. Death is usually before age 30, due to respiratory failure.

2. The disease is genetically determined, linked on the X chromosome (like hemophilia). So it is most common in males, with 1 in 3500 births.

3. Treatment is symptomatic (braces, wheelchairs, and ventilators). There is no good treatment and no cure. So it is urgent to find out what exactly is wrong with the muscles (the precise phenotype).

4. For decades, scientists looked for a protein difference between the normal and dystrophic muscle. They knew that the muscle fibers tended to fall apart and that they got replaced by fatty or other nonmuscle tissues. But with the methods they had, they could not find one. It was like looking for a needle in a haystack.

II. In reverse genetics, the gene is isolated before the protein.

A. Methods for analyzing DNA in chromosomes were developed during the 1980s.

1. By the 1980s, scientists were ready to take another approach. Why not try to isolate the gene first and then go after the defective protein?

2. At Harvard Medical School, Louis Kunkel and his colleagues saw a boy with Duchenne muscular dystrophy in the clinic. When they examined his chromosomes under the microscope, they saw that he was missing a small piece of the X chromosome. Figuring that the missing piece was the gene that is defective (in this case, missing) in muscular dystrophy, they compared the DNAs of X chromosomes of the affected boy with normal boys. They found that a piece of DNA was missing, and in 1985 they isolated the gene.

3. The gene was huge; in fact it turns out to be the largest in the human genome, at over 2.5 million base pairs. It makes an mRNA in developing muscle cells that is 14,600 bases long. Why is all that extra DNA in the gene? It is introns (the gene has 78 of them and so is in 79 pieces) as well as a complex of 9 promoters.

4. The protein coded for by the gene was indeed hard to find: It accounts for 0.002% of muscle protein. Appropriately called

dystrophin, it connects the inside of the muscle cells to the outside, running through the cell membrane. Without dystrophin, muscles tend to get injured by the shear forces of muscle contraction. Ultimately, this kills the muscle cell. This identified the primary phenotype—after the gene was isolated.

5. The discovery of the mutant allele and then protein responsible for this disease has led to molecular medicine, a targeted approach to treatment.

   a. A protein similar to dystrophin called urotrophin is already made by the body, and drugs are being developed to increase its synthesis so it can replace defective dystrophin.

   b. Gene therapy, adding the normal allele for dystrophin to muscle, is also being developed.

B. Nucleic acid hybridization is a key method to detect genes.

1. How can scientists compare two DNAs such as the normal X chromosome and the one that was deleted in the boy with muscular dystrophy?

2. A method to compare nucleic acids was developed by Sol Spiegelman in the 1960s. It is called nucleic acid hybridization.

3. Suppose a DNA has the sequence   AAAGGGCCCTTT
                                      TTTCCCGGGAAA.
   We have another DNA and want to know if it matches this sequence. One way to find out is to separate the DNA strands of the target DNA (a) AAAGGGCCCTTT and (b) TTTCCCGGGAAA and put these on filters. Now separate the strands of the unknown DNA and let them settle onto the filters. The unknown DNA will stick to the filters only if it has the complementary base pairs (A to T and G to C), that is, if it sticks to filter (a), then the unknown DNA must have the sequence TTTCCCGGGAAA. The double-stranded DNA that results comes from two different sources and is called hybrid DNA.

4. Now let's apply this to the situation with the X chromosomes from the muscular dystrophy patient and the normal boy. We try to hybridize the DNAs with the normal boy's DNA as the target. What will happen is that most of the two DNAs are very similar and will hybridize, but there will be a part of the X chromosome of normal DNA that does not have a partner

on the patient chromosome. That is where the gene for dystrophin is located.

III. DNA libraries and chips are used for rapid screening of a genome.

    A. Genome libraries can be made by cloning.

        1. Often only part of a gene has been isolated (for example, the deletion of the X chromosome in a patient with muscular dystrophy may be smaller than the huge gene).

        2. If we could make the isolated gene fragment into a hybridization probe, and if we could display the entire genome in fragments, the probe would bind to the fragment with the gene, and the gene could be "fished out" with this "hook."

        3. A genome library does this: The entire DNA of an organism is cut into small (gene-sized) pieces that are cloned into bacteria using the recombinant DNA method we described in the last lecture. So we have many colonies of bacteria, each having a different part of the genome.

        4. Now a mass DNA extraction of all the colonies is done, and the gene fragment is hybridized to all the colonies. The one it sticks to must have the whole gene, and so this bacteria colony can be grown and the whole gene isolated.

    B. A DNA microarray is the ultimate library.

        1. A major technological innovation in electronics in the 20th century was the silicon chip: a thin micro-wafer with circuits stamped on it.

        2. A DNA microarray is a small, glass microscope slide to which single-stranded DNAs are attached as targets for hybridization. The entire process is miniaturized so that the DNA chip can have thousands of genes on it.

        3. If the unknown DNA that is to be hybridized is colored, the spot location where it hybridizes will be colored, so detection is easy.

        4. DNA microarrays are being used to find genes and mutations, and in diagnosis.

        5. RNAs can also be hybridized, so that if all the human genes are present as DNAs on a chip, one can extract RNAs from a cell and ask which genes are expressed in a tissue at a certain time.

        6. For example, in breast cancer, it is important that the physician get an idea of what stage the tumor is in. If it is at an early stage, maybe the tumor is localized and surgery may "get it all," as surgeons sometimes (unwisely) say. Some early tumors may have already spread (metastasized), but the doctors don't know it. It would be good if the tumor had some sort of marker that would show whether it was the spreading type. If the physician had this information, only those patients who need chemotherapy and radiation after surgery would get it.

- **a.** But there has been no good way to tell the "spreading" from the "non-spreading" type of tumor, so the physicians play it safe and give most women the extra treatments.
- **b.** Enter gene chips. Dr. Laura van 't Veer at the Netherlands Cancer Agency took biopsies from both types of breast cancer, extracted their RNAs, and hybridized them to microarrays with thousands of human genes. She and her colleagues found that some genes were expressed more in the tumors that were found to spread, and others in tumors that did not. So she created a "gene expression signature." This may be very useful in targeting further aggressive treatments to only those who need them.

IV. Synthetic DNA can be used to make new genes and mutations.

- **A.** Chemists have developed methods to make DNA in the lab, base by base.
   1. Knowing the genetic code makes it possible to create mutations.
   2. This is a major advance in the use of genetics to ask "what if" questions. Previously, we needed to either look in nature for a mutation that arose spontaneously or treat the organism with a mutagen like X rays and look for the mutant phenotype (e.g., recall the prokaryotes that could not make an amino acid because they had a defect in a gene coding for an essential enzyme). With custom DNA in the lab, we can hypothesize that a certain gene is essential for the synthesis of an amino and then mutagenize it deliberately and see if an organism carrying the mutant now cannot make the amino acid.
- **B.** These lab techniques can be used to create useful mutations.
   1. For example, scientists found a naturally sweet protein that was too sweet. It stuck to the taste buds for hours.

2. The scientists determined that the three-dimensional fit for the sweet molecule was too tight, so they proposed changing the protein so that its amino acid sequence at the binding region was changed for less tight binding. Looking up the genetic code, they altered the DNA for the protein, cloned it into bacteria and—voila—sweet, but not lasting.

C. These lab techniques are being used in synthetic biology to create "life" and custom-made organisms.

Essential Reading:

Benjamin Pierce, *Genetics: A Conceptual Approach* (New York: W. H. Freeman, 2005), chap. 19.

William Thieman and Michael Palladino, *Introduction to Biotechnology* (San Francisco: Benjamin-Cummings, 2004), chap. 3.

Supplemental Reading:

Ricki Lewis, *Human Genetics*, 7th ed. (New York: McGraw-Hill, 2006).

John Smith, *Biotechnology*, 4th ed. (Cambridge: Cambridge University Press, 2004).

Questions to Consider:

1. This ability to make any DNA we want in the lab has implications on discussions of genetic resources. One argument for conserving nature has been the human-centered one: There are genes out there that we may be able to use for our purposes (making new drugs to cure cancer, as in the film *Medicine Man*). But if we can make any gene or mutation that we want, this reason becomes less compelling. Do you agree?

2. Compare the "old way" of doing genetic analysis by phenotype first and then isolating the gene to the "new way" of isolating the gene first and then the protein phenotype.

Lecture Eleven—Transcript
Isolating Genes and DNA

Welcome back. In the last lecture, I described how the technology of recombinant DNA makes it possible to amplify and express genes in other places. But you need to get the genes first, so I want to talk in this lecture about how we isolate genes. My opening story is about the genetic challenge of muscular dystrophy. In traditional genetics, scientists went from the phenotype to isolating the gene. Think of PKU, phenylketonuria. First we had the phenotype, mental retardation, on the large human scale. Then we had the phenotype at the protein level, the enzyme phenyalanine hydroxylase, remember, that catalyzes the conversion of phenylalanine to tyrosine. And we knew that that enzyme wasn't working in the children who inherited the bad alleles for phenylketonuria.

After finding out about the enzyme, and finding out that the enzyme didn't work, and getting the amino acid sequence of the enzyme, it was only then that we could isolate the DNA sequence or gene coding for that enzyme; because, of course, we could use the genetic code in reverse. We knew the amino acids; we could get the DNA base pairs. Muscular dystrophy was a challenge to this paradigm. The most common form of muscular dystrophy was first described by the French neurologist Guillaume Amand Duchenne in 1861. Duchenne noticed in some boys a progressive muscle wasting. The pelvic and calf muscles were the first to go before age 5, and they lost the ability to walk by age 12. The weakness then spread to other muscles, the breathing muscles, and death was usually in the 20s due to the failure of the respiratory system. The breathing muscles just would give out.

The muscular dystrophy Duchenne described is inherited as a recessive allele on the X chromosome. In that way, genetically it's like hemophilia, so it's most common in males. It's about 1 in 3500 births. If you think that that's a low number, 1 in 3500, think of the fact that there are about 4 million births a year in the United States, so that's going to be over 1000 young boys born with this disease. The treatment of muscular dystrophy remains symptomatic. That is, the children have braces and wheelchairs and ventilators to help them breathe. There is no cure, so it's urgent to find out exactly what's wrong in the muscles of these boys.

For decades, scientists had looked in the muscle tissue for a difference between the normal muscle and what we call dystrophic muscle, the muscle of a patient with muscular dystrophy. Now there's some overwhelmingly common proteins in muscle. I mentioned them in an earlier lecture, actin and myosin. They're the large proteins in the muscle fiber. They knew that muscle fibers in muscular dystrophy tended to fall apart very readily. They don't have good integrity, and they get replaced by fatty tissues and other nonmuscle fibrous tissues. But with the chemical methods people had, and even have now, they couldn't find a difference in the muscle of the patient with muscular dystrophy and the muscle of a patient without that disease. It was like looking for a needle in a haystack.

Methods for analyzing DNA and chromosomes were developed quite rapidly during the 1980s, and by the mid-'80s or so, scientists were ready to take another approach to muscular dystrophy. Their idea was, well, instead of trying to find the protein, let's get the gene first, and then we'll figure out what the protein is. This is called reverse genetics because it's not the traditional way of getting a gene. The traditional way was, like with PKU, find the protein, then find the gene. This time we're going to find the gene first. At the Harvard Medical School, a medical scientist, Louis Kunkel, and his colleagues, saw a boy with Duchenne muscular dystrophy in the clinic. When they looked at his chromosomes under a microscope, they saw that this boy was missing a small piece of the X chromosome.

You may recall in an earlier lecture that I described how we found out that a single gene called SRY on the Y chromosome determines maleness. Remember, there was a woman who was XY, and when the scientist said, whoa, you've got a Y chromosome, you should be a male, they looked carefully at her Y chromosome. She was missing a little piece, and that's how they isolated that missing piece as being the SRY, the maleness-determining gene. She was missing that, so she was a she. By the same token, Kunkel, finding a missing piece of the X chromosome in this boy with muscular dystrophy figured, whoa, that might be the gene that's responsible for normal muscle integrity that's missing in muscular dystrophy, in the case of this boy. So it became a case of using the techniques of molecular biology and DNA analysis to compare the DNA—this is long before genome sequencing—of an X chromosome that was intact and the DNA of the X chromosome that had the piece missing. They isolated the piece that was in the intact DNA but that was missing in the boy, and by 1985, they'd isolated the gene that was missing in muscular dystrophy.

The dystrophin gene, as they call it, is huge. In fact, it's the largest gene in the human genome. It has 2.5 million base pairs. That's a big gene. The average gene, I told you when discussing genome sequencing, is 27,000 base pairs. When you look at the messenger RNA, the copy of the gene that goes to the ribosome to make this protein, which is a pretty big protein as it is, it's 14,600 bases long. Wait a minute. The gene is 2.5 million; the messenger RNA, 14.6 thousand. Whoa, this is really a lot smaller. What's all that extra DNA? Well, of course, it's introns; it's intervening sequences. It's this extra DNA we have to get rid of at the RNA level by this splicing mechanism. In fact, this dystrophin gene has 78 intervening sequences. The gene is in 79 pieces, and we have to get rid of 78 things. That's a complicated splicing that goes on in the nucleus, but it does pretty well.

Once you have the gene, how are you going to get the protein? Well, last lecture I talked about recombinant DNA, didn't I? So you could take this gene and put it into a bacteria cell or a human cell that doesn't have the gene, and have it by a promoter that would allow it to express itself. Lo and behold, they had the protein, and now they knew the identity of the protein. They had a way of detecting it, and they found it in muscle. It turned out that this protein is 0.002% of muscle protein. It really is a needle in a haystack, but it's a very important protein. The protein called dystrophin is a protein that connects the muscle fiber to the outside of the muscle cell.

And so when the muscle contracts, if this connection is not there, the muscle loses its integrity because its connecting thing is not there, this dystrophin. This ultimately will kill the muscle cell, and then fatty tissue and other fibrous tissue come in to replace it. So what Kunkel and other scientists after him had done was identify the primary phenotype in muscular dystrophy—the protein that is either missing or defective, as this dystrophin protein—and they had done it by first isolating the gene and then using recombinant DNA technology. So you see the sequence of events. None of this could have happened 10 years previously, before the invention of recombinant DNA technology.

Now they identified the gene; so what? They've got the protein; so what? Because you read in the newspaper every day, "Scientists identify gene and protein responsible for X." And of course, then you say, then, then, then? Well, in the case of muscular dystrophy, the approach now is to try to get the body to make a protein it already has an intact gene for; that's one of the approaches. So there is a protein very similar to dystrophin; it's called urotrophin. It's different from dystrophin, but it's similar, and it actually can go in the muscle and replace dystrophin, but the body makes very little of it. So there is a huge effort now to develop drugs that will hype up, in these muscular dystrophy patients who can't make dystrophin, this replacement protein. So that's a promising development that never could have happened if we didn't know what dystrophin was.

The second approach is something I'll talk about in a later lecture, namely adding back the dystrophin gene, the intact gene, to the muscle. This is gene therapy, where we take the good gene and we add it back to the diseased tissue, and there is work going on there as well. Neither of these approaches could have been taken without isolating the gene and the protein responsible. This whole field is called molecular medicine, and it's really the subject of a good chunk of the last third of this Teaching Company course.

Back to comparing DNA. You remember what Kunkel's challenge was. He wanted to compare a DNA that has the dystrophin gene and a DNA that doesn't. Now you'd say, well, the easy way to do it would be a sequencing. Well, in those days, you couldn't sequence, and in many instances sequencing really doesn't work that well to do this. The way to do it was developed by a scientist named Sol Spiegelman in the 1960s. This technique is called nuclei acid hybridization. Suppose DNA has the following sequence—you've got to make a DNA of a certain length, so we'll make it easy—AAAGGGCCCTTT, the other strands to be understood. Opposite the As are three Ts; opposite the Gs are three Cs; opposite the Cs are three Gs; opposite the Ts are three As. I'll repeat: AAAGGGCCCTTT. Now we have a question. Is that gene present in some unknown sequence that we have? Is that gene present, that AAAGGGCCCTTT, in the sequence of unknown DNA that we have?

Here's the way to find out that was invented by Spiegelman in the 1960s. What you do is you take the original sequence, and you make the complement of it—not AAAGGGCCCTTT; that's our target. You make the opposite sequence, TTTCCCGGGAAA, the opposite sequence, the sequence that would recognize it. You take that sequence that is opposite, and you put it on a piece of filter paper, for example; you immobilize it in some way. Okay, so it's sitting there. Now we take our unknown DNA, and we unwind it to make it into a single strand. Now remember, we got our complement sequence, TTTCCCGGGAAA sitting there. All the DNA washes over it, and the only DNA—the unknown DNA—that will bind to it is going to be its complement. Guess what—our old buddy, AAAGGGCCCTTT. If nothing binds, then our outside DNA does not have AAAGGGCCCTTT. So we're looking for recognition. Because these DNAs—the one that's on the filter paper and the one that's unknown—come from a different source, they're called a hybrid DNA, and it's a laboratory phenomenon, the hybrid, right? Because half the DNA is from one place, half the DNA is from another place.

Back to Kunkel's dilemma and the dilemma of muscular dystrophy. Kunkel had an intact X chromosome, and he had a chromosome that was missing a piece of DNA. So he took a long part of the DNA of the X chromosomes, and he hybridized them to each other. So now he had one of the strands from one chromosome, from the muscular dystrophy patient, and the other strand from the normal DNA, and he hybridized them. Of course they matched. They're both X chromosomes, right? The DNAs will match, and they matched perfectly well except a loop happened because this loop meant that in one of the two halves of this DNA is a part that doesn't have a complement. Of course, that's the normal gene for dystrophin that was absent, in part or whole, from the patient with muscular dystrophy. So here was that loop. They struck out the loop, they put in a cloning vector, and they had the gene. That's exactly how they found this gene in muscular dystrophy.

Now you can take a probe for the dystrophin gene, and you can label it with fluorescence and then take human chromosomes and put them under a microscope when they are compact. What happens is the probe will bind, and you'll have little fluorescent dots where the DNA is. And this hybridization to a chromosome DNA—it's the same as in the test tube—can be done on a glass slide. You look through the microscope, and you say the dystrophin gene is—well, it turns out to be, glad we know this, on the X chromosome. Otherwise we'd be pretty embarrassed because everything we know about it genetically is it's on the X chromosome. You could do diagnosis with this. What if we're looking for multiple copies of a gene, or the presence or absence of a gene? You make a probe that is fluorescent. You bind it to chromosomes. You'll see multiple dots or fewer dots. In some cancers, for example, genes are amplified to large amounts, and you can make a diagnosis on the basis of where the dots land and how many dots there are.

Rapid screening of the genome for the presence of a gene, to isolate a gene, can be done by what are called DNA libraries. DNA libraries are not where you go look at books and you find DNA in it, or you find the genome sequence. It's a library—in other words, it's a bunch of volumes of the genome all displayed in some way. Genome libraries can actually be made by gene cloning. Now how do we do this, and why would we do it? Why we would do it is for the following reason. For example, in muscular dystrophy in these boys, sure, they were missing part of the X chromosome. Were they missing all of the dystrophin gene? When that little loop in hybridization was isolated by Kunkel, was that the whole gene? It actually wasn't. This gene is so huge. They were missing part of it. And of course, if you miss part of a protein, well, you're just missing too much of it. It won't be functional. If you have only half of a dystrophin protein, it doesn't fold right. It will not perform its function properly.

So, where was the rest of the gene, and how were they going to fish it out? Here's the idea. You take the genome, and you cut the genome into pieces—gene-sized pieces or whatever—and you take each one of these pieces and randomly put it into a vector for recombinant DNA cloning. Now consider we will have thousands of vectors, each of which has a gene in it; let's say a human gene. And so we'd have 24,000 vectors, each of which has a human gene in it. Now we infect those vectors into *E. coli*, our bacteria. Now we have 24,000 bacteria, each of which is carrying a human gene. Next step, we grow those bacteria up as colonies; not in a liquid form, but in a solid matrix so we can grow them up as little colonies of bacteria. You've seen colonies of funguses and things like this that grow in your kitchen if you don't watch it. Bacteria even grow as colonies, too, in your kitchen. So you have little colonies of bacteria.

Each one of those colonies has a human gene in it, so we can treat each colony chemically to take its DNA out as it sits there, and then we can separate the two strands of the DNA and then use a probe for the dystrophin gene. This probe might have only half of the gene because that half has been missing. We can take that probe and apply it, and it'll only bind to where the gene is, but it'll fish out the rest of the gene, too, along with it because it's got half the gene as the probe. The whole gene is in that bacteria cell, and you'll fish out the rest of the gene along with the half. It's a beautiful technique. The problem is, of course, you've got 24,000 bacterial colonies, and that's kind of a hassle to do.

Once we have identified the colony that has the entire gene, we can pick that colony out, put the colony cells into a liquid medium, and by tomorrow we have a lot of that gene because we grow up a lot of the cells that contain the vector that has the gene in it. Now we can re-isolate that vector, bust open the cells, take the vector out that has the human gene in it. And of course, since the vector was created by recombinant DNA techniques where you use a restriction enzyme, we take the same restriction enzyme; we can cut open the vector, and the human gene pops out. It's a terrific way to isolate a human gene that's intact. That's called a genome library.

Genome libraries have now been miniaturized into DNA microarrays. Now we don't even have to clone. We can do this hybridization in a miniature setup. The silicon chip was a major technological innovation in electronics in the 20th century. A silicon chip is a thin micro-wafer, if you've never seen one, that has electric circuits that are stamped onto it. A DNA microchip, or a DNA microarray, is a small glass microscope slide, and you put DNAs on it. Just put DNAs in teeny, tiny amounts, but in large numbers of DNA count, and a small droplet has millions of copies of a DNA probe. You can put these DNA probes on as single strands right beside one another on essentially a very small glass slide, a little rectangle about an inch in size. You put them in rows. In fact, you can get thousands and thousands of probes. In fact, they now have gene chips that have all of the human genome, all 24,000 genes, arrayed in rows on this microscope slide. You have probes for all 24,000 genes.

Now, why would you want to look at all 24,000 genes? Well, you can find whole genes there. You can find, in diagnosis, that a patient is missing a gene. You take the patient's DNA, and you make it single strand, and you try to hybridize the human genome. If one of those 24,000 genes doesn't hybridize, doesn't find its partner in this person's DNA, well, that person is missing that particular gene. So it's a way of doing a genetic diagnosis, especially in the case that they are missing. You can even screen for mutations in DNA that way. You can also hybridize RNAs to DNA that way. So let's say we have all 24,000 human genes on this microscope slide. You might say, well, how are they going to detect that? Of course, you use lasers and fancy detection techniques to do this at the miniature level. A scientist really is not looking under the microscope and seeing the

DNA. They're seeing little spots that are amplified, and a laser is scanning over them.

If we take a tissue at a certain time in its life cycle, and we take all the RNAs out of it that are expressed—all those messenger RNAs—well, those are the RNAs this tissue is expressing as the phenotype at that particular time. Different RNAs are expressed at different times. You know, the red blood cell makes the RNA for hemoglobin; the hair cell makes the RNA for hair. We take all those RNAs, and now they're single-stranded. We hybridize them to our DNA chip. We can find out which genes are being expressed. It's a gene expression signature, isn't it, of the particular tissue at this time. What you find when you do this, of course, is that not all genes are expressed in all tissues at all times. That's great. I don't have hair growing out of my bone marrow, and I don't have blood coming out of my scalp. It's nice we have genes expressed only at a certain time.

This has great significance, these DNA microarray gene expression signatures. Let me give you an example in clinical medicine. In breast cancer, it's essential for a physician to get an idea at the time of diagnosis of the stage of growth of a tumor. How advanced is the tumor, and is it localized, or is it going to spread? If a tumor is caught at an early stage— diagnosis is made at an early stage—surgery may "get it all." A surgeon likes to say, I got it all; got it all out. Surgeons shouldn't say that. That's not a wise thing to say, in most people's experience. Sometimes they don't get it all because sometimes tumor cells are hiding all over the body; the tumor has already spread. This phenomenon of tumor spread is called metastasis. I'll talk about this later on in the course. But if a tumor has spread already, the cells are hiding out. You really can't see them; they're single cells. You can't see them. A tumor is visible. Bear in mind, a tumor which is quite small—I just put my fingers together—has about a billion cells at the time of diagnosis. That's a lot of cells, so the likelihood of spread sometimes is profound.

Now what physicians would like to know, of course, is are they getting it all when they cut the tumor out at that point, or are there cells that have spread? In other words, if I look at this tumor cell at that particular time, is there something in that tumor cell that tells me I'm the spreading type; I'm the type of tumor that has spread, versus a tumor—no, no, I'm here right now; I'm not spreading. Is there something about it? Well, the cells look the same. When a pathologist, a doctor who deals with tissues, looks at a tumor biopsy at this time, very often—in breast cancer, for example—the tumor cells all look the same.

So, we don't know a difference just looking at them under the microscope of whether they're the same or not. Are there differences at the chemical level that we could detect from the spreading type and the nonspreading type? Because if there are—if we could identify the tumors that are the spreading type—then, of course, after surgery, you'll treat these patients with other therapies like radiation and drug therapy to kill cells that might be elsewhere in the body. If a tumor is not the spreading type, of course, you'll say, well, go home, you're cured.

Enter DNA microchips and a scientist at the Netherlands Cancer Agency, Dr. Laura van't Veer. She took biopsies from both types of breast cancer in retrospect; that is, types that had spread and types that had not spread. The biopsy cells looked the same under the microscope. It said breast cancer, breast cancer. Then she took their RNAs out and asked which genes have been expressed in the ones that spread and the ones that didn't spread later on. She found, with her colleagues, that some genes were expressed more in the tumors that were spreading, and other genes were expressed more in the tumors that didn't spread in comparison to the other group. She had a gene expression signature. There are about 70 genes that are involved in this particular signature.

So the idea now is to do a diagnosis of breast cancer in these particular cases very early on. If it's an early cancer where you don't know if it's spread or not, if it's the spreading type, then do this gene expression signature by DNA hybridization probes and the gene chip; find out which genes are expressed, and if it's the spreading type, you'll do the surgery and then treat the patient with radiation and drugs. If it's the nonspreading type, you'll do the surgery, and the patient can go home without having been treated. This is an example of the kind of work that is going on using gene expression and hybridization and gene chips.

Synthetic DNA can be used in the laboratory to make new genes and mutations. Chemists have developed, in the laboratories, ways of making DNA base by base. Knowing the genetic code, then, you can make any gene you want. I mentioned this in terms of the idea of synthetic genetics, where we were making the genes of a simple organism one by one in the laboratory. Well, if we can make the genes, we can make mutations. Now this is a very important aspect of genetics. Genetics tries to ask "what if" types of questions. If we want to ask a question—for example, if we have an enzyme, and we say, well, this enzyme has this function. What if this enzyme changes in a certain way? Will it have a different function?

Well, the only way to do that in the past was to look in nature for the mutation. We went out to nature to the organism that normally makes this protein, and we looked in nature for a mutation that had the mutant protein. Or we took an organism in the laboratory like bacteria, and we treated them with radiation to make more mutations and selected the mutation that we were interested in doing. We don't need to do that anymore. We don't need to look in nature for mutations; we can do it ourselves. We can say, I want to change that amino acid here. So instead of giving a genetic code—AAA; make me an AGA—at this point, send it to the synthesis lab, and they'll make you a gene that has AGA there instead of AAA there, and you have a different amino acid.

There are a number of examples by which this has been done, and it's a very powerful technology because all you've got to do is look up the genetic code, and you can change genes at will. We are no longer reliant on the accidents of nature, the mutations in nature. We can create mutations and better or worse genes in the laboratory. This synthetic biology is very powerful in this regard. In the next lecture, I'll turn to the products that have been made by the recombinant DNA revolution. Thank you.

Lecture Twelve
Biotechnology—Genetic Engineering

Scope: Biotechnology is the use of microbes (such as bacteria), plants, and animals to make products useful to humans. Agriculture was probably the first biotechnology, when people domesticated plants and used them as crops for food and fiber. Plant materials were used to make beer and bread, followed by yogurt, cheese, wine, etc. Microbes are grown for their products such as antibiotics and amino acids, an activity which became the fermentation industry. The discovery of genetic engineering by recombinant DNA, as well as knowledge from basic research of the conditions that maximize gene expression, led to the creation of a new biotechnology industry based on recombinant DNA. Proteins that are hard to get in usable amounts in nature, such as the clot-busting drug tPA and human insulin, are now made by genetically modified cells. Even whole animals and plants can be turned into factories for useful proteins.

Outline

I. Opening story: Biotechnology to the rescue.

    A. A stroke victim was saved by a genetically engineered drug.

        1. As he drove home from work, Bill first felt his face twitch, and then his speech became slurred. He was the latest of several million people a year in the U.S. who have a stroke, in which a blood clot blocks an artery leading from the heart to the brain. This deprives brain cells of oxygen, normally carried by the red blood cells, and irreversible damage can occur quickly.

        2. Normally, blood clots "go away" after some time. There is a clot-dissolving system in the blood that gets activated by cells near the clot. Of course, the time factor is important, because we want a clot to be there for a while to stop the flow of blood at an injury. Unfortunately for Bill, a stroke (as well as a heart attack) is not a situation where you want a clot around for long. Every minute that blood flow is blocked to the brain is harmful.

3. Lucky for Bill, he was near a hospital and drove his car into the ER parking lot, leaning on the horn. The staff ran out, got him into the ER, and immediately injected a drug right onto the clot. It quickly dissolved, and blood flow was restored with minimal permanent brain damage. Bill was home the next day.

4. The drug the ER staff injected was tissue plasminogen activator (tPA, also called PLAT). It is the protein that actually initiates the clot-dissolving process. In the normal course of events, this takes time (for good reason, as just stated). Adding it to the blood right at Bill's clot just sped up the process.

5. Thankfully for the typical blood clotting processes, tPA is made in small amounts and only when needed. So it is virtually impossible to get enough of it to store on the shelf of the ER, ready for injection when needed. Enter recombinant DNA.

6. First, DNA was extracted from human cells and the gene for tPA was isolated by the methods described in the last lecture. Then this DNA, with an appropriate promoter that stimulates active gene expression, was inserted into hamster cells growing in the laboratory by genetic engineering methods described two lectures ago. These cells containing the recombinant DNA churned out tPA in amounts far in excess of what could ever be extracted from blood. The tPA protein was purified and put into a vial, ready for a patient like Bill.

7. This scenario—of gene to useful protein by genetic engineering—has now been played out for dozens of products. It is part of a revolution in biotechnology.

B. Biotechnology is not new.

1. Biotechnology—the manipulation of microbes, plants, and animals to make produces useful to people—began long ago.

   a. Agriculture—harvesting, planting, and cultivation of plants and animals for food and fiber—was probably the first biotech. It may have begun about 10,000 years ago in what is now Iraq, when Sumerians learned that barley plants that grew near their settlements made seeds that could be mashed up and used to make beer, and later, bread. So they grew the seeds in plots near their settlement—the first farms. In ancient Egypt, the hieroglyphic symbol for food was a pitcher of beer and a loaf of bread.

    b. The process of making alcohol from mashed-up seeds (or grapes) was actually carried out by yeast cells and called fermentation (from Latin *fervere*, to boil; bubbles form because of the release of carbon dioxide).

    c. Fermentation under different conditions and by different organisms produced other products as well: wine, spirits, cheese, yogurt, vinegar, etc.

  2. By the mid-20th century, the industry called biotechnology was using microorganisms in huge vats, to make antibiotics, oils, amino acids, and enzymes for the food industry.

II. Modern biotechnology uses recombinant DNA.

  A. The invention of recDNA methods during the 1970s opened up two new horizons for the manipulation of organisms in biotechnology.

    1. First, the existing organisms could be genetically manipulated to be more efficient to make their products by deliberate mutations, addition of active promoters for gene expression, etc.

    2. Second, new genes could be inserted into productive organisms to turn them into factories for products that would ordinarily be inaccessible. This is the story of tPA.

  B. The key to production of a protein product is the promoter.

    1. Recall that the promoter is a DNA sequence adjacent to a gene that attracts RNA polymerase, the enzyme that makes mRNA and is responsible for gene expression.

    2. Biologists learned that promoters are specific for place (cell type) and time.

    3. So a promoter DNA would be added to the gene DNA appropriate to the cell type and environmental conditions. The vector DNA to which this was added is called an expression vector.

III. Human insulin was the first major product of DNA biotechnology.

  A. The problem: Insulin (from the Latin word for island—the type of tissue in the pancreas gland that makes it) is a protein that acts as a hormone to stimulate uptake of blood sugar into tissues. People with type 1 diabetes (from the Greek word meaning "passing through," referring to excessive urine production) don't make insulin and so need to inject it.

B. Previously, insulin came from slaughtered animals. But animal insulin is a bit different in amino acid sequence than the human one, and some people reacted against it, thus the need for human insulin. There was no supply of human pancreases.

C. So a team of scientists developed a way to make a lot of it by recombinant DNA.

    1. At City of Hope Medical Center in California, Keiichi Itakura synthesized the insulin gene (which has 51 amino acids).

    2. His colleague, Art Riggs, put the gene into an expression vector next to a high-expressing promoter.

    3. The recDNA vector was put into bacteria.

    4. The bacteria were grown in a large vat by the (then new) biotech company Genentech (founded by Herbert Boyer).

    5. The insulin was extracted from the vat, sent to a drug company, and then sent to physicians. This is the source of all insulin now used to treat diabetics.

IV. Other medically useful substances are produced by biotechnology.

A. Some proteins replace ones that are missing in genetic diseases. For example, in hemophilia (Talmud story in Lecture Three, etc.), a blood-clotting protein is missing. When the patient gets injured, it can be replaced by the clotting protein made by biotechnology.

B. Some proteins are used as drugs to treat diseases. tPA is one example. Another example is erythropoietin (EPO). This protein is made by the kidneys, enters the bloodstream, and goes to bone marrow, where it stimulates the production of red blood cells.

    1. People with kidney failure are treated with dialysis. This is very helpful, but it removes EPO, so the patients get very anemic (low red blood cells). They need transfusions, unless they get EPO. People with functional kidneys make very little EPO, so getting EPO for the patients from other people's blood would be very difficult.

    2. So the EPO gene was isolated and EPO made by recDNA. It is now used not just for dialysis but also for people undergoing cancer chemotherapy (which often destroys bone marrow cells).

       3. EPO became the first biotech drug of abuse: Athletes found it could increase their red blood cells by about 10%, and this gave them an edge in competition (e.g., the Tour de France).

V. Plants and animals can be genetically engineered to make products.

    A. Pharming results in transgenic animals.

        1. Dairy animals such as sheep, goats, and cows produce a lot of milk. Biologists have found that the expression of genes for major protein in milk is under the control of a lactoglobulin promoter that is expressed in the mammary gland.

        2. Idea: Take any gene you want expressed and put it in a DNA vector that has the lactoglobulin promoter. Then put this recDNA vector into a goat egg-cell nucleus. Allow the egg to develop to an embryo and insert the embryo into a surrogate mother. Result: a transgenic sheep that makes a desired protein in its milk.

        3. Example: Some people lack adequate human growth hormone (hGH). This is a protein made in the pituitary gland in the brain. Supply is extremely limited as a result. In Argentina, scientists put the gene for hGH into cows with high expressing lactoglobulin promoter. Ten cows can make enough hGH to supply the annual world demand.

    B. Plants can be genetically engineered to make products.

        1. As we will see, genetic engineering of plants is easier than animals because any cell can be used (you do not need an egg). In addition, plants grow a lot and produce a lot of protein in their leaves and fruits.

            a. Plants can be engineered to make proteins that are extracted. For example, tobacco plants (the farmers are always looking for new uses) have been modified by recDNA to make tPA in their leaves. This is a huge source.

            b. Plants can be engineered to make proteins in fruits that are eaten. For example, a "plantibody" project involves a gene for a vaccine against bacterial meningitis (see Lecture Nineteen on the immune system). This gene has been put into banana plants and is expressed in the fruits. This would be useful as it circumvents the need for vaccine administration by health professionals.

2. Plants can be engineered to make enzymes that create new biochemical pathways and new products.

   a. For example, a major component of detergents is lauric acid (look at a label). This molecule is made in a biochemical pathway in tropical plants such as the coconut and the palm tree. Palm kernel oil is a major source, and this must be imported from the tropical countries to those in more temperate climates. Recently, scientists pinpointed a key enzyme responsible for the biosynthesis of lauric acid in a tropical plant, cloned its DNA into an expression vector, and put the vector into a rapeseed plant (canola) that is grown widely in temperate climates. The transgenic plant makes oil that has 60% lauric acid (up from 0%).

   b. Tobacco mosaic virus infects, and reproduces in, but does not kill, tobacco plants. In a novel approach, the viral genome can be replaced in part with a new gene, in this case one for a vaccine, and instead of a lot of viral coat protein, the virus makes the vaccine protein in large quantities in tobacco leaves. This may be a new use for this widely grown crop.

Essential Reading:

Susan Barnum, *Biotechnology: An Introduction* (Belmont, CA: Thomson Brooks-Cole, 2005), chaps. 1, 6, and 7.

Maarten Chrispeels and David Sadava, *Plants, Genes and Crop Biotechnology* (Sudbury, MA: Jones and Bartlett, 2003), chap. 19.

Supplemental Reading:

Cynthia Robbins-Roth, *From Alchemy to IPO: The Business of Biotechnology* (Cambridge, MA: Perseus Group, 2001).

John Smith, *Biotechnology*, 4th ed. (Cambridge: Cambridge University Press, 2004).

Questions to Consider:

1. Why did drugs such as insulin, tPA, and hGH have to be made by biotechnology? What were the other ways to get these drugs, and why were they inadequate? Can you think of other useful proteins that need to be made this way?

2. Some people are opposed to genetically modified organisms in the food supply. How would these people react to finding out that drugs for human consumption such as insulin are made by genetically modified organisms (in this case, a bacterium making a human protein)?

Lecture Twelve—Transcript
Biotechnology—Genetic Engineering

Welcome back. In Lecture Ten, I described how recombinant DNA technology was invented. In the last lecture, I described how we could isolate genes for expressing in recombinant DNA technology. Now, in this lecture, let's see what was expressed when these DNA technologies were used. My opening story concerns Bill, a stroke victim. As he drove home from work, Bill first felt his face twitching. Then his speech became slurred and he got a really, really bad headache. Bill was the latest of several million people a year in the United States who have a stroke. A blood clot was blocking an artery leading from the heart to his brain. This would deprive brain cells of oxygen, which is normally carried by red blood cells, and irreversible damage to the brain could occur quite quickly.

Now, when you think of blood clots, you've got to think of the fact that clots do go away eventually. Now "go away" is not a really good biochemical term. We say that the clot dissolves eventually, but it better happen fairly slowly. The way this happens is the following. As the wound is healed—as the hole in the skin is healed, for example—a series of cells that is healing the wound actually makes a substance. The substance is called tissue plasminogen activator. I'll abbreviate it tPA so we don't need to talk about it again in its technical words. And tPA activates the blood clotting system that is all ready to go in the blood, and the clot then dissolves. This time factor is important, biologically speaking, because if the clot dissolved the minute it was formed, it's not going to do much good. The blood will continue to flow out, and you lose all of your blood.

So slow dissolving of the clot is a good thing, but not for Bill. Bill was having a stroke, and that's not a situation where you want a blood clot there for a long time. Every minute of blood flow that is blocked to the brain is harmful to the brain. Well, lucky for Bill, he was near a hospital and drove his car into the emergency room parking lot, leaned on the horn, and out came the emergency room staff. They got Bill into the ER and immediately injected a drug right on the surface of the blood clot. The clot dissolved right away, blood flow was restored, and there was minimal damage to the brain. Bill was home the next day, and he was fine. The drug that the emergency room staff had injected was tPA. It's also called PLAT in medical terms. This is the protein that actually initiates the clot-dissolving process.

As I mentioned, normally this takes a long time. So sure, the clot in Bill's brain would have gone away, but his brain would have gotten damaged in the meantime to an irreversible state. Adding this substance right away to the site of the clot activated the clot-dissolving system in the blood right there. Now the good thing about tissue plasminogen activator, tPA, is it's made in very small amounts and it's only made when it's needed. The bad thing is if we want to use that as a drug, a medication, as it was used in Bill, we better get a lot of it around. It's virtually impossible just to get enough tPA from the cells of a body, for example, to store on the shelf in the emergency room, ready for injection.

Enter recombinant DNA technology. First, DNA was extracted from human cells, and the gene for tPA was isolated by the methods I just described in the previous lecture. This DNA gene, with the appropriate promoter for stimulating its expression, was inserted. Well, the first technology did it in bacterial cells, and they found they weren't the best, so they used hamster cells growing in the laboratory. These genetic engineering methods caused those cells containing the recombinant DNA with our tPA gene to churn out human tPA in amounts far in excess of what you could ever extract from blood. The tPA protein was then purified, put in a vial, and set on the shelf, ready for a patient like Bill. This scenario of a gene to a useful protein by this genetic engineering technology has now been played out for dozens of products. It's part of a revolution in biotechnology.

Biotechnology is the manipulation of microbes, small organisms like bacteria and viruses, plants and animals, to make products that are useful to people. As such, biotechnology is not new. It began a long time ago. I will say that biotechnology really began with agriculture. Agriculture I can define as the harvesting, planting, and cultivation of plants and animals for food and fiber. This was really the first biotechnology, and estimates are that agriculture probably began about 10,000 years ago in what is now the region near present-day Iraq. We have evidence that Sumerians living there at the time learned that barley plants that were growing near the places they were living made seeds—we call them grains—that could be mashed up and used to make beer and, later on, bread. So they started growing these seeds in plots of land near their settlements; that is, they would use some of the seeds for mashing up to make beer and bread, and then they would grow the rest of the seeds nearby.

In ancient Egypt, the hieroglyphic symbol for food actually is a pitcher of beer and a loaf of bread, which reflects our barley domestication idea. You might say, well, bread first and beer? I mean, why were they drinking beer? Just to have a good time? Answer, no. When people began to live in settled places, they realized by trial and error that water purity was a big issue. They would be going to the bathroom in the same water they were drinking. People were getting sick. And alcoholic beverages do kill most of the bad things that are in water. Alcoholic beverages are sterile, and they're good to drink, so it's not surprising that they were invented quite early on by humans.

The process of making alcohol from mashed up seeds, or grapes to make wine, is actually not carried out by the seeds themselves, but by yeast cells that live in the mashed up grain or grapes. Or we can add them. This process is called fermentation. It's from the Latin word—and I'll mispronounce it— *fervere*. The "v" is not pronounced in Latin. I didn't take Latin in four years of high school for nothing; now I can show off, saying I know it. The Latin word *fervere* means "to boil." And the reason that it's used is that bubbles form in fermentation because of the release of carbon dioxide. Fermentation under different conditions, and by different organisms that have different genetic capabilities, produced other products as well, quite early on in human culture: wine in addition to other spirits, cheese, yogurt, vinegar— lots of things.

By the mid–20th century, there was a whole industry called biotechnology, using organisms for our purposes. It was using microorganisms in huge vats to make things like antibiotics—this is a major commercial enterprise—oils, amino acids, and enzymes for the food industry. Modern biotechnology, the biotechnology I will discuss now, is not necessarily the biotechnology I've just described, the fermentation industry. But keep in mind, it is still a giant industry that is quite a bit larger than the biotechnology I will now describe in terms of recombinant DNA. I'm going to talk about biotechnology and recombinant DNA in several ways. First, I'll describe the general strategies of using recombinant DNA to make things. Then I'll describe in a little more detail the first major product that was made; it was human insulin. I'll show you that there are a couple of other medically useful products produced by biotechnology, and finally I'll talk about genetically engineered animals and plants to make products of use. The general theme of this lecture is what products recombinant DNA makes for human use.

Now, biotechnology could be used to make products in two ways. First of all, we could take the existing organisms, the existing microbes, the existing plants and animals, and modify them genetically using recombinant DNA technology to make them more efficient. That is, we could, for example, add a promoter that was more active so more product would be made. We could genetically manipulate them to have a new biochemical pathway. The second use of recombinant DNA in biotechnology was, and is, that we could take new genes and insert them into productive organisms that have never had them before. We're not just manipulating bacteria to make things that they already make in a better way; we're having bacteria make things they've never made before, like tissue plasminogen activator—like tPA, for example.

The key to all of this technology is the promoter. Now let's recall what a promoter is. A promoter is a DNA sequence that is adjacent to a gene, that attracts the molecules that will express the gene, make the RNA copy, and the whole complex of molecules that will be involved in doing that. Promoters turn out to be specific for place—that is, what cell type is going to express the gene—and time. As I've said before, you don't have hair growing out of your bone marrow; you don't have blood cells growing out of your scalp, and the reason is the promoters. The genes are all there. The promoters are different beside those genes. It's a good example of basic research because all of the information we have on promoters was just derived from scientists who didn't want to do biotechnology, but really just wanted to see how things work in nature—what controls the expression of genes. This basic research led to this industry.

Now in tissue plasminogen activator, the gene for tPA was spliced into a vector that had in it already a selectable gene, of course, to find out if the gene was there, but also a promoter that will give high-level expression, that will attract the molecules involved in making messenger RNA. This vector with the recombinant DNA and the tPA was put into bacteria first, and then hamster, which then made a lot of the protein that we're interested in. A vector that has a promoter for high-level expression of genes is called an expression vector, not surprisingly. Although it's not the first product of biotechnology for humans, the first major product in widespread use was human insulin, about 25 years ago. Insulin comes from the Latin word— there we go again, all those years of Latin coming in handy for something— for "island." The reason insulin is an island is that this is the tissue of the pancreas that makes it; it's a little island of cells called the "islets of Langerhans."

Insulin is a protein that acts as a hormone to stimulate the uptake of blood sugar into tissues such as the liver and the muscle. In diabetes, people don't make insulin (in type I diabetes) or don't respond (in type II). But the insulin of type I diabetes where they don't make it is the one that we are interested in because this is the insulin we will have to replace. Previously in human medicine, insulin came from slaughtered animals. The insulin protein has 51 amino acids. It folds in a certain way, has a certain function, and the function is it goes to a cell in the muscle, or liver, and says, suck up the sugar from the blood. Fine. The insulin of the slaughtered animals will do this as well. It will go to the human cell and cause it to suck up sugar. But very often, the insulin, depending on the animal, is one or two amino acids different. It's not surprising that the gene in an animal for making insulin will be slightly different. Insulin is a protein; it's coded for by a gene. It's slightly different than the human gene, by one or two amino acids. But it still folds right. It still has the same function.

But, as we'll describe in a later lecture, the human immune system—the human system that recognizes things that are not self, that are not us, and reacts to them and causes an immune reaction to them—will recognize these one or two amino acid differences. So in some significant number of people who are diabetics, when they were taking nonhuman insulin, it worked, but eventually they reacted against it. These people were, of course, then in big problems because the insulin would be rejected by the body. So what do we need? We need human insulin. That's the real stuff. That's the 51 amino acids, it folds the right way, and you don't react to it. Every human makes the same insulin.

The problem in getting human insulin, of course, is that you have to get it from those islands in the pancreas gland. Insulin, first of all, is made in teeny tiny, itsy bitsy, very small amounts. You cannot detect the amounts, they're so small. In fact, later on I'll describe ways that biotechnologists developed to detect things in small amounts. So the only way to get this in reasonable amounts is by amplifying the expression of genes for insulin in recombinant DNA.

Here are the steps that were done. At the City of Hope Medical Center in California, a scientist named Keiichi Itakura went into the chemistry lab and made the insulin gene. Now, insulin has 51 amino acids, and you have three base pairs of DNA coding for each amino acid, so it's about 150 base pairs. It wasn't, even then, a big deal to make 151. It took time; now it's done by machine. It took time, but they made 151 bases for DNA. Itakura's colleague, Arthur Riggs, took this gene and put it into an expression vector right next to a high-expressing promoter. The expression vector now had the gene with a high-expressing promoter, and of course it had a marker so you could select the bacteria that had it. The expression vector was then put into bacteria, and the bacteria expressed human insulin. This is about seven or eight years after the first emergence of recombinant DNA technology.

Now, of course, the issue was we've got to grow a whole lot of this in a large vat, and this was done at a biotech company, Genentech, which was founded by Herb Boyer, one of the founders of recombinant DNA technology. The insulin was then extracted from the vat, sent to a drug company, and then sent to physicians. This is the source of all insulin now used to treat type I diabetics. It's really the paradigm, the great example, of a biotechnologically derived medication. Other medically useful products have been made by biotechnology, and I can classify these—I'm not going to name them all for you—in two ways. First of all, replacement proteins for ones that are missing in diseases: like insulin, for example. Insulin is replacing one that people can't make. Another example is the blood-clotting protein that is missing in hemophilia. In Lecture Three, I told you the story of the ancients who were missing a blood-clotting protein and the boys bled to death. This blood-clotting protein can now be supplied, so people no longer die of hemophilia and losing all of their blood. So this protein is now freely available, and these people can be treated with it so people don't die anymore.

Then you can have proteins that are used to treat diseases. I'll give you an example of that. There is a protein called erythropoietin (EPO). That's all I'm going to say; it's going to be called EPO from now on. So EPO is a hormone-like substance made by the kidneys. It enters the bloodstream. It goes to the bone marrow, and in the bone marrow it stimulates the production of red blood cells. Red blood cells only last about 120 days in the blood, so they must be constantly replaced, and they're replaced by cells in the bone marrow. Consider a patient with kidney failure, and there are many, many people with kidney failure for various reasons. These people, you may have heard, are treated these days with kidney dialysis. Kidney transplants are in limited availability, so they're treated with dialysis.

The kidney is a filter. It filters out the poisons, and it keeps the good things. Well, in this case, of course, in the dialysis machine, you filter out the bad things. Well, among the things that get filtered out is EPO. So these people in kidney failure have kidney function restored by dialysis, but they're not making EPO, so they have severe anemia. The only way to get around this is by massive transfusions—it's a major problem—or treating them with EPO.

So the EPO gene was isolated, and EPO was made by recombinant DNA biotechnology. This is now widely used for people who are undergoing kidney dialysis and also people who are being treated with cancer chemotherapy, drugs to treat cancer, because many of these drugs destroy bone marrow cells as well as destroying the tumor. So this is a very good drug for doing that.

EPO is also the first biotech drug of abuse because athletes found that if they take some EPO, they can increase their red blood cell count. Increasing the amount of red blood cells—because EPO does stimulate red blood cell production by about 10%, which is what EPO will do in a person who already has enough red blood cells—can give an athlete an edge in competition. There, of course, have been great controversies in bicycle races and elsewhere in the abuse of EPO.

Plants and animals can be genetically engineered to make products useful for us. The paradigm of this, the great example of this, is dairy animals. Sheep, goats, and cows, as you know, produce a lot of milk in their mammary glands, which are their version of breasts. Biologists, doing basic research, found that the expression of genes for the major milk proteins is under the control, not surprisingly, of a promoter, and this promoter is expressed—it's a sequence of DNA that causes the adjacent genes to be expressed—in the mammary gland. It's called the lactoglobulin promoter because lactoglobulin is the protein that is made. Well, this sets up a really nice biotechnology. You can take the gene you want expressed in milk and put it into a DNA vector, recombinant DNA vector, that has in it the lactoglobulin promoter, this promoter for the breast, the mammary gland. Then you put this vector into a sheep egg cell nucleus. If you put it into a sheep egg cell nucleus, the egg gets fertilized. The egg, then, can develop in the laboratory for a couple of days to an early embryo. You can insert the embryo into a surrogate mother, and the offspring that are born are sheep that will make not just milk, but milk that contains this extra protein, which is the protein that you want. As you'll see, this was actually behind the reason for cloning Dolly the sheep. I'll describe that in a couple of lectures.

For now, think of the following actual example. There are a significant number of humans—not a large number, but it is a number—that lack adequate amounts of growth hormone, human growth hormone. Many of these people are very short in stature. The growth hormone is a protein, so we can get that protein, of course, from the body, but it's made in the pituitary gland in extremely small amounts—like EPO, like tissue plasminogen activator, tPA—so we've got to get it by recombinant DNA biotechnology. So the gene was isolated, put into a vector, went into these animals—in this case, cows—and now there is a herd in Argentina of 10 cows that, in their milk, will supply the world need for human growth hormone every year. It's easy to isolate the protein from milk. This is much easier in terms of biotechnology than using bacteria; an amazing technology that's working really, really well. This process is called "pharming." It's not F-A-R-M-I-N-G; it's P-H-A-R-M-I-N-G, for pharmaceutical farming. It's kind of a fun word, but it's a major technology.

In addition to animals, plants can be genetically engineered to make useful products. Genetic engineering of plants is a lot easier than animals. We don't need to inject an expression vector into the fertilized egg of a plant because, as you recall from Lecture Four, plant cells are totipotent. We can take any plant cell growing in the laboratory, and we can put the vector in and then grow the plant up from that cell because we can manipulate the environment around it to have it be an embryo again. So it's really handy. Plants produce a lot of protein. They produce a lot of protein in their leaves; they produce a lot of protein in their fruits. So, for example, tobacco plants, in this case, have been genetically modified by recombinant DNA technology to make our first example, tPA, the clot-dissolving protein, in their leaves. This might be a huge potential source. Tobacco leaves are a very, very large leaf that has a large amount of protein in it, and it's easy to get the tPA out. This may be a new use for tobacco as the other uses of tobacco become less and less common in this country.

Proteins that are eaten—well, here's another cute word, a "plantibody." You probably have heard the term "antibody." Antibody is what the immune system makes to fight off disease, as in vaccines. A plantibody is a plant that is making a human antibody, so we can use recombinant DNA technology to have a plant make a vaccine. For example, the vaccine against bacterial meningitis has been expressed in the fruit of a plant such as bananas. And you say, now, wait a minute. It's in the fruit. These people still have to eat the fruit. That's true, but it doesn't have to be refrigerated. You can genetically modify the plants to grow where the people live. You don't need to administer it. You don't need health professionals administering it. It might be useful in remote areas.

We can create plants with new capabilities. For example, a major component of detergents—look on the label of a detergent, after the lecture, please—and you will see on that label of a detergent or a shampoo or a liquid soap, lauric acid. It's just detergent; that's all it is. It's soap. It's in almost every detergent product that you will see. This molecule is made in a biochemical pathway in tropical plants such as coconuts and palm trees, so a major source of it is palm kernel oil. Well, in America, we don't grow many palm trees. We grow lots of plants in temperate climates.

So scientists pinpointed one of the key enzymes, one of the major enzymes, that is in the biochemical pathway for making lauric acid. Lauric acid itself is not a protein, but it's made through a biochemical pathway. So scientists pinpointed this gene in palm trees. They cloned the gene into an expression vector, put the vector into a rapeseed plant, which makes canola. You've probably seen canola oil in the store. This is grown widely in temperate climates. The result is we have transgenic canola that normally, when it's not transgenic—when it doesn't have the new gene—makes oil that is 0% lauric acid. And now this particular strain makes 60% lauric acid. So they will be able to press the seeds and get lauric acid out.

There is a viral disease of tobacco plants called the tobacco mosaic virus. This is a major pest of tobacco, and what it does is it doesn't kill the plant, but it kind of destroys leaf tissues and spreads very rapidly. So this virus reproduces in the cells but doesn't kill the entire plant. The viral genome of tobacco can be replaced with other genes—in this case, genes for vaccines. Now instead of making a lot of viral coat protein and virus particles, these tobacco plants are making large amounts of a vaccine. This again may be a new use for what is a widely grown crop all around the world, and this crop, as used as smoking tobacco, is being reduced.

I've described in this lecture a number of products we can make through biotechnology. In the next lecture, I'll describe how biotechnology organisms can be used, especially in environmental cleanup. Thank you.

Lecture Thirteen
Biotechnology and the Environment

Scope: Some organisms have genes whose products can be used to sense or break down environmental pollutants. Other organisms can be genetically engineered to do so. A plant has even been made into a biosensor for land mines using a promoter from bacteria that is sensitive to the explosive and a gene from a jellyfish that makes a protein that glows. Biological control uses organisms to consume other organisms that we regard as pests. Many bacteria species have genes for using what humans think of as wastes for their energy and growth, and this forms the basis of such familiar processes as composting and wastewater treatment. Other bacteria have genes for enzymes that degrade pollutants such as oil and are used in cleaning up oil spills in a process called bioremediation. Still other bacteria can help extract minerals in mining. All of these species can be improved by genetic engineering. Creation of pollutant-digesting bacteria was the first example of patenting of a genetically modified organism.

Outline

I. Opening story: Biotechnology can be used to detect landmines.

    A. Landmines are a sad legacy of recent history.

        1. Mines have wreaked havoc both during and after recent wars. They are cheap, plastic casings filled with an explosive such as TNT (trinitrotoluene) that are triggered to explode when disturbed. The UN estimates that over 100 million unexploded mines lie on or below ground in many countries, from Angola to Cambodia. This makes plowing the fields for farming or other uses a risky business.

        2. Encased in plastic, the mines avoid metal detectors. The best way to find them is the most dangerous: A person gingerly walks around, poking the ground with a long stick and jumping out of the way of any explosion.

    B. Neal Stewart at the University of Tennessee is trying to use plants to remedy this ecologically adverse situation—this is an example of bioremediation. He is making plants that will tell us where the mines are.

1. The idea is to make the plant a biosensor, making a detectable protein wherever the landmines are. This requires two genetic components.
   a. A gene whose protein product can be visualized. Certain deep-sea jellyfish glow in the dark of the depths because they make a protein that fluoresces in weak black (ultraviolet) light. In the 1990s, the DNA coding for this green fluorescent protein (GFP) was isolated and biotechnologists put it into vectors and used it as a marker for the presence of recombinant DNA in many organisms. Glowing organisms were the result (glowing fish were sold for a while).
   b. A promoter that turns on a gene in the presence of TNT. Microbiologists found a bacterium, *Pseudomonas putida*, that could digest TNT and use its breakdown products. The genes coding for the enzymes responsible for this metabolism have promoters that become active for gene expression in the presence of a very low amount of TNT.
2. Stewart has put the two together: a TNT-sensitive promoter and the DNA coding for GFP. He added them to a vector and made transgenic plants. When they are around TNT, they glow under ultraviolet light. A biosensor is born.
3. A major challenge is detecting the glowing plants. Stewart and his colleagues propose remote sensing and seeding from airplanes.

II. Organisms have long been used to solve environmental problems.

    A. Biological control uses the pests of pests.

       1. An old biology poem says:

> Big things have little things
> Upon their backs to bite 'em
> And lesser things, still lesser things
> And so ad infinitum.

       2. This is the food chain in ecology. Knowledge of this chain has allowed biologists to use it to introduce pests that eat pests.
   a. For example, in my first job as a student biologist, I described the tiny insects that preyed on the bud moth caterpillar, a worm that eats up the leaves of apple trees. We introduced this insect to reduce populations of the

harmful worm, thereby reducing the need for pesticides. This is called biological control.

   b. This method is now widespread and works with traditional ways of pest control in a process called integrated pest management.

B. We can use bacteria as nature's recyclers. Bacteria have the genetic capacity to thrive on all sorts of nutrients, including what we refer to as wastes.

   1. Composting uses bacteria that break down carbon-rich stores such as cellulose in wood chips, paper, straw, and hay, as well as nitrogen-rich sources, such as protein wastes, coffee grounds, and fruit and vegetable scraps.

   2. Wastewater treatment uses a variety of bacteria to act on human wastes, paper products, and household chemicals.

III. Bacteria and plants have genes for environmental cleanup.

   A. In addition to being nature's recyclers, bacteria can break down many human-made pollutants. They have been discovered simply by mixing soil or water, or some other source of bacteria, with the pollutant and seeing what survives, and thrives.

   1. The first bacteria developed for cleaning up oil spills were developed by Ananda Chakrabarty in the 1970s. He contaminated soils separately with various components of crude oil and isolated bacteria that survived. Then he mated the bacteria sequentially to get a single stain that could break down multiple substances (this was before genetic engineering, which is the way it is done today). Importantly, he applied for and was awarded a patent for this "super-bug." This landmark decision led to a flood of patents for genetically modified organisms.

   a. In 1989, the oil tanker *Exxon Valdez* ran aground near the Alaskan shore, releasing 11 million gallons of crude oil over 1000 miles of shoreline. Physical methods, such as skimming the water and spraying the rocky shore, were used first. This dispersed about two-thirds of the oil. Bacteria did the rest: Nitrogen and phosphorus salts were sprayed on the shoreline and rocks to stimulate the growth of *Pseudomonas* bacteria already there; other strains were added. Soon, the bacteria became active and worked quickly to degrade the oil. The process is ongoing.

  b. The government of Kuwait is using bioremediation to try to clean up the 250 million gallons of oil that was spilled onto the desert in the Gulf War of 1991. This may be the single largest bioremediation project.

 2. Extremophiles have many useful genes.

  a. These are microbes that live in very hot or cold or pressured or salty environments. They are part of a separate group of organisms called archaea because they resemble the organisms thought to be the first on Earth. In archaea genomes, half of the genes do not resemble genes in bacteria or eukaryotes.

  b. *Deinococcus radiodurans* is a microbe that lives in the most dangerous environment of all, high levels of radiation. Normally, radiation kills cells by damaging their DNA and overwhelming the cell's ability to repair the damage. It gets around this by having the most efficient radiation DNA repair system in nature. The genes from other extremophiles are being engineered into *D. radiodurans*. No matter what the environment, it keeps coming back. No wonder it is called "Conan the Bacterium"! It is being used to clean up the most toxic sites.

B. Plants can be genetically engineered for environmental cleanup.

 1. The bacterial genes that allow environmental cleanup can be put into plants. Thus there are transgenic plants that can break down oil, convert solid mercury and arsenic into harmless substances, etc.

 2. Why use plants when the microbes are available? The issue is getting the bacteria out of the soil when they are done. This is very energy-intensive. Plants can just be harvested by conventional agriculture.

IV. Biomining uses bacteria to help extract metals.

 A. Mining for minerals is an old human activity that has changed little for millennia.

  1. The earth is dug up, ores are taken out, and minerals such as copper and gold are extracted from the ores by harsh methods such as chemicals or heat.

  2. It is environmentally damaging.

B. The bacterium *Thiobacillus ferrooxidans* uses copper sulfide (instead of carbohydrates, for example) to get energy.
   1. This process releases the copper. Ores are sprayed with sulfuric acid and, if necessary, the bacteria. They grow and leach out the copper. This accounts for 25% ($1 billion) of all copper mined in the world.
   2. The bacteria release a lot of heat as they break down the ore, and this slows down the process. Scientists are now using recombinant DNA technology to transfer the genes for copper release into an extremophile bacterium from a hot spring to make the process more efficient.

Essential Reading:

George Acquah, *Understanding Biotechnology* (Upper Saddle River, NJ: Pearson Prentice-Hall, 2004), chap. 18.

William Thieman and Michael Palladino, *Introduction to Biotechnology* (San Francisco: Benjamin-Cummings, 2004), chap. 9.

Supplemental Reading:

John Smith, *Biotechnology*, 4th ed. (Cambridge: Cambridge University Press, 2004).

Sharon Walker. *Biotechnology Demystified* (New York: McGraw-Hill, 2007).

Questions to Consider:

1. Have you visited a water treatment plant? Your water company's Web site or plant brochure can give you an idea of the role of bacterial genes in this process.

2. Ecologists have been surprised by the rapidity of recovery of ecosystems after the disastrous oil spills in Santa Barbara (in 1969) and Alaska (in 1989). How important are bacteria in the recovery processes? Would genetic engineering help?

Lecture Thirteen—Transcript
Biotechnology and the Environment

Welcome back. In my last lecture, I described how biotechnology and recombinant DNA have been used to make products using gene expression and vectors, and these products are useful to us in things like medicine and, later on you'll see, agriculture. I'd like to describe how the organisms themselves can be used to clean up the environment where we have environmental problems; in other words, how these organisms can do things for us after they are genetically modified. My opening story is about land mines. Land mines are a sad legacy of recent history. These mines have wreaked havoc both during and after recent wars in many locations around the world. Land mines are cheap. They've got plastic casings filled with an explosive such as TNT, and "TNT" stands for trinitrotoluene. That's the end of "trinitrotoluene"; from now on, it'll be "TNT," which is the explosive. These mines are triggered to explode whenever they're disturbed, vibrated in some way.

The United Nations estimates that there are over 100 million unexploded land mines lying on or below the ground in countries ranging from Angola to Cambodia, to countries in Europe as well. This makes plowing fields for farming or other uses a risky business. If you're a farmer, and you want to use your field after a recent war, plowing it or digging it up and planting seeds is not going to be a thing you want to do if there are land mines in the area. So you'd like to detect them: very important. You'd like to detect them and then explode them or get rid of them some other way. These mines are encased in plastic, so they avoid conventional metal detectors. The best way to find land mines, unfortunately, is the most dangerous. A person gingerly walks around, poking the ground with a long stick, and if they hear a mine about to explode, [they] jump out of the way. Not a terrific occupation, and a very dangerous one.

At the University of Tennessee, Neal Stewart is trying to use plants and biotechnology to remedy this ecologically adverse situation. This is an example of bioremediation: the use of biological organisms to improve the environment. What Stewart is trying to do is to use biotechnology to make plants that will tell us where land mines are located in a certain region. Specifically, he's trying to make a plant biosensor. The biosensor is going to require two things. First of all, it's going to require a gene that makes a protein that's detectable. That is, he's going to have a plant growing in the ground, and that gene is going to make a protein we can see. And second, that protein should be under the control of a promoter, and this promoter would be expressed when land mines are around. Now, how are we going to get those two things? Well, the 1990s saw the isolation of the gene and the promoter that might be useful. Biotechnology allows us to put both the gene and the promoter into a plant.

First, a gene whose product we can see. In the deep sea, there are some jellyfish that glow in the dark because they make a protein that fluoresces. "Fluorescence" means that a chemical absorbs energy—electrical energy or light energy—and then emits that energy as a flash of light. A fluorescent light, for example, emits energy in the form of light when in the presence of electrical energy. Here we have a fluorescent protein that fluoresces green in the jellyfish and emits its fluorescence in the presence of the very small amount of high-energy light, ultraviolet light, that reaches the ocean depths. It's kind of like the ink that is stamped on my wrist when my students take me to one of their favorite nightclubs in Hollywood. You stamp the thing on your wrist saying you're okay, and they shine a black light on it, and it glows, and the letters "OK" are flashed, and I can get by the bouncer into the nightclub.

In the 1990s, the gene for this green fluorescent protein, made by the jellyfish, was isolated. Biotechnologists started putting this gene into vectors, to use it just like antibiotic resistance would be, to detect the presence of the vector when it's in a cell. So you'd put the gene into a vector as a marker for the presence of recombinant DNA in host cells. And the result was glowing organisms or cells. Glowing fish, at one time, for example, were sold as a novelty. They were taken off the market because people didn't like it. I use, for example, a vector that expresses green fluorescent protein in teaching, even teaching students who are nonmajors, as you are—those who are listening or watching this series of lectures. I teach a laboratory where we will take bacteria and have them make the green fluorescent protein. It's quite a sobering exercise for a nonscientist to realize that they, in a very simple experiment, put a gene for a jellyfish into a bacterium. So that's our gene that we're going to be able to see, and hopefully the plant, then, will fluoresce green.

Second, we need a promoter, and we need the promoter that will turn the gene on in the presence of TNT. In the 1980s, microbiologists found a bacterium called *Pseudomonas putida*—interesting name—that had genes for enzymes that will break down TNT and use its breakdown products for their own purposes. There are bacteria out there that will make genes to break down almost anything in nature. We don't have a lot of those genes. There are certain species of bacteria that do. Into the 1990s, these scientists looked at the genes coding for these enzymes responsible for this metabolism, for this breakdown, of the TNT, and they found that these genes, not surprisingly, had promoters that became active for turning on the gene in the presence of TNT. Very interesting; they were TNT-sensitive promoters. You can envision the TNT binding to a protein—and it does—that goes to the promoter and turns the gene on. In fact, just being near the TNT in the soil or the air was enough to set off these genes. They were that sensitive.

So now we had the promoter, a TNT-sensitive promoter, and the DNA coding for a green fluorescent protein. Stewart then took these two together, the promoter and the gene, added them to a vector, and made some transgenic plants. The result was whenever these plants are around TNT, these plants will glow under ultraviolet light. A biosensor is born. Now, life is not that simple. Challenges remain for this to be a feasible technology in regions of the world where there a lot of land mines. Well, first of all, you have to spread the seeds around a field and have them grow. Well, that's not a big deal. You can actually do that from an airplane. The seeds will sprout. The transgenic plants will grow, and they do express the green fluorescent protein.

But you know, walking around the field with a black light at night, like we would at the nightclub when finding you have a wrist that glows—find this glowing plant, there's TNT around—I think that's not what you want. It's just as dangerous as poking the ground with a stick. So Stewart and his colleagues are proposing using what is called "remote sensing" from airplanes that can detect ultraviolet light, and we have many examples in our defense industry of using remote sensing. This might be combined with seeding from airplanes, so this technology moves along. I bring up this story as an example of bioremediation: again, using organisms to solve environmental problems.

There's an old biological saying that I learned when I was an undergraduate, and that is, "Big things have little things upon their backs to bite 'em; and lesser things, still lesser things, and so ad infinitum." Another way of looking at this is the great food chain in ecology, right? Plants are eaten by animals, we eat the animals, and other creatures eventually eat us; genes of parasites and hosts and energy going through a food chain. Knowledge of the food chain allows biologists to use it. We use it in agriculture, of course, but we can use it, for example, to introduce pests of pests. One of my first jobs as a biologist was, when I was an undergraduate, working with the agriculture department, and my job was to describe the life cycle and ecology of tiny insects. These insects—related to wasps, only they're extremely tiny—make their living by reproducing inside of pupae, which are the immature stages—or caterpillars, which are other immature stages—of a bud moth; of the apple bud moth, in my case.

Now, this particular bud moth, the apple bud moth worm, the caterpillar, eats up the leaves of apple trees and causes significant damage to the apple tree such that the yield of apples goes way down. If you don't have leaves, trees are not going to produce many apples. The objective was to try to, and we did, introduce this insect pest—this lesser thing that would dine on this lesser thing, this bud moth—to reduce the populations of the worm. It would reduce the need for pesticides, and the pesticides weren't working well anyway on this particular caterpillar. This is called biological control. It has a genetic basis. The host worm, the caterpillar, has genes for molecules it happens to make for its own purposes; some of them are defense molecules. They go up in the air, and the parasite, this small wasp-like insect, has glands that detect this worm. The parasite flies around and says, oh, dinner. It goes over to the worm, lays its eggs, and reproduces, thereby killing the worm. So there are genes for both the host and the parasite that have been well described. It's a sensor system.

Biological control like this is now widespread, and it works, along with traditional ways of pest control—using pesticides in much-reduced amounts—in a process called "integrated pest management." We can use bacteria as nature's recyclers. Bacteria eat things, just like our insect that I just described eats things. Bacteria eat things as well, and they thrive on all sorts of nutrients, including things that we refer to as wastes. There are species of bacteria that have the genetic capacity to produce, as I've mentioned, enzymes—and therefore biochemical pathways—that humans don't. As an example, composting. A compost pile uses bacteria to break down the carbon-rich stores such as cellulose, which is the cell walls, or indigestible parts of wood chips, paper, straw, or hay, as well as nitrogen-rich sources such as protein wastes—coffee grounds even, right? What's a coffee ground? A coffee ground is ground-up coffee seeds; that's part of the coffee plant. Some of that are things that we don't digest, that don't form part of coffee. And so these grounds contain the cell walls of plants, which contain cellulose, and the seed coating of the coffee seed. Those are indigestible except, believe it or not, by some bacteria.

Fruit and vegetable scraps, also digestible by bacteria even though we, as I mentioned before, can't digest them. So, in a compost heap, what happens is the bacteria work on these things and produce four things. Carbon dioxide and water—that's the end products of the respiration, so the bacteria are thriving. They're getting energy out of it. And heat; if you'll notice, a compost pile gets pretty warm because the energy comes off. Remember thermodynamics? Energy is neither created nor destroyed, so the energy from these wastes ends up in the bodies of these bacteria, some of it; some of it comes off as heat. Then there's indigestible parts even the bacteria can't eat, and that ends up as what is called humus. Humus can be spread over the soil to provide nutrients for other bacteria that are in the soil. So these bacteria are doing a job for us, right? They're digesting things to make simpler components.

Wastewater treatment uses bacteria to act on human wastes and paper products and household chemicals. The liquids and solids here are treated differently. There's one group of bacteria that digests harmful substances in the solids of our wastes. The remaining sludge that they don't digest is used to fill up landfills or as fertilizer. Some of these bacteria, by the way, that digest human waste make a gas called methane gas, which you may have heard of, as a by-product, and this gas is used for energy. Liquid and solid wastes, where solids are dissolved in the liquids, are digested by still other bacteria. There's a whole series of bacteria now that will digest different substances that are in things that we call waste.

I'll give you one example: ammonia, which is a toxic thing that is in urine. Ammonia, up until now, has been digested by a group of bacteria that are in the wastewater treatment plant, and it is digested to various molecules, ultimately to nitrogen that goes up in the air as nitrogen gas. You'll recall ammonia, amine groups, are breakdowns of proteins. Toxic to us, ammonia, but not to the bacteria. Different bacteria break it down in different steps. Recently, a single bacterium, a new species, was discovered, called *Candida Brocadia anammoxidans*, which will break down ammonia to nitrogen in a single step. And this is now going to be used widely in wastewater treatment. So we're still discovering more efficient and better ways to use bacteria for our purposes—this is bioremediation—in wastewater, for example.

Bacteria and plants can be given, or have, genes that remove pollutants. So in addition to being nature's recyclers, bacteria break down many, many human-made pollutants. Well, how do we discover this? We can discover this ability by bacteria in the following experiment. We can take some soil with water and we take the pollutant that we're interested in, like oil, and then we look and see whether any of it gets broken down. Those bacteria that live in the presence of that pollutant are the ones that are thriving on it. And then we grow up those bacteria, and we know that's a bacterium that likes to break down this plastic or this oil or whatever. For example, there were bacteria that were isolated first from soil in this type of experiment— we would add oil to them and see whether the bacteria would thrive—that were essentially isolated on each component of oil by a scientist named Ananda Chakrabarty in the 1970s.

Now what Chakrabarty did was contaminate soils separately with all the different major components of crude oil, and there are about a dozen of them. So you take component number one, chemical number one; he'd add it to the soil and see whether there were bacteria that eat it. Then component number two and component number three, so he had a whole bunch of bacteria now that would break down each component of crude oil. Then he did bacterial genetics at the time—this is the 1970s—and mated them. This is before gene cloning was really invented, just the beginning of it. And so he did traditional bacterial genetics to get a single genetic variety—a "super-bug," we call it—that would break down multiple substances, a whole bunch of different components of crude oil.

Chakrabarty was working for a company, so he applied for, and was awarded, a patent for this super-bug in 1980. This case was argued for a number of years and was decided by the U.S. Supreme Court, and the Supreme Court ruled, and I will read, that "a live, human-made microorganism is patentable subject matter under [Title 35 U.S.C.] 101"— that's legal stuff. "Respondent's [Chakrabarty's] microorganism constitutes a manufacture or composition of matter within that statute." This was a landmark decision by the Supreme Court. It essentially said a genetically manipulated organism could be patented, and the case led to a flood of patents for genetically modified organisms as well as genes.

You'll recall in a previous lecture I described how the scientists Cohen and Boyer, and their universities, who invented the method of making recombinant DNA, patented it and reaped great rewards from it. Now we're seeing things like patenting genes that people are finding. Every university now, of substance, has a patent office, and they are busily patenting every gene and every process that biotechnologists find, in the hope that they'll hit a home run and get something valuable. I'll say that very few home runs have been hit, as is true in baseball. There have been a lot of strikeouts. One example that's going on is that, for example, the patent for human embryonic stem cells was filed by the university where it was discovered, the University of Wisconsin, and that is being argued now in lower courts because scientists are worried that it could limit the research that people could do on stem cells because they would have to pay expensive royalties for any experiment they want to do.

In 1989, the oil tanker *Exxon Valdez* ran aground near the Alaskan shore, releasing 11 million gallons of crude oil over 1000 miles of shoreline. This was an environmental disaster of major proportions. Cleanup by physical methods such as skimming the water and spraying the rocky shore with detergents was used first. And the result? This dispersed about two-thirds of the oil. Bacteria did the rest by bioremediation; these genetic strains that can eat up oil that Chakrabarty and others had patented were used. Nitrogen and phosphorus salts were first sprayed on the shoreline to get the bacteria to thrive, so it gave them a nice growth medium because they normally don't live on oil; they need other things. Then the *Pseudomonas* bacteria that were already there would grow, and other strains were added so that all the oil would be digested. They worked very quickly to digest most of the remaining oil. This process is ongoing. The government of Kuwait is using bioremediation to try to clean up 250 million gallons of oil, way more than the *Exxon Valdez*—20 times more—that was spilled, probably deliberately in a number of cases, by exploding oil wells, onto the desert during the Gulf War of 1991. This is probably the largest single bioremediation project in the world, and it's going on as I speak.

There is a type of bacteria called extremophiles that have many, many genes that are useful in bioremediation. What are extremophiles? "Phile" means "you like," right? "Extreme" means these are microbes, bacteria, that love the extremes of nature. They're kind of the ultimate; the ultimate athletes of the biological world. These are bacteria, usually, that can live in very hot places like hot springs, or the ice in Antarctica, or high pressure deep in the ocean, or very salty environments like the Dead Sea. In fact, these organisms form a separate group of organisms called the archaea, a word for old. They're called archaea because they resemble the organisms that, sometimes it's believed, were the first living cells that were on the earth.

The archaea genomes have been sequenced, and half of the genes of the archaea do not resemble anything in other types of bacteria or eukaryotes. They're prokaryotic cells, but they are really different. For instance, some of them have genes that use carbon dioxide, just like plants do, not to make sugars, but to make methane gas. Archaeans are by far the major producer of this methane gas; it's one of the greenhouse gases.

The granddaddy of all archaeans is a bacterium called *Deinococcus radiodurans*. *Deinococcus radiodurans* is a bacterium that lives in probably the most dangerous environment of them all: extremely high levels of radiation. Now normally, radiation kills cells by damaging DNA. And when a human's, or any cell's, DNA is damaged by radiation, we can repair it. We have a system of repairing the type of damage that radiation does to DNA. But large amounts of radiation overwhelm that, and you get, as we've mentioned before, permanent mutations and cancers as a result. Now, *Deinococcus radiodurans* gets around this by having the most efficient and sensitive radiation repair system in nature. It's a phenomenally good system, way better than we do.

Now genes from other extremophiles that live in high salt, high temperature, etc., are being engineered into *Deinococcus radiodurans*. No matter what the environment, this microbe keeps coming back. People call it "Conan the Bacterium," after a movie called *Conan the Barbarian*. It's used to clean up the most toxic sites we know of. For example, in America, there are these Superfund sites, which are a group of sites around the world that are extremely contaminated with extremely bad stuff. These *Deinococcus* bacteria that have all of these genes for cleanup are being used there.

Plants can be genetically engineered for environmental cleanup. For instance, bacteria genes that allow environmental cleanup can be put into transgenic plants to break down oil. There are plants that will convert solid mercury and arsenic into harmless substances. Now you might ask, why use plants when microbes are available and around? Well, the issue is you want to get the microbe out of the soil when you don't need it anymore. You don't want extra microbes; it upsets the ecology of the soil. Getting bacteria out of the soil in the environment is quite difficult once they're established. A plant is easy. You plant it, it does its thing; then you take it out, you harvest it. So that becomes a lot easier. So this might be a better way of doing bioremediation in some cases than bacteria.

Mining is another industry that is using bacteria, some of them genetically engineered, to extract metals. Mining for minerals is an old human activity, and it's changed very little over the millennia of time that humans have been mining. You dig up the ground, ores are taken out—ores are complexes of our mineral of interest with other things—then the minerals, like copper and gold, are extracted from the ores. But this requires, to extract the minerals, very harsh methods such as really toxic chemicals and a lot of heat. You may know that mining is environmentally a very damaging process. There is a bacterium called *Thiobacillus ferrooxidans*. This bacterium uses a chemical called copper sulfide to get energy. We use carbohydrates to get energy. We break down sugars to get energy, and we convert them to CO_2. In these bacteria, copper sulfide, which is an inorganic chemical, is used for energy.

What happens? They use it, and then they release copper. Well, that's what we want in mining, isn't it? And so now what is happening is the ores that are extracted, the complex, are sprayed with sulfuric acid to make copper sulfide. The bacteria come in. The bacteria then grow and leech out and give us the copper. This now accounts for about one-quarter's worth, $1 billion, of all copper mined in the world. Bacteria are doing some of the mining for us. The problem with this is the bacteria—and they do this—grow very rapidly. They release a lot of heat. It's a breakdown product of metabolism as they break down the ore, and this slows down the process. So scientists are now using recombinant DNA technology to transfer the genes for the release of copper into other extremophile bacteria from a hot spring. These extremophile bacteria in the hot spring live in hot environments, so they can tolerate the heat. So these bacteria will be heat tolerant and will be able to break down the copper to release it for our use. As we will see in the next lecture, the bacteria in hot springs figured prominently in another story of DNA manipulation, development of the polymerase chain reaction. Thank you.

Lecture Fourteen
Manipulating DNA by PCR and Other Methods

Scope: The book and film *Jurassic Park* brought DNA to public attention. Although the story is fictional, it was based on the science of DNA. Three major ways to manipulate DNA are described in this lecture. The first, the polymerase chain reaction, allows any DNA sequence—even in tiny amounts in a single cell—to be amplified in the test tube, obviating the need for recombinant DNA cloning. This method uses an enzyme from a heat-loving bacterium that lives in hot springs. The second method, DNA sequencing, uses chemical modifications to determine the sequence of any short DNA. This can be automated, and computers analyze the sequence for its biochemical and genetic meaning. The third important technique, RNAi (i = inhibition), is a way to specifically block the expression of a single gene. It came from accidental observations in petunia plants and is now the subject of intensive research for drug development to treat diseases involving gene expression.

Outline

I. Opening story: DNA manipulation in *Jurassic Park*.

    A. Science fiction can be based in science facts.

        1. In 1990, author Michael Crichton, trained as a physician and scientist, published *Jurassic Park*, a best-selling novel that brought the letters "DNA" into public consciousness as never before.

        2. Dr. Raul Cano, a microbiologist, had announced that he had extracted some intact DNA from a bee preserved in amber, the preserved resin of a tree that lived about 40 million years ago. Crichton then extended this idea into fiction.

        3. In the novel, a mosquito was trapped in amber after sucking up some dinosaur blood during the Jurassic period of geological time. Dinosaur DNA fragments were extracted from the mosquito and spliced together with DNA from current reptiles, birds, and frogs to fill out complete genomes of dinosaurs. These were then inserted into special egg-like

structures, and the dinosaurs of the book—and the 1993 film—were cloned.

B. Crichton's book sparked interest in the science involved, even to the extent of sparking debates about dinosaur cloning.

    1. Although the presence of undegraded DNA is deemed unlikely by most scientists, the techniques of DNA manipulation continue to be developed.

    2. These powerful lab methods have come from increasing knowledge of DNA in nature.

II. The polymerase chain reaction can amplify any known DNA sequence.

    A. In 1956, Arthur Kornberg described the first enzyme that can catalyze DNA replication, a DNA polymerase.

        1. He showed this in an experiment. First, the two strands of DNA had to be separated to expose their bases for base pairing with the new strands. Recall that this process is called semiconservative replication. When Kornberg added the enzyme extracted from cells, along with nucleotide building blocks (A, T, G, and C), to DNA in the test tube, the DNA was duplicated. For this tour de force of biochemistry he was awarded the Nobel Prize three years later.

        2. The discovery of DNA polymerases (there are several) opened up the possibility of continuously amplifying DNA in the test tube. This polymerase chain reaction (PCR) could be useful in many types of genetic studies. In Kornberg's experiments, DNA was replicated once. Why not let it go on for more rounds … 2, 4, 8, 16, 32 … ?

        3. The problem was that separating the two strands of DNA takes energy, since the opposite bases (A with T and G with C) fit together exactly. Weak chemical interactions called hydrogen bonds must be broken. This separation is usually done with heat, up to over 80°C (175°F). So in the DNA doubling experiment, after the DNA doubled, the two new DNA molecules had to be separated into their four component strands by heat before being cooled down for polymerase action.

        4. Heat destroys the three-dimensional structures of most proteins irreversibly (like boiling an egg), and since Kornberg's bacterial DNA polymerase is a protein, it would be irreversibly destroyed. So, new DNA polymerase would have to be added to the mixture for each round of replication. Not only is this a hassle, it is prohibitively expensive.

5. Meanwhile, microbiologist Thomas Brock had been studying the first extremophilic bacteria that live in the hot springs in Yellowstone National Park. Appropriately named *Thermus aquaticus* ("hot water"), these prokaryotes thrive in water above 70°C that would kill most other organisms. Brock and his colleagues wrote research papers that described how these bacteria survive by having heat-resistant biochemical machinery. Brock and his student, Hudson Freeze, described the first DNA polymerase enzyme that survives heat.

6. At a biotechnology company in San Francisco, a group of scientists led by Kary Mullis came up with the idea in 1983 of using *Thermus aquaticus* DNA polymerase in PCR. Heating and cooling cycles could process without the need to add new DNA polymerase. They published it in 1985, and it was an immediate hit. The Cetus Corporation sold the patent rights for $300 million to a larger corporation. They gave Mullis a $10,000 bonus. In 1993, he won the Nobel Prize.

B. PCR is a major technique in basic and applied biology.

1. The most important advantages of PCR to amplify DNA over cloning by recombinant DNA is that PCR is fast. Typically, it takes just a few hours to amplify a DNA sequence a millionfold.

2. Another advantage of PCR is that is it extremely sensitive. The DNA of just a single cell can be amplified for analysis or use. As we will see in the next few lectures, this makes PCR valuable in forensics and diagnosis.

III. DNA can be sequenced and analyzed.

A. In 1968, Robert Holley was awarded the Nobel Prize for leading a team that determined the sequence of the first nucleic acid. It took his team five years (1959–1964) to get the 80-nucleotide sequence of a transfer RNA. Today, this is done by machine and takes a minute.

1. The widely used method for DNA sequencing, 800 base pairs at a time, was developed by Frederick Sanger in 1977.

2. DNA sequencing is similar to PCR—with a twist. The two strands of the DNA to be sequenced are separated, and DNA

polymerase is added, along with the four bases, A, T, G, and C. DNA replication begins. Say our DNA has the sequence:

TTGTGCATTAAACT ...

Replication will add: AA ... and continue.

3. But now comes the twist: Included in the mix is normal C but also a modified C (C^*), which terminates replication at that point. Now, the next base in the parent DNA is a G. So the next base to be added to the growing new chain is C, making it AAC. But instead of normal C, DNA polymerase, which doesn't know the difference, might add C^*, making the new strand AAC^*.

4. The fate of these two new strands is now different. If normal C is added, replication continues: AACACGTAATTTGA ... But if C^* was added, the strand stops right there and ends up much shorter: AAC^*.

5. At the end of replication, the new DNA strands are separated. Suppose C^* has a dye attached so that it shines red under laser light. The various DNA strands are separated by size and detected by laser light. The only one that shines red is AAC^*. So we know that the third base is C!

6. In separate reactions, modified T, G, and A are used in the replication, each base with a different colored dye: T (green), G (blue), and A (yellow). So in our example, when there are fragments that end in A, they will shine yellow; these will be 1, 2, 4, 8, and 14 bases long. So there is an A at positions 1, 2, 4, 8, and 14!

7. The whole process is now automated. The scientist puts the DNA in one end and gets the sequence on a computer at the other.

B. There are powerful methods to examine sequences.

1. Getting the DNA sequence isn't enough. We want to know what it means. What is the sequence of a protein-coding region, and what is the amino acid sequence of the protein? What are the sequences of gene control regions, like promoters? Where are the noncoding introns?

2. We know the genetic code, so with a DNA sequence we can surmise the coding sequences. But this too is now done by computer. The DNA sequence is entered in a DNA search program (there are several available), and the information comes out.

3. But there is more: The program also checks to see if the DNA sequence has ever been seen before in nature. All new sequences are sent to a central database (and there are millions of sequences out there now). If the sequence has been seen, you now know what the protein might be.

IV. RNAi is used to inhibit gene expression.

A. In the early 1990s, scientists in the Netherlands discovered that the expression of several genes for flower color in petunia plants could be turned off simultaneously. They called this "gene silencing."

B. Scientists soon found this phenomenon in other organisms. In 1998, Andrew Fire and Craig Mello found out how it works in a tiny worm. (This was the same worm whose genome was sequenced, as we described in Lecture Nine.)

1. Gene silencing occurs when the cell makes a double-stranded RNA, with one of the strands complementary to the mRNA for the gene. To be clear: If the target mRNA that wants to be translated to protein has the sequence:

AAAUGAAGUU,

the anti-RNA will be UUUACUUCAA,
and its other strand AAAUGAAGUU.

After being made, this double-stranded RNA gets bound up with an "escort" enzyme complex that guides it to the ribosome and peels off the "anti" strand. Once the "anti" strand binds to a target mRNA, the expression of that mRNA is blocked.

2. Fire and Mello's explanation soon was found to be true for other animals as well. Gene silencing is a way for cells to turn off genes in humans, flies, and petunias.

3. This science has led to technology: If most eukaryotes have the machinery for RNAi, we can introduce RNA against any gene and use it to silence that gene, and only that gene.

a. This is powerful manipulation for asking "what if" questions: If we hypothesize that the expression of gene A causes phenotype B, then we can turn off gene A by RNAi and see if B does not occur.

b. This extends to diseases caused be gene expression. Suppose cancer is caused by a gene being inappropriately expressed; we can use RNAi as a drug to turn the gene off, and shut off the cancer as well. No wonder Fire and Mello won the Nobel Prize.

c. In my own research on lung cancer, I have shown that if I add RNAi directed against the mRNA for a protein that removes life-saving drugs from tumor cells, the protein is no longer made and the cells become once again sensitive to tolerable doses of chemotherapy.

Essential Reading:

Harvey Lodish, Arnold Berk, Paul Matsudaira, Chris Kaiser, Monty Krieger, Matthew P. Scott, Lawrence Zipursky, and James Darnell, *Molecular Cell Biology*, 5th ed. (New York: W. H. Freeman, 2005), chap. 9.

David Sadava, Craig Heller, Gordon Orians, William Purves, and David Hillis, *Life: The Science of Biology,* 8th ed. (Sunderland, MA: Sinauer Associates; New York: W. H. Freeman and Co., 2008), chaps. 11 and 16.

Supplemental Reading:

Kerry Mullis, *Dancing Naked in the Mind Field* (New York: Vantage Books, 2000).

William Thieman and Michael Palladino, *Introduction to Biotechnology* (San Francisco: Benjamin-Cummings, 2004).

Questions to Consider:

1. Two ways to manipulate DNA are technological advances that came from basic scientific research. Can you trace the flow from basic to applied for PCR and for RNAi? What does this tell you about the need for public support of basic research?

2. Recently, DNA fragments that are 400,000 years old were isolated from specks of permafrost in Siberia. The DNA is both from plants (28 species) and from animals (mammoth and bison). Does this bring the *Jurassic Park* scenario any closer?

Lecture Fourteen—Transcript
Manipulating DNA by PCR and Other Methods

Welcome back. In the last four lectures, I've described gene cloning and recombinant DNA technology as a way to amplify or get more copies of a DNA sequence using living organisms. Recently, science has developed a new and faster way to do this, and this and other DNA-manipulating technologies have changed biology profoundly. My opening story is about science fiction that's based on science fact. In 1990, author Michael Crichton, trained as a physician and a scientist, published his novel *Jurassic Park*. This novel brought "DNA" into public consciousness, and the film even more so. Like all of his novels, Crichton based his science fiction on some science fact.

Amber is the fossilized remains of resins from a tree often has trapped insects inside of it, just circumstantially. These insects that were living on the tree and somehow got trapped in the amber can be, like the amber, tens of millions of years old. In the 1980s, Raul Cano, a microbiologist who happens to be an expert on bioremediation, as we described in the last lecture, had published a paper describing that he had extracted some intact DNA from a bee that had been preserved in amber about 40 million years ago; quite a sensational finding. Crichton, a novelist, then extended this idea into fiction. In Crichton's novel, a mosquito was trapped in amber after sucking up some dinosaur blood during the Jurassic period of geological time. We measure geological time in these names of periods. Jurassic was when the dinosaurs lived.

DNA, in the novel, was extracted from this mosquito, and some of it was identified as reptilian. That means the mosquito may have sucked up some dinosaur blood and has dinosaur DNA inside it. So these dinosaur DNA fragments were then spliced together, along with DNA in the laboratory, with current reptiles, birds, and frogs. Why those things? Because reptiles, birds, and frogs are the closest relatives, we thought at the time—we still do—to dinosaurs. So gradually, this would complete the genome of a hypothetical dinosaur. So we started with a little fragment and completed the genome. These genomes, in the novel, are then inserted into special egg-like structures, and the dinosaurs of the book and the 1993 film were cloned, and the result was pretty exciting. There are the dinosaurs that were in the movie, and you can recall they were pretty scary, and they kind of snapped back at us in ways we didn't expect.

Now Crichton's book is really a cautionary tale, as many of his novels are, about the limits of scientific tinkering with life. We've got to watch out what we're doing when we're dealing with life. In this case, he's talking about biotechnology. This is much in the tradition of Mary Shelley's *Frankenstein*. *Jurassic Park* sparked a lot of interest in the science involved, even to the extent of sparking debates about dinosaur cloning, which were kind of silly because people really haven't isolated dinosaur DNA. The presence of undegraded, intact DNA to any extent in amber is hotly debated. It's deemed actually unlikely by most scientists. It's possible that what Cano was seeing was contamination. But the techniques of DNA manipulation continue to be developed. These powerful lab methods have come from increasing knowledge of what DNA is, increasing knowledge of the molecular biology of DNA in nature.

I'm going to talk about a couple of these methods in this lecture. First is the polymerase chain reaction to amplify DNA, any known sequence. Second, I'll describe how DNA can be sequenced, amplified, and then analyzed after amplification. Third, I'm going to talk about a new technique called RNAi, or RNA inhibition, to inhibit the expression of specific genes.

In 1956, three years after the announcement of the DNA double helix, Arthur Kornberg described the first enzyme that can catalyze DNA replication. This is called—and I've mentioned this before—DNA polymerase. DNA is a polymer, and the enzyme is called DNA polymerase. Now Kornberg showed this as an experiment in the test tube. Recall that DNA replicates semiconservatively. Each old strand acts as a template for a new strand.

What happened was Kornberg took DNA in a test tube, and he added the four building blocks for DNA—our letters A, T, G, and C, the monomers of DNA—in large amounts, and he added an extract of bacteria cells that contained DNA polymerase, the enzyme. This was a cell-free or test-tube system. What happened was the two strands of DNA were separated, and semiconservative replication occurred. This was a tour de force in biochemistry, and three years later Kornberg was awarded the Nobel Prize. The discovery of DNA polymerases, and there are several in the cell, opened up the possibility of continuously amplifying DNA in the test tube. We'd call this a polymerase chain reaction. Now I'm going to call it PCR, polymerase chain reaction. I don't have to say that again.

PCR could be useful in many types of genetic studies. We could take a gene in the test tube and just replicate it—1, 2, 4, 8, 16, 32—just in the test tube, just like Kornberg did. In Kornberg's experiments, DNA was replicated once. Why not let it go on for more rounds—2, 4, 8, 16, 32, etc.? The problem is the way we separate the two strands of DNA. Let me describe that. The two strands of DNA are held together by the base pairs fitting. Remember, A fits with T, G fits with C. They kind of fit together, and they're weakly held together. The actual name of this weak attraction is called a hydrogen bond. These weak interactions have to be broken for the DNA to unzip. Now to do that requires heat. It's usually done by heat, and it's kind of like boiling an egg, right? You have to heat it to about 80° centigrade, which is about 175° Fahrenheit.

So in our experiment where we want to amplify DNA by polymerase chain reaction, after the DNA has doubled, we want the two new molecules—we want to replicate them in the test tube, so we separate them by heating, and then we add the DNA polymerase, and it replicates. But the problem is adding DNA polymerase, because the DNA polymerase that's already there was destroyed by heat—remember, boiling an egg. You're destroying the DNA polymerase protein by heat, so we have to add DNA polymerase again. We add DNA polymerase, add the four bases, and we have four strands of DNA. So repeat it, right? Now we have four strands of DNA, and we have to separate them. We heat it up, destroy the polymerase, and we have to add polymerase again. This can be a real hassle, adding polymerase each time, and it's extremely expensive. The DNA polymerase we have to add is a pure protein. It's very expensive to get a lot of that stuff around. You can't make a lot of it, even by gene cloning, and keep it stable.

In science, basic research discoveries in one subject unexpectedly influence another. This is something we've seen repeatedly in science. From the 1960s onward, an eminent microbiologist, Thomas Brock, had been studying extremophilic bacteria. Do you remember what these are? These are bacteria that live in weird places. In this case, they were bacteria that live in the hot springs in Yellowstone National Park in the United States. Appropriately, these bacteria are called *Thermus aquaticus*. Isn't that a great name? "*Thermus*" is hot; "*aquaticus*" is water. Hot water; isn't that a great name? *Homo sapiens*: "*Homo*," we're all alike; "*sapiens*," we're wise. I don't know if that's a great name, but *Thermus aquaticus* is one of the great names of species in biology, hot water.

These bacteria live in water above 70°, about 150° Fahrenheit, that would kill almost any other organism because the proteins would be destroyed. Over the next 20 years, Brock and his colleagues described how these bacteria survive. They discovered the way they do it is they have a biochemical machinery that is heat resistant. Where heat normally destroys the three-dimensional structures of proteins, these proteins are held together so tightly that their three-dimensional structure stays intact in heat. In the late 1960s to early '70s, Brock and his student, Hudson Freeze, described the first example of a DNA polymerase enzyme that survives heat. Brock published it in the 1970s, and it was a very interesting enzyme, and he was a very famous microbiologist. It was an interesting example of nature adapting to an extreme environment.

Move a little bit forward to 1983, to a biotechnology company in the San Francisco Bay Area called the Cetus Corporation. Scientists at the Cetus Corporation were interested in revving up the idea of polymerase chain reaction, but the problem again was we've got to add polymerase every time because of the heat. A scientist, Kary Mullis, in this group who were interested in developing PCR read Brock's papers and said, here is a DNA polymerase that likes heat, has no problem with heat. So we could just add it once and heat all you want. This thing will not get destroyed, so we could do heating and cooling cycles without the need to add new polymerase. When you look back in retrospect, this is an obvious idea. But that's what great scientists see when other people don't, obvious ideas. Cetus and a group, of course, published it in 1985, and it was an immediate hit, this technique of polymerase chain reaction, amplifying DNA.

Cetus, the company, patented it, of course, and sold the patent rights for $300 million to a larger company. Mullis got a $10,000 bonus. The $300 million patent rights gave him a $10,000 bonus, but he got his reward in 1993. Kary Mullis won the Nobel Prize for the polymerase chain reaction. Now the polymerase chain reaction is essentially a way of amplifying DNA again and again and again and again. The DNA strands are separated and amplified and amplified and amplified, repeatedly. It has two great advantages over cloning by recombinant DNA as a way of amplifying a DNA sequence, a gene. First of all, PCR is fast. It just takes a couple of hours of heating and cooling to essentially amplify a DNA a millionfold, a couple of hours; whereas it would take days, and then you'd have to do all the purification steps of getting the DNA out of bacteria.

Second, PCR is very sensitive. DNA of just a single cell—now, a single cell has one trillionth of a gram of DNA. That's 11 zeroes and a 1 after a decimal point. It's one trillionth of a gram. You can't do much with a trillionth of a gram of DNA in terms of analyzing it for sequencing or for other reasons. You can't do much with it. We need about a millionth of a gram. Going from a trillionth to a millionth is a millionfold amplification, and that can be done by PCR in a couple of hours. So this makes PCR very valuable in forensics—identifying people; you'll remember the story of Jim, our bank robber from the very first lecture—and in diagnosis, as you'll see in later lectures.

PCR is also extremely sensitive—all you need is a single cell, and you can amplify it—so it's very susceptible to false results. We know that from PCR used in court cases, very famous court cases, where people are worried about contamination. If any DNA, just a teeny, tiny amount, from anywhere else is in this test tube that houses a PCR reaction, you'll get false results. So when I do PCR in my own laboratory, I'm wearing gloves, and I'm using it in a separate location that's only being used for PCR and no other purpose. This is an amazing and powerful technology. That's the first technology that I've described to you, and I'll describe many uses of it in subsequent lectures.

The second technology is technology of DNA sequencing and the DNA sequence and analysis. In 1968, Robert Holley was awarded the Nobel Prize. During the late '50s and early '60s, he and his team of six scientists determined the sequence of the first nucleic acid polymer. It was a transfer RNA, one of these RNAs that bring amino acid, but it was a small one. It took five years, and six people, for 80 nucleotides. It was a landmark achievement. You can do it in a minute now by machine. It's just trivial to do 80 nucleotides, so things have developed pretty rapidly. The widely used method for doing DNA sequencing was developed by a scientist named Frederick Sanger in 1977. In Lecture Nine, I described how it's possible to sequence 800-base-pair fragments of DNA at one time. Now let's see how that is done.

DNA sequencing is very similar to PCR. You have DNA, and you're amplifying the other strand. You're doing DNA replication, but it's done with a twist. The two strands of DNA to be sequenced are separated, and DNA polymerase is added as normal—with A, T, G, and C, just like in the normal way—and then replication begins. Let's say we have a DNA sequence that starts with the letters TTG. Now I'm going to kill the answer, right? The DNA opposite TTG will be AAC. Remember T goes with A, G goes with C, so TTG will replicate AAC. Now how are we going to tell that those are the letters that are there? That's my key question.

Now here's the twist. In the mixture of A, T, G, and C—this is the invention of people who invented DNA sequencing, including Sanger—is not just the normal nucleotide, for example for A. But instead of the normal A, there is also a modified letter A. So the first letter that goes in will be either A or modified A. It'll be random. So when we separate out the DNA, there will either be an A there or a modified A. Now here's the real hooker in the whole process. If there is a modified A, the DNA replication stops at that point. So if our DNA replication stops at that point and we separate the strands, we will have only a single base there, A, right? That modified A happens to be colored a certain color; let's say it's red. Wherever there's a red nucleotide at position one, DNA that's one nucleotide long, we know that's an A.

Now supposing a regular A went in there instead of our special A. If regular A went in there, then the replication proceeds. If special A went in there, replication stops. That's the specialness of the special A. So if regular A goes in there, replication proceeds—and remember there were two Ts in the opposite strand (TTG)—so it's going to be A followed by another A. Now maybe we'll get the colored A there instead, so now we'll have a normal and colored A. Now we'll have a two-base sequence that has an A in it. That means A is in position number two; by the same token, C, G, etc. This is now completely automated; machines do it. It used to be that we did DNA sequencing manually, and we looked at all the colors and the sizes of DNA. Now it's all done by automation, and you feed the whole thing into a computer. So this ingenious idea of having fake A and regular A, fake C and regular C, was invented by Sanger and other people, and that's how we got DNA sequencing.

So a scientist puts in DNA at the one end and gets out a genome sequence at the other end. Along with laboratory-based DNA synthesis, as I described earlier on and will describe later, this sequencing technology has been revolutionary. Most research institutes or laboratories have a core lab, it's called, that does all the sequencing for you. Or you can mail DNA to a company and get the sequence by e-mail. Where I work, for example, we just take a DNA we want to sequence, we send it up to the core lab, and the next day they have the sequence for us. Scientists have stopped doing sequencing. They just send it away now.

We just get sequences. Is that enough information? Of course, as I described in Lecture Nine, what's the meaning of DNA sequences? Well, we want open reading frames, sequences that code for proteins, amino acid sequences of the proteins we can determine from the genetic code. We can get gene control regions like promoters, and we can do comparative genomics with DNA sequences, comparing to other genome sequences in the data bank. All of this is done now by computer. I mentioned the field; it's called bioinformatics, and it's very sophisticated. Very often you don't even see your own sequencing data. You just see the comparisons. This is a huge information issue. DNA sequencing has led to a huge information issue in biology where we are accumulating information and sequences faster than we can analyze them.

RNAi is a very potent technology that I want to describe now. In the early 1990s, Dutch scientists were trying to use DNA technology to change the colors of petunia flowers. I think I mentioned before in the course that flowers are a big business in Holland. Surprisingly, these scientists got a bunch of white flowers that had no color at all. They said, what's going on in these plants? We've added some genes, and now we're getting nothing. Everything's been turned off. All the other color genes, as well as our new color genes, have been turned off. These scientists gave a name for this, and they called it gene silencing. They believed it was going on at the transcription level somewhere, or at the protein translation level, at the ribosome. You'll recall DNA is transcribed or expressed as messenger RNA, and then it's translated at the ribosome into protein. These scientists thought that all of these color genes have somehow been suppressed in some way, and they thought it had something to do with the copy, the messenger RNA that was made, but they didn't really know how this was happening.

In 1998, two scientists, Andrew Fire and Craig Mello, found out how silencing works in a model organism. The model organism was the tiny worm I've described earlier in the course. You'll recall I described the genome of this worm as being a model organism for what goes on in all complex eukaryotes such as us and other creatures. What Fire and Mello found was something very interesting. They found that silencing occurs when the cell makes a double-stranded RNA, and that one of the strands is complementary, the opposite strand, to the messenger RNA of the gene. Now let's go back a minute to the Dutch scientists. The Dutch scientists had—and this is actually what happened—all of their color genes, and when they looked at the messenger RNAs of the color genes, somehow the addition of the new gene had caused a downregulation, had caused an opposite RNA to all of those colored genes to bind to them and block them from being translated.

You'll recall that when the copy or messenger RNA goes out to the ribosome to make a protein, the bases must be exposed in order for the genetic coding to work, to bring in the right amino acids. If those bases are covered up by other bases to make a double-stranded RNA, then we're not going to get any expression of that particular gene. To be clear, if the target RNA that we want to translate has—the protein has the sequence AAAAA, that's the target sequence. The anti-RNA will be the opposite, and in RNA it's U instead of A, so it'll be UUUUU, the base that binds to A. Now the RNA inhibition is not single stranded; it's double stranded. So the RNA that's double stranded will be AAAAAUUUUU. There's a mechanism in the cell to take this double-stranded RNA (AAAAAUUUUU). Some proteins literally escort it to the ribosome where its target messenger RNA is, peels off all those As, and lets the Us bind to the As that are in the messenger RNA. So it peels off this anti-RNA and allows it to bind. That's called RNA inhibition.

This mechanism happens to be universal, and Fire and Mello's explanation was soon found to be true for other animals and plants, and all over nature. Gene silencing is a way for cells to turn off the expression of genes in all organisms from humans to flies to petunias. Fire and Mello won the Nobel Prize in 2006 for this discovery. This science that they found, this way of turning off genes by specific sequences that will bind to messenger RNA, has led to technology. If most eukaryotes have this machinery to use this RNAi to silence genes, then we can introduce this RNA ourselves and silence any gene we want that the organism is not silencing itself. If we know by genome sequencing the sequence of any gene, we can introduce a double-stranded RNA that will peel off to a single strand that will silence that gene in particular. We can specifically silence any gene we want.

First of all, in research this is very, very powerful. We can ask "what if" questions. For example, we could hypothesize the expression of gene A causes phenotype B. Oh yeah? I'll do an experiment. I'll turn off gene A by RNAi. I'll block its expression at the RNA level and see if B doesn't occur. If B doesn't occur, then A must cause B. If B does occur, then I'm wrong— my hypothesis is wrong. Applications? Take human welfare. There are many diseases that, as you'll see when I talk about molecular medicine, are caused by abnormalities in gene expression. Supposing cancer, in an instance, is caused by a gene that is inappropriately expressed. We can use RNAi as a drug, a pharmaceutical, to turn that gene off and shut off the cancer as well.

To show you what's going on here in the industry, there was a small company I know of that had RNAi expertise. This company was literally almost going out of business, and in 2000 a group of investors gave them $55 million just because they had the RNAi expertise. Remember, 1998 was when RNAi was discovered, even as a basic research tool. But people saw right away you could turn off genes specifically and target them, so they gave them $55 million. A major pharmaceutical company bought this company for $1 billion in 2006 right after the Nobel Prize was announced. I say that not to say it's a great investment for those people who put in $55 million and turned it into $1 billion, but to say that major pharmaceutical companies are very interested in this.

In my own research, I'm using RNAi. Let me just briefly describe that. I am working on a type of human lung cancer called human small cell lung carcinoma. This is a particularly devastating disease. It has a dismal prognosis after it is diagnosed. It accounts for about 20%, approximately, of lung cancer worldwide. About 90% of people are dead within five years after diagnosis. The tumor cells express many, many genes that are newly expressed. Among them is a protein at the cell boundary that allows them to pump out cancer-fighting drugs. So whenever a drug tries to get in the cell, the tumor pumps it out. It's called drug resistance, a horrifying idea because then you have to flood huge doses of the drug into the patient. If you know anything about chemotherapy and cancer therapy, these drugs have very toxic side effects. Giving 100 times that will not be permissible for the patient, so the patient will die at that point. So it's intolerable.

A tumor with this type of drug resistance is untreatable. Recently I did some RNAi experiments in the lab because I knew that this pump—I knew what the gene was for this pump from the human genome sequence. So I took some drug-resistant cells, and I added RNAi against the expression of this pump in the tumor cells, hoping that I could have the pump not expressed and bring the tumor cells away from drug resistance. Indeed, the hypothesis was correct, and the cells did become once again sensitive to tolerable doses of chemotherapy. Has this reached the clinic? No, this was in cells that came from patients. But it's a promising avenue for reversing drug resistance. I use it as an example because of the specificity at the gene level of being able to selectively turn off the expression of a single gene that's clinically relevant.

We turn in the next lecture to the use of DNA technologies such as PCR to identify individuals. Thank you.

Lecture Fifteen
DNA in Identification—Forensics

Scope: Genetic identification of people has been done by analysis of the expression of genes, such as blood typing. There are few genes for blood type, so many people share the same genes. As a result, this method can only eliminate the identity of a person but not positively identify an individual. Short tandem repeats (STR) are DNA sequences a few base pairs long that are repeated side by side in an inherited pattern. There are thousands of STRs scattered throughout the human genome. They are polymorphic, meaning that there are rare and common alleles (in this case, repeat number). With many STRs and alleles, the probability that two people are alike is extremely low, and so this can be a positive identification. A tiny amount of tissue, even a single cell, can be the starting point for DNA identification. It has many uses, including in criminal investigations, in historical analysis, and in the case of disasters where there are human remains, among other places.

Outline

I. Opening story: Baby 81 was identified by DNA.

    A. The tsunami of December 26, 2004, left thousands of dead bodies in its wake.

        1. A baby, Abilass Jeyarajah, was torn from his mother's arms when the tsunami hit Sri Lanka. Amazingly, he survived and was brought to a local hospital while his parents frantically looked for him.

        2. Because he was the 81st infant brought in that day, he was called "Baby 81."

        3. A few days later, his parents came to the hospital, where they heard there were unclaimed babies, both dead and alive. Joyfully, they were reunited with Abilass.

        4. However, in the previous two days, other couples had come to the hospital searching for their missing babies, and eight had claimed Baby 81 was theirs. The question ended up in court.

> **5.** In court in February 2005, Judge M. P. Mohaiden had not just wisdom to rely on to find out the true parents: He had the evidence from genetics and DNA.

B. The genetic evidence in DNA clearly identified Baby 81's parents.

> **1.** As described in Lecture Nine, we humans are over 99% identical in our 3.2 billion base pairs of DNA. That leaves a lot of room for variation.
>
> **2.** A major source of variation is in repeated sequences, with individuals having different numbers of repeats in an inherited pattern.
>
> **3.** When Baby 81's DNA was examined for these repeats, he had a pattern that was shared by his true parents but not by any of the other eight couples.

II. Genetics by phenotype can be used to identify individuals.

A. Phenotypes that reflect alleles have been used for identification.

> **1.** In genetics, it is possible to predict genotypes and phenotypes from inheritance patterns.
>
> **2.** Think back to Mendel: If short pea plants are recessive to tall, we can predict that two short parents will produce short offspring and not tall ones. That is, tall plants would not ordinarily come from short parents.
>
> **3.** Now consider human genetics and identifying Baby 81. One phenotype that is clearly inherited and not subject to environmental variation is blood type. This is due to proteins expressed on the surface of red blood cells. Which protein is expressed is determined by the genetic alleles present. There are three alleles: A and B are codominant, and O is recessive.
>
> **4.** For example, a person with type A blood either inherited an A allele from each parent or A from one parent and O from the other. A person with type AB blood inherited A from one parent and B from the other, etc.
>
> **5.** Consider Baby 81. We don't have the real data, but suppose Baby 81 was type AB. That would mean that his parents would have to pass on A and B, and neither of them could be type O. Blood type analysis could eliminate parents in some cases. But a real problem is that there are many people in Sri Lanka with A or B alleles. There has to be a better method, and there is.

B. The HLA (human leukocyte antigen) system has more alleles.

1. This genetic system codes for proteins on the surfaces of cells, including white blood cells. It is used in transplants, since the cell surface is recognized by the immune system if it is different.

2. There are many more alleles: HLA-A has 23, HLA-B has 47, HLA-C has 8, and HLA-D has 23. A person might inherit A11 B16 C3 D11 from one parent and A9 B12 C3 D20 from the other parent.

3. With more alleles and four genetic systems, it is more likely that people will be different and parents and children can be matched.

4. Problem: You need well-fixed tissues or blood; the HLA proteins are not always present on all cells; there is a lot of mixture of the genes in gamete production.

III. Genetic analysis of DNA variants is the best identification.

   A. To match Baby 81 with his parents, DNA fingerprinting was done. It works as follows.

   B. The human genome contains short sequences, 2–10 base pairs long, that are repeated in tandem: The STR might be TCAT; and the sequence might be TCATTCATTCATTCAT, repeated four times.

   1. There are about 10,000 different STRs in the human genome. The repeat number is inherited.

   2. Of the many STRs, 13 scattered throughout the genome are used in DNA identification. These are short sequences repeated up to five times, and they have common and less common alleles (repeat numbers). We call a gene with common and less common alleles polymorphic. A population survey must be done to find out the frequencies of these alleles in a population before we do identification.

   3. Suppose we are dealing with two of the STR loci and they have alleles (repeat numbers) that I will call A, B, and C.

   4. For STR 1, A is 1 in 100 (0.01), B is 1 in 5 (0.2), and C is 4 in 5 (0.8).

   5. For STR 2, A is 1 is 10 (0.1), B is 1 in 2 (0.5), and C is 2 in 5 (0.4).

   6. Here is the key argument, and it comes from Mendel and probability. For a person to be carrying alleles A and B of STR 1, the probability is the product of the two probabilities,

or 0.01×0.2, which is 0.002. For a person to be carrying A and B of STR 2, the probability is 0.1×0.5, which is 0.05.

7. Now comes the important number: For a person to have A and B from both STR 1 and STR 2, the probability is once again the product, which is 0.002×0.05, or 0.0001, which is 1 in 10,000.

8. With 13 gene STR systems, the probability of two people having the same genetic markers is vanishingly low. That is why DNA matches are used in identification.

C. DNA profiling is done by cutting DNA with restriction enzymes and sizing the region that has the STR for the number of repeats.

1. For this, about 1 ug (microgram; 1 millionth of a gram) of DNA is needed. A single cell has 1 millionth of that—about 1 trillionth gram of DNA.

2. To get information from this, PCR is used and the millionfold increase in that cell's DNA makes it ready to analyze. A single cell of hair, skin, or blood is enough to get going.

IV. There are interesting examples of DNA identification.

A. Sir Alec Jeffreys developed DNA fingerprinting.

1. In the early 1980s, Professor Alec Jeffreys at the University of Leicester, UK, was studying genetic differences between individuals. He was looking at the genes for the muscle protein myoglobin and compared DNA from seals with humans. To his surprise, there were common, short, repeated sequences in many animals. When he examined the STRs in a human family, the parents and children had them. But he noticed that the children's sequences were a composite of the parents, indicating that they were inherited. Realizing he had a way to identify people by DNA, he published his findings in spring 1985. The genetic floodgates opened.

2. The first case involved immigration. A family from Ghana had immigrated to the UK. When one of the four sons visited Ghana, he was detained on return by British immigration officials because he had a forged passport. They refused readmission, claiming he was not the son from the UK but a cousin from Ghana sneaking in. Jeffreys did DNA analyses of the mother and the three undisputed sons (the father was missing), as well as the son in dispute, and this showed that he was definitely her son.

3. Soon, Jeffreys was called to a criminal case in Leicestershire. Two girls had been raped and murdered in the same area in similar circumstances, two years apart. A man in jail had confessed to the second crime, but claimed innocence of the first one. Jeffreys did DNA analyses of the victims, the suspect, and the semen found on the victims. It showed that the same man had probably committed both crimes, as police suspected—but it was not the man in custody who had confessed!

    a. The police asked all men in the area to give a blood sample for DNA, and 5000 men did so. Over 90% of them could be eliminated by blood typing (HLA on the semen). When DNA analyses were done on those samples remaining, there was still no match. Then, a woman overheard a man saying that he had given two blood samples, one for himself and one in the name of a friend. That friend, when truly tested, turned out to the killer.

    b. DNA is now used widely in forensic cases.

B. An interesting use of DNA identification is in historical analysis.

    1. In July 1918, with the Russian Communist Revolution raging, the last Romanov Emperor, Tsar Nicholas II, his wife, and three of their children were killed in a town in the Ural Mountains and buried in a shallow, unmarked grave. Seventy-three years later, in a new Russia, two amateur historians found what they thought was the grave. The sizes of the skeletons were consistent with the family, and gold dental fillings certainly suggested that they were rich. But the skeletons were too damaged for further identification.

    2. Fortunately, the bones had cells with DNA that could be analyzed. STR alleles in the bones were compared with those of survivors from the Romanov family. DNA from a great-granddaughter of the Tsar's sister and a great-grandson of his aunt, as well as the body of the Tsar's brother (buried in 1899), were tested and showed the same alleles as the dead family. This proved that they were the Romanovs. They were reburied in a state funeral.

C. DNA identification has many other uses.

    1. DNA was used to identify the victims in the World Trade Center terrorist attack.

2. The military genotypes the DNA of all personnel to aid in identification in battle. There are over 3 million DNA types stored in the U.S. military database.

3. DNA databases, with stored STR genetics, are being built up all over the world. For example, in the UK, people arrested for serious crimes are DNA typed, and there are now over 3.5 million people in the database. This has led to a great increase in "cold hits," where criminals are identified for arrest only on the basis of DNA left at the crime scene. In the U.S., the FBI has about 3 million DNAs stored and typed of people convicted—first of sex crimes but now of all serious crimes.

Essential Reading:

Ricki Lewis, *Human Genetics*, 7th ed. (New York: McGraw-Hill, 2006), chap. 14.

David Sadava, Craig Heller, Gordon Orians, William Purves, and David Hillis, *Life: The Science of Biology,* 8th ed. (Sunderland, MA: Sinauer Associates; New York: W. H. Freeman and Co., 2008), chap. 16.

Supplemental Reading:

Robert Massie, *The Romanovs: The Final Chapter* (New York: Random House, 1995).

Philip Reilly, *Abraham Lincoln's DNA and Other Adventures in Genetics* (Woodbury, NY: Cold Spring Harbor Laboratory Press, 2000).

Questions to Consider:

1. In 1994, Californians voted to have mandatory DNA identification testing not just of people convicted of felony crimes but of those arrested as well. This will create a similar database to that in the UK, which has been doing this for some time and gets many "cold hits" of suspects police never would have sought from DNA left at crimes. Are there privacy issues about the government holding DNA samples?

2. Trace the evolution of genetics in the courtroom from using phenotypes such as blood types to exclude people to using DNA to identify people. What are the genetic-statistical arguments used? Are they convincing?

Lecture Fifteen—Transcript
DNA in Identification—Forensics

Welcome back. In the last lecture, I described the development of polymerase chain reaction (PCR). In this lecture, I want to show you how it can be used to help identify organisms, and especially people. My opening story is about Baby 81. Abilass Jeyarajah was a baby who was torn from his mother's arms when the tsunami of December 26, 2004, hit Sri Lanka. Amazingly, Abilass survived. He was washed up on the shore half a mile away. While his parents frantically looked for him, the baby was picked up by a local teacher and brought to the regional hospital. It was the worst day imaginable for the hospital staff, that day of the tsunami. Hundreds of dead and dying children were everywhere, as well as adults. When Abilass was brought in, the nurses and the doctors perked up. This kid was alive. He was healthy. He was a true miracle, and he quickly became a celebrity in the hospital. Because he was the 81st infant brought in that day, they called him—they didn't know his name—"Baby 81."

A few days later, his frantic parents came to the hospital, where they heard there were unclaimed babies, both dead and alive. Joyfully, they were reunited with Abilass. Not so fast, said the hospital staff. In the previous two days, other couples had come to the hospital searching for their missing babies. Eight couples had claimed Baby 81 was theirs. The question ended up with a judge named Mohaiden. Remember the story in the Bible, in the Old Testament, King Solomon faced a dilemma of ruling on which of two women was the true mother of an infant. Remember, what Solomon, the wise man, decided to do. He said I'm going to cut the infant in two, and then you can each have a half. Of course, the real mother was immediately revealed. In Sri Lanka, a couple of months later, in February 2005, Judge Mohaiden had this worst case. He had nine married couples claiming the parentage of a six-month-old boy. Unlike Solomon, who just had wisdom, the judge had DNA for identification. Testing by molecular biologists soon found the real parents.

I want to describe genetic testing in this lecture, and I'll describe it first by using the phenotype to identify one individual from another. By the phenotype, then, we can infer what the genotype or genes are. Then I'll describe how we can analyze DNA variants, the genotype, directly, and that's the best identification, of course, because you're no longer reliant on the environment that may influence the phenotypic expression of genes. Finally, I'll give you some interesting examples of DNA identification.

First, doing genetics by phenotype analysis. Well, phenotype analysis is the way that most people identify genotype, isn't it? A blue-eyed, red-haired person; a plant with wrinkled pea seeds; a short plant versus a tall plant. In genetics, we can infer genotypes from the phenotypes and their inheritance patterns. Think back to Mendel and Mendelian genetics. In Mendel's experiments, if short pea plants were recessive to tall pea plants, we could predict which of the two short parents will produce short offspring and not tall ones. That is, tall plants would not ordinarily come from short parents. Now let's consider human genetics and identifying Baby 81. As I described in Lecture Nine, we humans are 99% identical in our genomes, one person to another; 3.2 billion base pairs, 99% identical. There's lots of room for variation. So we can identify people that way if we had a way of doing DNA. But let's go back to Baby 81 and do it by phenotype instead.

Now one phenotype that's clearly inherited is the blood type. You'll recall the blood type is due to proteins that are expressed on the surface of red blood cells, and you can determine which proteins are there by an antiserum test, and that will identify which alleles are present. You remember what those alleles are? They are A, B, and O. You'll recall from the previous lecture, A and B alleles are codominant. When they are together, they are both expressed, and O is recessive to both of them. So, for example, a person who is type A, like I am, can presume to have inherited an A allele from one parent, and from the other parent either an A or an O allele. A person who is type AB would have inherited an A allele from one parent and a B allele from the other parent.

Let's consider hypothetically Baby 81. Now we don't have the real data. I don't have it. But supposing Baby 81 was type AB. That means that his parents would have had alleles A and B, right? One would contribute A, and the other B. Neither parent could be type O. So I think you can see that this blood type analysis could have eliminated some of the parents in some cases, correct? Of those many couples, what if one of the couples, in one of their cases, was type O? Well, they're eliminated. But there are probably many people in Sri Lanka who have A and B alleles, and there might be a number of the couples who had both A and B alleles, so it's possible to find lots of them. There has to be a better way than doing blood typing to identify, or even eliminate, parents; and there is.

The other way is called the HLA, or human leukocyte antigen, system. This is a system that codes for proteins on the surfaces of many, but not all, cells, including white blood cells. That's where it got its name, human leukocyte antigen. Antigen means it provokes an immune response; that is, the body reacts to it if it's different. HLA phenotyping, and therefore genotyping, is used in transplants. This was revolutionary because this was a way that people could match transplants genetically so that a transplant from one person to another wouldn't be rejected by the recipient as being outside of the body by the immune system. You'll recall from the last lecture, and you'll hear in a future lecture, the immune system's job is to recognize things that are foreign, that are different genetically, and then reject them. So if I receive a transplant from a person who has similar ABO or similar HLA types, I could receive the proper transplant that's similar to me.

Well, in contrast to ABO blood type, there are four different HLA genes, labeled nicely A, B, C, and D. HLA-A has 23 alleles. HLA-B has 47, and these are codominant alleles. HLA-C has 8, and HLA-D has 23. So a person could be—I have from one parent HLA-A11, B16, C3, and D11; that's one chromosome from one parent, and A9, B12, C3, D20—it sounds like bingo—on the other chromosome from the other parent. Well, with more alleles and these four genetic systems, it's more likely that people will be different from one another, and that parents and children can be matched a little bit better. There are a couple of problems with the HLA system. First, you need well-preserved tissues or blood, and that's a little bit difficult sometimes because the HLA proteins stick out of cells, and they tend to ruin their structure. They're not going to be easy to see.

Second, HLA proteins are not always present in all cells. Third, a lot of mixture of these genes goes on when gametes are produced; and fourth, there are some pretty common HLA alleles and some extremely rare ones. And so it's likely that in the case of Abilass, the young boy, some of the parents had the same HLA alleles. That's a little bit more likely than not. Let's talk now instead about phenotype analysis to include genes. Phenotype analysis, as I said, has its limitations. Genetic analysis, of course, is far better because there we're analyzing DNA. We're not worried about expression or anything like this. It's the DNA. It's in every cell, so we can analyze any cell we want at any time of the lifetime of the organism. This DNA fingerprinting was done to match Baby 81 with his parents.

Now, human genome sequencing has revealed that the genome contains short sequences, about 2 to 10 base pairs long, that are repeated many times in tandem. These are appropriately called "short tandem repeats." It's nice; molecular biologists don't use as many Latin words as other scientists. That's nice; we tend to just call them as we see them—short tandem repeats, right alongside. Let's do the sequence TCAT in DNA. Remember the other strand is understood; TCAT would be AGTA. Our TCAT sequence is going to be present four times, so here is our four base pair sequence of TCAT: TCAT, TCAT, TCAT, TCAT. There, I said it four times. It's repeated in sequence in tandem, right by each other. Looking through the whole genome, there are these different short tandem repeats, and the repeat numbers are inherited.

So you might inherit one chromosome that has TCAT repeated five times, and the other chromosome from the other parent might have TCAT repeated seven times. Again, we have two chromosomes, one from each parent, and you've got these block repeats. You might ask, how does block repeat happen? People wave their hands. Molecular biologists, believe it or not, wave their hands, and they say the DNA polymerase enzyme that replicates stutters. "Stuttering" is not a chemical term, is it? So the DNA polymerase is replicating a TCAT, and it does it again, or it does it three or four times. It's just not clear exactly how it happens. We have some ideas, but it's not clear.

There are 10,000 of these scattered throughout the genome, but for identification purposes, we use typically 13 of them that are scattered all over the genome. These 13 repeated sequences, short tandem repeats, which have, again, a different repeat number, are located on different chromosomes throughout the genome. These are, again, short ones that are repeated up to five times. These repeats are polymorphic. What does that mean? It means that—"poly" means "more," and "morphos" means "form," so there are more than one type. As I mentioned, I might inherit five from one parent, at a certain location in a certain chromosome, and seven from my other parent.

Now if we were all the same for this repeat number, it wouldn't do any good, right? These polymorphisms, these different number repeats, are what set us apart because I might have a different collection than you would. It does no good to say, who was the robber? The robber had two eyes. That's just a terrific way to identify a person. Two legs, that's just great. Better to say the robber had, according to our evidence, repeats of the following numbers. But to do this type of analysis, to analyze DNA this way, we need first to find out what the population has for these different alleles. What does the population survey tell us? What are the frequencies of these alleles in the population? For example, supposing I have, again, my five and my seven, from both parents, right? And supposing 5 is present 50% of the time in the population, and 7 is present 50% of the time in the population in the United States of America. If somebody comes across and has 10, they're really different, right? They're a unique individual. That's totally different than anyone in our population.

Let's go through this reasoning. Supposing we are dealing with 2 of these 13 short tandem repeat genes, and supposing both of them have three alleles. I'll call those alleles A, B, and C. Now let's look at short tandem repeat 1, the first one. The A allele, let's say, is frequent in our population in 1 person in 100; 1 person in 100 has this allele. The B allele is more common, 1 in 5. The C allele is the most common, 4 in 5. Okay, 1 in 100, 1 in 5, 4 in 5; those are A, B, and C's frequencies in the population. For the second short tandem repeat, the A allele might be 1 in 10. Don't memorize the numbers because we're going to do a calculation. The B is 1 in 2, very common; half the people. The C is 2 in 5. So here B is the most common one; the other is C. A, B, and C are just levels of repeats, right? So A might be five repeats, and B might be seven in my example. I just called it A, B, and C. I'm just giving you frequencies now in the population.

Now here is the key argument for doing DNA identification in this way, and it comes from Mendel and from probability. For a person to be carrying both the A and B alleles of short tandem repeat 1, the combined probability of having both of them—A and B of short tandem repeat 1—is the product of the two probabilities. Do you remember? Flip a coin, heads or tails: one half. Flip two coins, heads or tails; if you want two tails, $1/2 \times 1/2$, or $1/4$ of the time, you'll get two tails. Okay, so what is the probability of A and B? The probability of A in short tandem repeat 1 was 1 in 100, and B was 1 in 5. So the total probability is 1 in 500. The probability for short tandem repeat 2, 1 in 10 times 1 in 2, so that's 1 in 20. So for A, for the first one, the A and B, there's a probability of 1 in 500; the second one is 1 in 20. So the probability of having both of them at once is the product of their probabilities or 1 in 10,000. Now we're getting a pretty low probability of a person carrying those four alleles; alleles A and B of short tandem repeat 1, and A and B of short tandem repeat 2.

Now think about it. We have 13 different systems we're dealing with for identifying people. So you can see now that if we've got these different alleles, the probability of two people having identical abnormalities, unless they're identical twins, is vanishingly low. It turns out we are all virtually unique in these sequences. That's why DNA matches are so useful in identifying people. For Baby 81, it means not just identifying his DNA. That doesn't do you any good, right, identifying Baby 81 as being a unique person? But we want to get a connection between Baby 81 and something, which of course was his parents. Once you knew Baby 81's short tandem repeats, you could get what his parents were. And so to put it in more genetic terms, if Baby 81 had AA for short tandem repeat 1, he just had two copies of allele A, then both parents must each have AA, and so they tested the parents as well. It turns out the parents matched the child's DNA type, and so they were the only parents that would do it. This is a way, because the probabilities are so low that two people are identical, of positively identifying people rather than eliminating people.

DNA profiling is done by cutting DNA with restriction enzymes to cut it and then sizing the region that has a short tandem repeat between the two cuts. So we'll take a DNA piece from a chromosome, and we'll cut it. And between the restriction sites might be five or two, and then we can use a method of separating them out. Does it have five repeats or three repeats or seven repeats? We'll be able to find out the alleles that way. To do this analysis, we need about a millionth of a gram of DNA, 1/1,000,000 of a gram of DNA. A single cell, as I mentioned in the last lecture, has one millionth of that, or a trillionth of a gram of DNA, so we have to amplify it. How are we going to do that? Of course, by PCR. So we can take a single cell, amplify the DNA a millionfold; then do our little cut, find out how many repeats there are for each of these 13, and we can essentially identify that person's DNA type and then do what we want with that particular information. All you need to do this is a single cell, and it's easy to get lots more cells than that.

There are a number of interesting examples of DNA identification. In the early 1980s, Alec Jeffreys, who because of the work I'm going to describe became Sir Alec Jeffreys, developed DNA fingerprinting at the University of Leicester in the United Kingdom. He was studying genetic differences between individuals of various species, looking at various short sequences of genes. Whole genomes had not been sequenced at that time. He was comparing the genes, looking at seals from the ocean and humans. To his surprise, he noticed these common short repeated sequences, these blocks of repeats in these animals. When he looked at the human ones, he found these short human repeats that were similar between parents and children. He noticed that the children's sequences were a composite of the parents, and he thought, wait a minute. Maybe that means that they were inherited from the parents. When Jeffreys realized he had a way of identifying people, he published his findings in the spring of 1985, and the genetic floodgates, as they say, opened.

The first case that came to his attention, he was called up to study, was a case involving immigration. A family from Ghana in Africa had immigrated to the United Kingdom. When one of the four sons of these parents went for a visit to Ghana, he tried to come back, and he was detained at the airport by British immigration authorities because his passport just wasn't right. The authorities then claimed he wasn't the son at all, but he was a cousin from Ghana who was trying to sneak into the country. Jeffreys did DNA analyses of the mother and the three undisputed sons that were remaining—she had four sons; this was the fourth—as well as the son in dispute. And the result was it was definitely this mother's son, and they let him into the country. So this solved an immigration identity issue.

Soon Jeffreys was called to a criminal case in Leicestershire. Two girls had been raped and murdered in the same area under similar circumstances two years apart. A man in jail had confessed to the second crime, but claimed innocence of the first one. He said, I did the second one, not the first one. So Jeffreys did DNA analysis of the victims, the suspect, and semen that had dried that was found on the victims, the two victims. As a result, Jeffreys did conclude the same man had committed both crimes, but it wasn't the man in custody who had confessed. Why this guy confessed, no one will ever know. So the police now asked all men in the area to give a blood sample for both HLA typing, and if that didn't work, DNA typing, and 5000 men did so.

Over 90% of the men were eliminated by HLA typing right away. Now, HLA turns out to be expressed on semen if it's preserved reasonably well, so they could eliminate 90% of the men. When DNA analysis was done on the men remaining, there was still no match. Now, circumstantially, a woman overheard a man saying, yeah, I gave a sample—I gave two blood samples. I gave one for me and one for a friend who didn't want to give a sample. Police said, uh oh, maybe that's the guy who did it. So the police asked the friend to please give a sample, and when they tested the friend, done by DNA, that turned out to be the killer. As a result of this case, DNA is now widely used in forensic cases and is very widely used in criminal law, as we saw in the opening story of the course.

DNA in history. In 1918, with the Russian Communist Revolution raging, the last emperor of the Romanov dynasty, Tsar Nicholas II, his wife, and three of their children were killed in a town in the Ural Mountains in what was then the Soviet Union, now Russia, and they were buried in a shallow, unmarked grave. In 1991, in a new Russia, no longer communist, two amateur historians found what they thought was the grave. There were two older people and three younger people. The sizes of the skeletons were consistent with a family. There obviously was a husband and a woman and three younger people. There were gold dental fillings. Well, at that time, they said, these people were pretty rich. Not everyone in Russia could afford gold fillings at the time of the Revolution. Maybe that's one of the reasons they had a revolution.

The skeletons were unfortunately too damaged for further identification, but fortunately the bones that were there had DNA in their bone marrow, dried up blood with DNA, and the short tandem repeats—the DNA identification—from the bone were compared with those of survivors from the Romanov family. There are survivors from the family. For example, a great-granddaughter of the tsar's sister was still alive. The great-grandson of the tsar's aunt was still alive. The body of the tsar's brother, buried in 1899, was actually exhumed—we knew it was the tsar's brother—and some DNA was there, enough for identification purposes. The result? The same alleles were present in the dead family, so it proves they were the Romanovs.

What do I mean by the same alleles? For example, in the large skeletons, the parents, for one of the short tandem repeats, they had alleles 15 and 16 in one parent and 15 and 16 in the other parent. Guess what? The children all had 15 and 16; that's good. For another short tandem repeat, there were alleles 8 and 8 in one parent and 7 and 10 in the other parent. Guess what? The children had alleles 8 and 10—that's possible, right—7 and 8—that's possible—and 8 and 10, that's possible. So the chromosomes and the short tandem repeats all were consistent with these being the children of those parents, and the alleles were consistent with being in the Romanov family, so there was a huge military funeral with full honors later on, a state funeral.

DNA identification has been used in many, many other instances now. For example, it was used to identify victims in the World Trade Center terrorist attack in the United States in 2001. Many of those victims were beyond identification by any other means. In some instances, there were just little fragments of bone, but there was enough DNA to identify these people. The military in many countries in the world—the United States most notably—is now genotyping the DNA of all personnel to aid in identification in the field of battle where a person may die in a circumstance that will not allow identification by other means. There are over 3 million DNA types stored in the U.S. military database. DNA databases with short tandem repeats are being built up all over the world. For example, for some time in the United Kingdom, everyone arrested for serious crimes—arrested only for serious crimes—has been DNA typed, and there are now over 3.5 million people in their database.

I mentioned in the very first lecture the idea of a "cold hit," where you just have DNA evidence from a criminal, and you have no other way of connecting that person to the crime. This had led to such an increase of cold hits in Britain that there are so many cold hits going on that they're behind in arresting people, and they have to prioritize the cold hits for the most serious crimes. They have a backlog of arrests to make. In the United States, there have been a number of ballot propositions where I live in California recently that are dealing with DNA typing for people not necessarily convicted, but even arrested. In the United States, the Federal Bureau of Investigation (FBI) has 3 million DNAs stored and typed—as is Jim's, our opening bank robber—of these people. First it was done on people convicted of sex crimes, but now all serious crimes are stored and typed.

Identifying organisms genetically by their DNA has also rewritten the book of evolution, as we'll see in the next lecture. Thank you.

Lecture Sixteen
DNA and Evolution

Scope: Charles Darwin looked at nature and the environment and proposed two ideas that unified biology. First, he related organisms by descent with modifications from a common ancestor. Second, he proposed that these modifications become a permanent part of organisms by natural selection. In his view, confirmed not only by his extensive observations but by much data since then, many organisms of a species are born, and they differ slightly in terms of genetics. Those genetic characteristics best adapted to the environment at the time are passed on (selected) to the next generation. Both spontaneous and induced DNA mutations provide genetic variations. Organisms carrying advantageous protein phenotypes are selected for reproduction. Genetic bottlenecks, in which a few organisms are responsible for a large population, can lead to a special set of genes in a population. Some organisms evolve by DNA changes that are neutral to selection. These changes can serve as a molecular clock to determine relatedness of organisms.

Outline

I. Opening story: Darwin proposed natural selection to explain evolution.

   A. Charles Darwin was born on the same day as Abraham Lincoln, February 12, 1809.

      1. The son of a society doctor and a mother from the Wedgwood family, Darwin was sent to medical school in Edinburgh but dropped out and transferred to Cambridge to study for the ministry.

         a. He studied botany under Professor John Stevens Henslow and was fascinated by natural history.

         b. When Darwin graduated in 1831, Henslow recommended him to Capt. Robert Fitzroy, who was looking for an amiable companion and naturalist for his ship the *Beagle*, which was about to leave on a surveying voyage first to South America and then around the world.

2. Before they left, Fitzroy gave Darwin a copy of a recently published book on geology that explained the very slow changes in rocks over time.

B. Darwin changed biological science.

    1. The *Beagle* left Plymouth Harbor on December 27, 1831, and returned to Falmouth after a round-the-world voyage on October 2, 1836.

    2. While Fitzroy did his job, Darwin did his—and changed biology forever. Darwin made careful observations of both the organisms he saw and the environment. He saw animals and plants that appeared specifically adapted to their environments. This was not new; people had seen this since ancient times and attributed it to special creation.

    3. Darwin noticed resemblances between organisms in different places.

        a. Organisms on the Galapagos Islands in the middle of the Pacific Ocean were similar to ones of that type on the coast of South America (Chile).

        b. Organisms in the temperate regions of South America more closely resembled those in the tropics of South America than their temperate counterparts in Europe.

        c. Fossil organisms in South America resembled living organisms he saw on that continent more than fossils and living organisms in Europe.

        d. How could this be if organisms were specially created for each environment? Wouldn't all the organisms living in all the temperate climates be the same?

    4. Darwin proposed his first idea: The organisms in South America had a common ancient ancestor (that had traveled to the Galapagos). He called this "descent with modification." His geology book and observations confirmed the idea that the Earth was very old.

    5. Darwin then proposed his explanation for descent with modification (evolution): natural selection.

        a. Many members of a species (type of organism) are born.

        b. There are inherited variations among these organisms. These occur randomly.

        c. The changing environment selects those organisms with the best adapted variations for survival and reproduction. In this way, organisms change over generations of time.

6. Note that genetic changes are random, but selection is directed to the environment at that time (and not any future time, when the environment may change). Evolution is not progress; it is not linear, but branched.

II. There is a lot of evidence for evolution by natural selection.

A. Agriculture: In the Book of Ruth in the Hebrew Bible, Naomi sent her daughter Ruth to lie with the rich man Boaz on the barley threshing floor.

1. Before barley became a crop, its stalks would shatter when harvested. This is good for the plant (seeds on the ground) but not the farmer (seeds on the ground!). Better to pick up the stalk and then thresh it to separate out the seeds.

2. Humans harvested barley plants that did not shatter and threshed them. They ate most of the seeds and planted some for next year's crop. Thus, they selected for the characteristic of not shattering.

3. Much of agriculture has been more conscious selection. For example, a wild mustard plant (*Brassica*) grows like a weed with flat leaves. Selection led to different vegetables from genetic variation of the same species:

For terminal growth: cabbage	For leaves: kale
For lateral growth: Brussels sprouts	For stems and flowers: broccoli
For stem: kohlrabi	For flowers in clusters: cauliflower

B. In England in 1842, the bison moths were 2% dark color, 98% white. In 1898, they were 95% dark. Dark color is due to a dominant allele, so the frequencies of the alleles were not related to whether they were dominant or recessive. What happened for this change through time (evolution)?

1. Black was a dominant allele but was selected against because the dark-colored moths on the light tree trunks would get picked off by birds.

2. Industrial plants during the 1800s in that region spewed out black smoke that coated the tree trunks; now the light moths were picked off by birds. So the dark moths were selected for reproduction.

3. In the 1950s, this hypothesis was confirmed experimentally.

C. On the Galapagos, Darwin famously saw finches with big beaks (that eat big and small seeds) and small beaks (that eat only small seeds).

    1. In 1977, there was a severe drought, and fewer seeds were produced. Both big and small seeds were affected. With fewer seeds, big-beaked birds were favored because they could eat any size, but the smaller ones could eat only small ones—and these ran out. The population of finches fell from 1200 to 200.

    2. Over the next decade, there was evolution to big-beaked birds, because when there were few seeds, there were equal numbers of big and small seeds, and the big-beaked birds had a selective advantage because they could eat both kinds.

D. Fossils show evolutionary change over long periods.

    1. As explorers went to new lands and dug for canals and mines, they saw rocks in layers, with the top rocks the most recent. There were bones and plant impressions in these rocks, the remains of ancient organisms. The deepest (oldest) rocks had fossils that least resembled modern organisms.

    2. When these fossils were examined, in many cases there was a progression over time: evolutionary change.

E. Homologous structures are evidence for common ancestry.

    1. Examination of anatomy of current organisms shows homologous structures that have been adapted for different functions: For example, the front limbs of vertebrates all have a large bone, then smaller ones, and tiny ones at the end. In humans, these are the arms and fingers. But the same pattern is adapted in birds (for flying), seals (for swimming), and sheep (for running).

    2. The biochemical unity of life (same DNA, genetic code, etc.) also can be explained by common ancestry.

III. Protein changes due to DNA mutations explain natural selection.

  A. Mutations are the raw material of evolution, and they are nondirected.

    1. Spontaneous mutations are due to errors in DNA replication.

      a. They are rare: The usual rate is 1/100,000. But with millions of germ line cells there is a good chance of it occurring: Germ line cells produce eggs/sperm.

      b. Duplications are an important mutation source: One or more copies of a gene are made by DNA polymerase "stuttering," as was mentioned earlier. Extra copes of a gene mean that one copy can mutate and not cause adverse effects because there is still a good copy.

2. Induced mutations are caused by environment—most are natural factors (e.g., ultraviolet radiation from sunlight damages DNA). The damage can be repaired but not always, and this can end up as a mutation. Most mutagens are natural, such as substances in our diet.

B. The phenotype protein is selected.
1. Antibiotic resistance in bacteria is inherited.
   a. All bacteria have an enzyme that breaks down certain waste products.
   b. Penicillin, an antibiotic made by molds, binds to and inhibits another bacterial enzyme that makes the cell wall.
2. Some bacteria have a mutation in the gene coding for the first enzyme such that it breaks down penicillin.
   a. This makes these cells antibiotic resistant.
   b. In a normal bacterial population, this mutation is rare. But in the presence of penicillin, the few bacteria carrying it are selected for.

IV. Some DNA changes in evolution are not selected.

A. Some DNA mutations do not lead to phenotypic changes.
1. Hemoglobin—There are hundreds of DNA changes that:
   a. do not lead to a different amino acid (the genetic code is redundant) and
   b. lead to an amino acid change that is not selected for because the reproductive fitness does not change (e.g., at position 7 there is a change of:

   A to G
   T   C

   with amino acid change but no effect).
2. Many DNA mutations in genes are of this type.

B. Some DNA changes lead to evolution but not by natural selection.
1. There used to be tens of thousands of elephant seals in the North Atlantic.
   a. Hunting reduced the population to about 20 in 1890.
   b. The species was conserved, and now there are 30,000. They are genetically almost the same because they all came from a few ancestors. So the genes that were in

those seals in 1890 are present in all of their descendents. This is an example of a population bottleneck. It is one way that evolution can occur without selection.

2. In 1968, population geneticist Motoo Kimura proposed that evolution can occur by neutral mutations that are not subject to natural selection but accumulate in a population of organisms.

   a. This can occur in small populations (see the seals, above).

   b. The rate of accumulation of mutations in this case is equal to the mutation rate of the allele (or vice versa). For example, for a protein, one can trace relationships from fossils and give an age when the last common ancestor lived (e.g., for insects vs. vertebrates this was 600 million years ago). Then look at a protein (e.g., cytochrome c) that both insects and vertebrates have and at gene changes. Then calculate changes per year: It turns out to be one per 20 million years. Now, if there are two organisms and we want to see when they last had a common ancestor for this gene, we look at the differences between them and then calculate based on 1/20 million years. This is called "molecular phylogeny."

Essential Reading:

Benjamin Pierce, *Genetics: A Conceptual Approach* (New York: W. H. Freeman, 2005), chap. 23.

David Sadava, Craig Heller, Gordon Orians, William Purves, and David Hillis, *Life: The Science of Biology*, 8th ed. (Sunderland, MA: Sinauer Associates; New York: W. H. Freeman and Co., 2008), chaps. 23–26.

Supplemental Reading:

Charles Darwin, *The Origin of Species* (New York: Random House, 1979).

Richard Dawkins, *The Selfish Gene: 30th Anniversary Edition* (Oxford: Oxford University Press, 2006).

Douglas Futuyma, *Evolution* (Sunderland, MA: Sinauer Associates, 2005).

Questions to Consider:

1. Compare evolution (change in allele frequencies in a population through time) by natural selection, a genetic bottleneck, and neutral

mutations. Which do you think accounts for most evolutionary changes?

2. Mendel published his experiments on genetics (1866) after Darwin published his book *The Origin of Species* (1858). In fact, Mendel read Darwin, but there is no evidence of the reverse. How do you think Darwin would have used Mendel's gene concepts to support the theory of evolution by natural selection?

Lecture Sixteen—Transcript
DNA and Evolution

Welcome back. In the first lecture of this course, I described three major ideas that form the underpinnings of biology and of genetics. Those three ideas were the cell theory, mechanism, and evolution by natural selection. Most of the lectures up to now have dealt with cell theory and mechanism, and now we turn to evolution by natural selection. What I'll show you is that DNA analysis has made great strides in understanding evolution, and the use of PCR and the analytical techniques that I've described in recent lectures have essentially rewritten the book of evolutionary theory. My opening story concerns a great biologist. Charles Darwin was born on the same day as Abraham Lincoln, February 12, 1809. Darwin was the son of a prominent physician. His mother was one of the Wedgwoods from the English china family. So Darwin's life, in terms of his wealth, was quite assured throughout his life, and he never really had to get a regular job.

Through his father's influence, Darwin was sent to medical school at the University of Edinburgh, but he got disgusted by it—he really didn't like surgery, especially at that time—and dropped out and transferred to the University of Cambridge to study for the ministry. At Cambridge, Darwin studied botany under the tutelage of Professor John Stevens Henslow, one of the great botanists of the time, and became fascinated by natural history, the study of organisms in nature. When he graduated in 1831, Henslow recommended Darwin to Captain Robert Fitzroy, who was looking for what he called an amiable companion and a naturalist for his ship, the *Beagle*. The *Beagle* was about to leave on a surveying voyage around South America and then around the rest of the world. Before they left, Fitzroy gave Darwin a copy of a recently published book on geology, the study of rocks, and this book explained very, very slow changes that occurred in the earth's crust over time.

The *Beagle* left England, Plymouth Harbor, on December 27, 1831, and returned to Falmouth Harbor on October 2, 1836, almost five years later. It was a long trip. The purposes of this voyage were to survey the coast of South America, the Falkland Islands, and the Galapagos Islands for the British War Department and commerce. Those were the days when, as the song went, Britannia ruled the waves, and Britain was a major naval power. You'll recall the Falkland Islands. This is a group of islands off the coast of Argentina, and they'd been claimed by the Argentines for a long time. Most recently, in 1982, Argentina tried to invade the Falklands, but the British repelled them. The Galapagos Islands in the central Pacific were deemed important strategically. They're on the equator off the coast of Ecuador. After the Galapagos, the *Beagle* proceeded across the Pacific to New Zealand and Australia, stopping in Tahiti, then around Africa, and then home. It was a long five-year trip.

While Captain Fitzroy did his surveying job, Darwin did his and changed biology forever. Darwin made careful observations of the organisms he saw, the plants and animals, and the environment in which they existed. He saw animals and plants that appeared specifically adapted to their environments. We'd say now the genome produced an "adaptive phenotype." This wasn't anything new. People had seen this since ancient times and noted it, and they always attributed it to special creation. Organisms were created to be adapted to their particular place where they were living. But here's a great advantage Darwin had. He was traveling, and Darwin noticed resemblances between organisms in different places. This is the great significance of the voyage of the *Beagle*.

First, Darwin noticed that organisms on the Galapagos Islands—the birds in the Galapagos Islands, the plants, the tortoises—in the middle of the Pacific were similar to the same type of organism, the same type of birds, on the coast of South America. He said, that's kind of interesting. Second, Darwin noticed that the organisms in the temperate regions, the temperate climates of South America, more closely resembled the similar organisms in the tropics of South America, in a different climate, than their temperate counterparts in Europe. This was puzzling to him. Third, Darwin saw fossil organisms in South America. He saw organisms in rocks, in strata of rocks, beneath the ground when he went digging, and in canyons, he would see layers of rocks in South America. These fossils resembled living organisms in South America more than the fossils and living organisms in Europe. There seemed to be a commonality.

Now, Darwin asked himself, how could this be if organisms were specially created for each environment? Wouldn't all the organisms living in the temperate climates be similar to each other, rather than organisms in a location being similar to one another? Darwin proposed his first idea. He had two of them. His first idea was that the organisms in South America had a common ancient ancestor, and this ancestor had somehow traveled and gotten to the Galapagos. And then this common ancestor had given rise to organisms over many generations, and these had changed. He called this "descent with modification." Not dissent, no argument; descent with modification. The organisms descended from one another, and they were slightly modified.

Now, Darwin's geology book and observations that he saw in the rocks confirmed the idea that the earth was very old, and there might be a long period of time for these modifications to build up. Now how did these modifications build up, and how did we get to the organisms that we have now? Darwin then proposed his second idea. His second idea was an explanation for descent with modification. Descent with modification means change through time. Change through time is evolution, and Darwin explained evolution by his theory of natural selection. When Darwin went around the world, he made these observations and came up with his idea of descent with modification, and then he explained descent with modification by evolution, by natural selection. Now, biologists today say evolution is the same as natural selection, but bear in mind evolution just means change through time—things evolve. Humans evolve throughout their lives; that's just a word. But evolution in biology very often is assumed to mean Darwin's idea of evolution by natural selection.

Darwin's idea had several aspects to it. First, he said, many members of a species or type of organism are born. Second, there are inherited variations among these organisms, and these variations occur randomly with no preconceived notion. So there might be tall giraffes and short giraffes just through what we would say now is genetic mutation. But remember Darwin is writing even before the time of Mendel. Third, the changing environment selects those organisms at that time with the variations that are best for survival, and most importantly, reproduction—and then these variations are passed on to the next generation. In this way, organisms change through generations of time.

Now it's very important to note several things about Darwin's idea. First, genetic changes, in his theory, are random. There's no preconceived idea of what changes are going to occur. But natural selection is directed by the environment at that time. Second, selection is not predictive. What is adaptable at one time may not be adaptable in the future. Third, evolution is not progress. It's not linear, going from simple to complicated. If an adaptation is not needed, an organism may just not have it anymore; they may lose it. I've described in the course a number of instances where humans lack genes that many other organisms have. Many organisms make vitamin C. Many organisms make all 20 amino acids. We only make 12 of them, and we don't make vitamin C. It's possible that our ancient, ancient, ancient ancestors made all of those things. We've lost them because we didn't need them to survive and reproduce. We could get these things other ways.

Darwin published his book in 1859; it's called *The Origin of Species*. What's interesting is it took over 20 years from the time Darwin's trip ended on the *Beagle* until he actually published his book. He had published a number of articles before then. He was a prominent scientist by then, although he never really had a university professorship. He hung around groups of scientists and collaborated with people. After the publication of *The Origin of Species*, he published many, many more books. Darwin was a phenomenal scientist. He published books on, for example, the descent of man, the human evolution. He published a book on plants called *The Power of Movement in Plants* that described endless experiments that he did that set the stage for what we know now about how plants work, plant physiology. He published the greatest description, until that time, of barnacles; little creatures that live on ships and near the seashore. He published books on the emotions. He published books on geology. I mean the guy was an absolutely phenomenal scientist. When he died, he was buried in Westminster Abbey right near Isaac Newton, the great physicist, and it's really a sobering thing for a scientist like me to visit the burial sites of these two people right near each other.

There's a lot of evidence for evolution by natural selection, a lot of evidence that Darwin's theory is probably correct. Darwin's theory is a way of explaining biology. It's a way of tying together the diversity of organisms we see. My first line of evidence I'll describe is agriculture. In the book of Ruth in the Hebrew Bible, there's the story of Ruth and Naomi. Naomi sent her daughter Ruth to lie with a rich man, Boaz, on the barley threshing floor; that's the story. Now when I was a kid and I heard this story, there were a couple of things I always asked about it, and I never got the answer. First of all, what was lying with a rich man, and what went on when they lay together? No, I wasn't allowed to find out what that was. And second, what's a barley threshing floor? Is that a place where people lie around together? No one ever told me what that was either.

Well, it turns out that both of these are genetically important, and I want to describe the barley threshing floor. Before barley became a crop, these plants were growing, and I've described earlier on in the course the domestication of barley, the importance of barley in terms of beer and making bread. Before it became a crop, the characteristic of the plant was that there was a stem, and of course, seeds would form attached to the stem. When the wind blew, the seeds would fall off. The cells that attached the barley seed to the stem were very weak, and they would fall off, and the seed would fall to the ground. Great idea; the seeds get spread over the ground, and they sprout, and you get more barley plants. So, for the plant, this is, we might say, evolutionarily a very adaptable characteristic because it will allow the plant to grow and then reproduce.

For the farmer, this is a bad idea because a farmer can't go around picking up individual seeds off the ground. So we can envision that when farmers wanted to harvest barley early on, they would cut the stem and carry the stem with its seeds to a room called, believe it or not, the threshing floor. Now the only stems that would survive this transport were ones that had the seeds very tightly attached, that wouldn't fall off readily. And so they would carry this stalk to this threshing floor; then they would thresh it—they'd beat it on a cloth—and they would separate the stems from the seeds. That's what threshing means. It's now done by machine; in the old days, it was done by hand. So the seeds now would finally fall off. Well, that's very convenient for the farmer. We're dealing here with a mutation. The mutation is a mutation in the cells that attach the seeds to the stem. Once the farmers harvested those seeds, they chose some of those seeds for growing the next generation, and I think you can see that over a period of generations this strong attachment was selected for. And so the ideas of seeds and stems shattering was bred out of the barley plant.

More recently in agriculture, there has been more conscious selection. For example, the wild mustard plant is a plant that grows like a weed; it has flat leaves. Conscious selection by people of mutations that came up from this plant has led to different vegetables from this same species. Selecting for terminal growth produces cabbage. Selecting for broader leaves gives kale. Selecting for lateral growth, on the sides, gives brussels sprouts. Selecting for stems and flowers gives broccoli. Selecting for the stem, this thicker stem, gives kohlrabi. Selecting for flowers in clusters gave cauliflower. These are all mutations of a single plant called *Brassica*, the mustard plant. So agriculture is powerful evidence of natural selection where humans, either consciously or unwittingly, select for mutations and then propagate those mutations in subsequent generations.

A second example of natural selection is in moths in England. In 1842 in England, the bison moths were 2% dark color and 98% white. Wait a second, now. Dark color is a dominantly inherited allele. There's a lesson in this, and the lesson is just because an allele is dominant or recessive doesn't mean it's going to be the most common one in a population. Dark color was very rare in 1842. In 1898, the same species of moth was 95% dark and 5% white. What happened for this change through time, evolution? Black, again a dominant allele, was selected originally because the dark moths landing on light-colored tree trunks would be picked off by birds. So birds were the selective agent, and the dark moths would not survive to reproduce, and so they were light colored.

During the 1800s, industrialization happened in this region in England, and the factories spewed out black smoke. The black smoke coated the trees, and now the dark moths would survive better than the light moths, which would be picked off by birds. And so that's how we got a change through time. In the 1950s, this hypothesis I've just described based on this past history was tested by experiment. The two genetic strains of moths were reared in the laboratory and released either in the woods in heavily-polluted Birmingham or lightly-polluted Dorset. So in the heavily polluted area, the trees were black; in the lightly polluted, they were white. The result? In the polluted area, the dark moths survived twice as well. In the less-polluted area, the light moths survived twice as well, as one would predict from natural selection, and birds were seen eating the moths as a selective agent.

The third line of evidence for evolution—and there are a bunch of them; I'll just describe some outstanding examples—are finches. These are birds that Darwin famously saw on the Galapagos. He saw birds with large beaks and birds with small beaks, and he surmised they all came from an original ancestor that had mutated. They had mutated to large beaks that could eat large seeds and small beaks that could eat small seeds. So Darwin would draw a family tree of these finches that he found in different regions of the Galapagos. In 1977, this hypothesis of Darwin was tested. There was a severe drought, and fewer seeds were produced all around; fewer large seeds and fewer small seeds were produced by the plants. With fewer seeds, the big-beaked birds would be favored because they could eat any size of seed, whereas the smaller ones can only eat the small seeds. Both big and small seeds were running out. The result? Over the next couple of years, the population of finches fell from 1200 in the Galapagos to just 200. Initially, big- and small-beaked birds were equal, but over time in the next decade, because of this reduction in seeds, evolution to big-beaked birds happened. It confirmed Darwin's idea.

Line of evidence number four: fossils. Fossils show evolutionary change over long periods of historical time. As explorers went to new lands and dug canals and mines, they saw rocks in layers. The top rocks are the most recent; the bottom rocks are the most ancient. There were bones and plant impressions in these rocks, the remains of ancient organisms, and people could compare these impressions on rocks with current organisms and with each other. By the 1800s, geologists recognized the same fossils in the same strata of rocks. This is the kind of evidence that Darwin had read about before his trip on the *Beagle*. The deepest rocks, the rocks that were deepest in the Earth's crust, had the fossils that least resembled modern organisms, so there was a progression. The deepest, oldest rocks had the least similar organisms to current, and then on upwards.

An outstanding example of this is the horse. If you look at the oldest horses, they're very small. Younger horses get larger and larger. Their legs get larger; obviously the selection is for speed and for running away from predators. Their teeth get larger so they can graze better over time. We surmise those are selective agents. So, the first tiny fossil horse 40 million years ago is quite small, and now we have the modern horse, which arose about a million years ago in rocks. A fifth line of evidence for Darwin's theory of natural selection is homologous structures. Homologous structures are nice evidence for common ancestry. Homologous structures are structures that are similar in lots of organisms but have different functions. In other words, selection selects for slight mutations of the same structure to have a different function.

So, for example, the front limbs of vertebrate animals—animals with backbones. All of them have a large bone—think of your arm—and two smaller ones, and then tiny ones at the end. The large bone, the two small ones, and the tiny ones—the hands and the fingers. Humans have arms and fingers, as I've just said. Birds have wings for flying. Seals have flippers for swimming. Sheep have legs adapted for running, etc. A sixth line of evidence, more for common ancestry of organisms, is the biochemical unity of life. We spent a lot of time in this course so far talking about DNA and the genetic code and the amazing universality in life of the same rules for making proteins and expressing genes and behavior of genes. This can be explained by common ancestry.

Protein changes can explain natural selection, and now I'm going to turn to that at the molecular level. Darwin knew nothing about what the gene was. He wrote even before Mendel. And by the way, there's no evidence that

Mendel read Darwin, or vice versa, when they were alive. But now we can look at the gene as DNA and its phenotype as protein. Protein changes can explain natural selection. Mutations are the raw material of evolution, and they are nondirective; they're random changes in DNA sequences. Spontaneous mutations, as I've described earlier in the course, are errors in the replication of DNA when it duplicates. They're pretty rare. The rate might be 1 in 100,000 changes. Some of them get repaired, but sometimes they can slip through the repair system and end up as mutations. If they're in germ line cells, producing eggs and sperm, they get passed on to the next generation.

An important source of mutations is gene duplications, where two copies of a gene are made. I described repeated sequences, but this also happens with gene duplications. So if I had two copies of an important gene, one of the copies can mutate, and that's not going to be harmful to the organism if it mutated because you've got one good copy there that's making a protein for functioning in the biochemical pathway. So we have gene families arising in evolution where a bunch of similar genes are there, and then those second and third and fourth copies of the gene can evolve over time. How do gene duplications happen? People wave their hands, and they say the DNA polymerase stutters, as I indicated before. We're not quite sure how that happens.

The environment can cause mutations as well, induce mutations. For example, ultraviolet light from the sun—you probably know if you're concerned with sunburn—damages DNA. This can be repaired, but if it's not, it can end up as a mutation. We are surrounded by chemicals in our environment, all organisms are, and these chemicals can cause mutations, and many of these, as I'll describe later on, are natural selective agents. What is selected? What is selected is the phenotype. Natural selection doesn't select DNA; it selects the phenotype. The phenotype, of course, is protein.

Let me give you an example of that. The example I'll describe is antibiotic resistance in bacteria. Bacteria have an enzyme in their genome, coded for by their genome, that breaks down certain waste products in the bacterium. It's just an enzyme that does certain things in metabolism, coded for by a gene. Penicillin, you may know, is an antibiotic, but it happens to be something made by a fungus that kills bacteria. This is an antibacterial chemical. Some bacteria have a mutation in the gene coding for this enzyme that normally breaks down chemicals that has the enzyme fold differently, and now, lo and behold, it can break down penicillin. So these bacteria, with this rare mutation, are penicillin resistant. Fine, that's okay. That's a phenotype caused by a genetic mutation. In a population of bacteria just out there in nature, in the absence of penicillin, this particular mutation to break down penicillin is rare. It's just there; it happens randomly.

In the presence of penicillin, of course, penicillin now is a selective agent. It negatively selects all the bacteria that aren't resistant to it, kills them; and the ones that survive, of course, are the penicillin-resistant ones. Now, note mutation is random, as I've described. The mutation is a random event; it just happens. It is not driven by a purpose. Penicillin didn't come into the environment and say, a-ha, I challenge you to become resistant to me. It didn't happen that way. There were already bacteria that randomly were resistant. This is the reason, by the way, a physician shouldn't prescribe an antibiotic unless a diagnosis of a bacterial infection has been made. Otherwise, of course, you're going to select for resistant strains, and then when you get a really bad infection, it'll pass that resistance on to the bad infective organism.

Now I've described natural selection as the way of evolution; that's how organisms change through time. It turns out that it's not quite the whole story. In fact, it may not be even all of the story. There are DNA changes in evolution that are not selected. There are DNA mutations, for example, that don't lead to phenotypic changes. Now, first of all, let's look at DNA that codes for protein. People found quite some time ago that hemoglobin—the protein involved with hemoglobin—has hundreds of DNA changes in its gene that, for example, don't lead to a different amino acid. There are 64 code words in the genetic code in DNA, 64 code words, and there are only 20 amino acids. So there are multiple code words for an amino acid. If I change one code word for—I'll give you the name of an amino acid— glutamic acid, and I change it to another, that other code word is going to be redundant, and you won't get a mutation. Or you can get an amino acid change that's not selected because the fitness doesn't change. So you can get an amino acid that's at a different location.

Some DNA changes lead to evolution, but not by natural selection. For instance, there used to be tens of thousands of elephant seals in the North Atlantic, and that was reduced by hunting to a population of 20 in 1890. Then the species was conserved, and now all of the elephant seals—there are thousands of them now, about 30,000—are almost the same genetically because there were 20 left in 1890, and all of them came from those 20. This is an example of what is called a population bottleneck, where there are few survivors and the organisms that come from those few survivors are the ones that survive.

In 1968, population geneticist Motoo Kimura in Japan proposed that evolution can occur by neutral mutations that have nothing to do with natural selection. These just accumulate over time in the DNA that doesn't code for protein. We can begin to compare organisms by these neutral mutations. So, for example, for a protein, we can look at amino acid sequence differences between organisms that are alive now; for instance, we can trace relationships from fossils. If we compare, for instance, insects with vertebrates, we had a common ancestor 600 million years ago. If we compare the same protein, they're different because those differences have accumulated over time. We can get a rate of that difference over that period of time. We can say so many changes happened per million years in this particular protein, or this particular gene, or this particular DNA sequence.

Now, if we have two other organisms, we can compare those organisms by this clock. We don't know how long ago their common ancestor was. We can say, we already know the rate at which the clock works. If those two organisms have this amount of difference, their common ancestor must have lived a certain number of millions of years ago, etc. This is called molecular phylogeny; it's a way of comparing DNA sequences or protein sequences of organisms and inferring the last common ancestor. In the next lecture, we'll see how evolution—and these principles I've described—works in humans. Thank you.

Lecture Seventeen
DNA and Human Evolution

Scope: The mechanisms that explain evolution in the rest of the living world apply to humans as well. In sickle cell disease, a harmful genetic variant (allele) has been subjected to natural selection because it affords protection against a more serious disease, malaria. There are many examples of population bottlenecks in humans, which lead to distinctive frequencies of certain alleles. Molecular clocks can be used to trace human origins through DNA markers on the Y chromosome (males) and mitochondrial DNA (females). The origins and spread of human populations can also be traced in this way. Comparisons of the human genome with the recently sequenced chimp genome reveal some hints of the evolution of humans. Some gene differences as well as inserted sequences may be important. This is underscored by the findings of evolutionary developmental biology, in which a relatively small set of genes appear to trigger key events in the fascinating processes that occur in the embryos of many complex animals.

Outline

I. Opening story: Sickle cell disease is an example of natural selection in humans.

    A. People often think they are "above nature"—in control of their destiny. Sickle cell disease proves that natural selection acts on humans, as on any other species.

        1. Sickle cell disease is a disorder affecting the structure of red blood cells. It is inherited as an autosomal recessive, meaning that of the 1100 children born in the U.S. every year with the disease, in most cases their parents were healthy carriers for the harmful allele.

        2. Normally, red blood cells, which have the red oxygen-carrying pigment, hemoglobin, are donut-shaped and flexible so they can pass through narrow blood capillaries. They have a lifetime of about 120 days and are replaced by new cells that are made in bone marrow.

        3. People with this disease have red blood cells shaped like sickles. They are brittle and tend to block narrow capillaries, starving the tissues involved of life-giving oxygen. So patients tend to have lung, spleen, and kidney damage, and pain in the abdomen, legs, and chest. The abnormal shape targets the cells for early destruction (after about 16 days), so patients have a low blood count (anemia).

4. There is no cure for this chronic disease. Treatments include pain medications, antibiotics (the spleen damage makes them especially vulnerable to transfusions), and blood transfusions. A new drug, hydroxyurea, appears to prevent sickling and has had some success.

5. Sickle cell disease was the first human genetic disease whose molecular nature was described. In 1948, Linus Pauling and Harvey Itano pinpointed the abnormal phenotype on the protein hemoglobin. A DNA base-pair change in amino acid coding position 6 of 141 in the gene coding for the protein portion of hemoglobin:

$$A \quad to \quad T$$
$$T \qquad\quad A$$

leads to a single amino acid change in the protein. This results in abnormal hemoglobin folding, which leads to bad binding of oxygen and sickle-shaped red blood cells. Knowing this precise phenotypic description led to the development of hydroxyurea.

B. The population distribution of sickle cell disease is unusual.

1. The sickle allele is not universally distributed among humans. In fact, it is relatively common in some populations, but rare in others. The disease apparently originated in Africa, and is still relatively common there: In the U.S., 300 million have the disease, and about 1100 babies are born with it annually. In Nigeria, 120 million have the disease, and 80,000 babies are born with it annually. The transatlantic slave trade brought people carrying the allele for sickle cell disease to the U.S., where it occurs mostly in African Americans.

2. The appearance of such an allele in a certain populations prompted geneticists to ask how it happened and why it is maintained there. The first question is easily answered by a founder effect, where a spontaneous mutation occurred in some people that spread to their descendents. The second question is not so easy. Why is a clearly harmful mutation,

which certainly lowers reproductive fitness, maintained at such a high level?

3. In 1954, geneticist Anthony Allison noticed a similarity in the geographic distributions of people with the sickle cell disease and of malaria, which continues to be a scourge of Africa and other tropical regions. The organism that causes malaria lives in human red blood cells during part of its life. Allison proposed that if cells were sickled the parasite might not reproduce. So people with this disease were resistant to malaria, a far more harmful one. In fact, it is the heterozygous carriers for the allele that are at the greatest advantage against malaria.

4. The term "balanced polymorphism" describes this situation.

II. Population bottlenecks lead to unusual allele frequencies in humans.

A. Hereditary asthma is frequent on an island.

1. In the middle of the South Atlantic Ocean is the island of Tristan de Cunha. The island was fist settled by a Scot, William Glass, who brought his family there in 1817. They were joined by a few settlers from another island, but after Glass's death in 1856, most of the 120 or so descendents left for the Americas. The 300 or so people on the island today all came from 12 of the group in 1850s.

2. The group of 120 that had descended from Glass had many different alleles. The 12 who remained on the island and "begat" the subsequent population had their own subset of these alleles that were then passed on.

3. For instance, the current islanders have the highest rate of hereditary asthma in the world, due to a group of alleles that affect their respiratory system. This is an example of a population bottleneck. It is one way that evolution can occur without selection.

B. There are some "Jewish diseases."

1. The Jewish people have been subjected to many genocidal population reductions over the centuries. After each of these events, a small population remained, and this caused bottlenecks.

2. It is not surprising that there are a number of "Jewish genetic diseases," more common in them than in other groups of

people. These include Gaucher disease, Tay-Sachs disease, dystautonomia, and Canavan disease.

III. Molecular clocks can trace evolutionary relationships.

    A. In the previous lecture, we saw how alleles can accumulate in organisms without selection, just driven by the mutation rate, and that this can serve as a molecular clock. If we compare two organisms, we can estimate when they had a common ancestor and thereby gain insight into how closely related they are.

        1. The human Y chromosome is inherited through males and has over 30 regions that are nonselected and mutate at a constant rate. If we compare males around the world with one another, we can determine when they had a common ancestor. My brothers and I probably have identical Y markers: Our common ancestor is recent. My third cousins and I have different Y markers: We have a common ancestor longer ago. And so on, to the most diverse humans. This analysis traces Y chromosome "Adam" to about 80,000 years ago. Note: "Adam" is not the first man or the only one living at that time, just the male whose DNA alleles end up in males today.

        2. DNA in the mitochondrion, a part of the cell outside the nucleus that is passed on through the female, can also be used as a molecular clock. In this case, mitochondrial "Eve" lived about 150,000 years ago.

        3. Molecular markers can be used to trace migrations of populations.

            a. As the human population has spread over the Earth, those starting the new populations have specific genetic markers (e.g., skin color over time).

            b. DNA markers (Y and mitochondrion) can be used to identify populations and, along with the clock, when they diverged.

            c. This has set up the "genographic" and other projects to trace human origins and migrations by DNA markers.

    B. Genealogy can be done by genetics.

        1. In Jewish tradition, priests called Cohens (hence the common surname) are males descended from Aaron, brother of Moses, who lived 3300 years, or 100 generations, ago. A Cohen, Dr. Karl Skorecki, was attending synagogue services, and when a Cohen was called for, a visitor named Cohen with very different skin color, eye color, facial features, and hair color than Skorecki's stepped up. "Can we both be descended from the same man?" he wondered.

2. Analysis of Y chromosomes of Cohens from around the world provided an affirmative answer. Virtually all had a distinctive genetic marker on the Y chromosome.

3. The use of such DNA sequence markers to trace the origins of human groups has become a major effort. Web sites invite people to send in a tissue sample and have their DNA analyzed to find their family, ethnic group, or geographic origins.

IV. Genome sequences highlight human evolution.

   A. Several phenotypic characteristics make us human.

      1. Culture: the use of tools; genes have not yet been found for this.

      2. Walking upright: A single gene, AHI1, appears to control placing one foot in front of the other. Humans have it; chimps have a mutated sequence of it.

      3. A large brain: A chimp gene, MYH16, is mutated in humans. In chimps, this strong muscle protein in the jaw prevents skull growth to accommodate the brain. In humans, the mutation prevents the strong jaw and the brain can grow.

      4. Thought: The human genome has repeated sequences for a number of genes expressed only in the brain. Chimps do not.

   B. The chimp genome was sequenced in 2005; it is 2.9 billion base pairs (like the human genome).

      1. According to both fossil and molecular clock data, humans and chimps had a common ancestor that diverged about 6 million years ago.

      2. Comparison of the two genomes shows that in humans the average protein differs by two amino acids, there are 35 million single base-pair changes, and there are 5 million insertions and deletions that account for 70 million base pairs. The latter may be key (see below).

      3. Human genes that show the most differences with the chimp include ones involved in brain chemistry, speech, and disease resistance.

      4. This is only the beginning of this comparative effort.

   C. The evolution of development is surprising.

1. Development is the process by which an organism goes from fertilized egg to birth. In humans, it involves expression of about one-third of the total genes.
2. The amazing aspect of development is that the basic tool kit for making a complex organism is similar throughout biology. A limited number of genes is involved in making a worm or fly or mouse or person.
3. The first hint of this came with the discovery that genes that control which segment of a fruit fly developed which structure are similar to the genes that control the development of the body plan in humans. This initiated a new field: evo-devo (evolutionary developmental biology).
   a. Example: Over 90% of animals have eyes, but there are very different types. We have camera eyes, but insects have compound eyes (many eyes in a single structure). In 1915, a mutant fruit fly was discovered that had no eyes. This remained a lab curiosity until developmental geneticist Walter Gerhing found that the actual protein phenotype was a protein that stimulates transcription of eye genes.
   b. When the DNA sequence for the fly eye factor was compared by computer to other genomes, a similar gene was found in the human genome. Gene swapping experiments by recombinant DNA showed that the fly gene could stimulate mouse eye formation in the embryo and vice versa. So the mechanism for control is the same throughout the animals.
4. This leads to rapid evolution: Just adding (or mutating) a promoter of a transcription protein can activate a gene that was not active before. Since the human and chimp genomes have lots of inserts and deletions, this may be the key difference.

Essential Reading:

Ricki Lewis, *Human Genetics*, 7th ed. (New York: McGraw-Hill, 2006), chap. 16.

David Sadava, Craig Heller, Gordon Orians, William Purves, and David Hillis, *Life: The Science of Biology*, 8th ed. (Sunderland, MA: Sinauer Associates; New York: W. H. Freeman and Co., 2008), chaps. 20 and 23.

Supplemental Reading:

Elof Axel Carlson, *The Unfit: A History of a Bad Idea* (Woodbury, NY: Cold Spring Harbor Laboratory Press, 2001).

Linda Stone, Paul Lurquin, and Luca Cavalli-Sforza, *Genes, Culture and Human Evolution: A Synthesis* (Malden, MA: Blackwell, 2007).

Questions to Consider:

1. Can you think of human populations that have a specific set of alleles? How do you think these alleles ended up in the population?

2. In the molecular evolution story, "Adam" and "Eve" did not live at the same time. How can this be so?

Lecture Seventeen—Transcript
DNA and Human Evolution

Welcome back. In the last lecture, I described evolution, the change of organisms through time, and I described how the phenotype, which can be protein, is selected. There are also nonselected types of evolution where genes and changes of genes just accumulate over time. Now I want to show you how all of this applies to humans. My opening story concerns thinking we're "above nature." You know we humans often think we're in control of our destiny. Natural laws don't really apply to us. Sickle cell disease proves that natural selection acts on humans just as it does on any other species.

Let's go back to our previous lecture, Darwin and evolution by natural selection. Remember Darwin had two big ideas. The first was descent with modification—change over time—and the second was modifications becoming permanent, as we've passed them on from one generation to another by natural selection—the environment selecting those modifications that are best adapted and reproduced, passed on, to the next generation. Sickle cell disease is a disease affecting red blood cells. The allele for sickle cell disease is inherited as a recessive. Of the 1100 children born in the United States every year who have sickle cell disease, in most cases their parents were healthy carriers. That is, they were healthy carriers of the harmful allele, and they had a normal allele as well. Of course, they have a one in four chance, if they are carriers, of having a child with disease.

Normal red blood cells carry hemoglobin and they're donut shaped. They're flexible so they can pass through narrow blood channels called capillaries, so they can kind of squeeze their way through. I remember when I was a student I saw one of my favorite movies, *Fantastic Voyage*. It was a real '60s flick, and in this movie some scientists were miniaturized to a very small size. So, they went into the blood stream to eliminate a blood clot in a nuclear scientist, as I recall. The plot is not important. The acting was not great, but the important thing was the special effects. Here is this little ship in the blood stream, and we saw these red blood cells. You saw them changing their shape and squeezing through blood capillaries. I will always like that movie for that vision. Red blood cells have a lifetime of about 120 days in the bone marrow, and then they die and new cells are made afterwards to replace them.

Sickle red blood cells are very different. Sickle red blood cells are brittle. They block the narrow capillaries because they are brittle. They are shaped like a sickle so they can kind of clump together, and by blocking capillaries, they're going to starve tissues of the life-giving oxygen that red blood cells carry. So, people with sickle cell disease have lung damage, spleen damage, and kidney damage. They have abdominal pain. They have pain in the legs and in the chest. What's more, the sickle cells are selected for killing after 16 days. So, rather than 120 days in the blood stream, these cells only last 16 and the bone marrow can't keep up replacing them. So people with sickle cell disease have a low blood count. They have a low number of red blood cells. They have what is called an anemia. It used to be called sickle cell anemia. There is no cure for this disease. It's a chronic disease. Treatments include pain medications, antibiotics—the spleen damage makes these patients vulnerable to infections—and blood transfusions. There's a new drug that's being used to treat these patients called hydroxyurea, and it prevents sickling. There has been some success with this drug. Sickle cell disease is the first human genetic disease whose molecular nature was fully described down to the DNA level.

In 1948, the great chemist, Linus Pauling, and his student, Harvey Itano, pinpointed the abnormal phenotype of sickle cell disease on the protein hemoglobin. This is the first time a specific protein had been identified as being abnormal in a mutation. The DNA base-pair change is at amino acid coding position number 6 of 141. There are 141 amino acids, beads on this chain, to make this protein in hemoglobin, and only one of them is changed. That single change leads to a single amino acid change, and that single amino acid change results in the hemoglobin folding abnormally. It stacks up, and you get this sickling, etc. This precise knowledge of the phenotype, by the way, and the folding of the molecule has led to the development of hydroxyurea, this drug to treat sickling because it can bind to certain parts of the hemoglobin. This is an example of molecular medicine, to which we will turn in the next set of lectures.

The population distribution of sickle cell disease is rather unusual. Sickle cell disease is not universally distributed among humans. It's relatively common in some people but rare in other groups of people. Sickle cell disease originated in Africa and is still relatively common there. Of 300 million Americans, as I mentioned, 1100 newborns a year have sickle cell anemia, sickle cell disease. Of 120 million Nigerians, a third the size of the American population, 80,000 babies are born with this disease a year—it's really common in Africa, in Nigeria. By the time of the transatlantic slave trade, sickle cell disease had spread to southern Europe. It occurs to some extent in Portugal, Spain, Italy, and Greece, and the slaves brought it to the United States, where it occurs now mostly in African Americans.

Now, the presence of such an allele in certain populations prompted geneticists to ask two questions. First, how did it happen that this allele is present only in certain populations—not only, but largely, in certain populations? Second, why is it there? How is it maintained there? Why does it still exist? These are really questions of evolution. First—how it happened. Well, you can think of bottlenecks, or founder affects, where you began with a small group of people, some of whom might have had this mutation. And then the population expanded from these people, right? Do you recall late in the last lecture I described the example of the elephant seals, most of whom were killed off? We had 20 seals left, and now all of the 30,000 seals look like those 20 because they have that selection of mutations. Well, in this case, there was a small group of Africans and many of them had this particular allele, and now this allele is in the population.

Second question—how is it maintained? Well, that's a real evolution question. This is pretty clearly a harmful mutation that certainly lowers the reproductive fitness of a person. A person might not even survive to reproductive age sometimes with this disease. In 1954, a geneticist, Anthony Allison, found a similarity in the geographic distribution of sickle cell disease in Africa and Asia and malaria. Malaria has been and continues to be a scourge of tropical regions. Knowing that the organism that causes malaria reproduces in part inside of red blood cells, this is a complicated life cycle—an insect bites a human, the organism gets into the blood and then burrows into a red blood cell. Well, knowing that fact, Allison proposed that people who are carriers of the sickle cell allele, or are homozygous for the allele, would be at a selective advantage for being resistant to malaria because their hemoglobin in part or in whole would be sickled, and the cell would be abnormally shaped. So, maybe the parasite can't get in and reproduce.

This is called a "balanced polymorphism." As you recall, "*poly*" means "many," "*morph*" means "forms." This is a balanced polymorphism, which is a balance between the good and the bad. The good in this case, resistance to malaria, outweighs the bad, carrying the sickle cell allele. So, here we have evolution, natural selection, affecting humans. What about some of those other things I talked about in the last lecture? For example, population bottlenecks—you remember you wipe out a population to a small number and then you see the alleles in that small number greatly expand in that population. Can we see this in humans?

Tristan da Cunha is an island in the middle of the South Atlantic Ocean. It was first settled by a Scot, William Glass, in 1817 when he brought his family there. He was joined by a couple of settlers from another island. Now, Glass died about 40 years later in 1856, and by that time there were 120 people on the island, descendents of the original family. Ninety percent of them left after Glass died. He was kind of a dominating figure, and after he died, they said, let's get out of here. This is not a place to make a living, so most of them left for the Americas. Twelve people were left after Glass died. The population on the island now is 300. Those 300 all came from those 12 original settlers in the 1850s because Tristan de Cunha does not have an immigration issue. People just don't want to go there. Well, since mutations are random, this group of 120 before the great emigration from the island had a large variety of alleles, but the 12 who "begat" as the saying goes the current population of 300 had their own selection of alleles. We might have a bottleneck effect, and indeed we do. The current islanders on Tristan de Cunha have the highest rate of a very rare gene for hereditary asthma. They have the highest rate in the world that we know of for hereditary asthma, and it's a group of alleles that affect their respiratory, or breathing, system. So, scientists are studying this because they want to know all about asthma. Medically, this is a very important population to study, but I'm using it as an example of genetic bottleneck where we wiped out a lot of a population through emigration in this case and then the survivors gave rise to the rest of the population.

Another example of a bottleneck would be what are called the "Jewish diseases." The Jewish people have been subjected to many genocidal population reductions over the centuries. One estimate is that if it were not for these genocides, instead of 15 million Jews in the world today there'd be 250 million. After each of these events, well, a small population remained, and this caused a genetic bottleneck. That population then expanded their alleles. So, as a result, it's not surprising that there are a number of these Jewish genes in the case of genetic diseases that are more common in them than in other people.

An example is Gaucher disease, which in terms of carriers—that is people who have one dominant and the recessive—these are all recessively inherited allele carriers. For Gaucher disease, overall in the United States its carrier frequency is 1 in 200. In Jews, it's 1 in 16. For Tay-Sachs disease, overall in the U.S. it's 1 in 250. For Jews, it's 1 in 25. So, these two examples I've described show how genetic bottlenecks and evolution as a result of that can occur in humans just as it occurs in other organisms.

What about molecular clocks and evolutionary relationships? In the previous lecture, I described what a molecular clock is. A molecular clock looks at differences between DNA sequences of proteins between two organisms and then calculates back if we have fossil evidence to their last common ancestor. So, if we have 20 differences between these two organisms, and their last common ancestor lived, as far as fossil evidence goes, 20 million years ago, there's one difference per million years that's piling up because these are nonselected differences. These are not subject to natural selection. They're just accumulating because mutations happen. I've seen that bumper sticker, "Mutations happen."

Okay, so now we have two new organisms, and we compare them, and instead of 20 differences they have 5 differences. If there's one difference per million years, we can say, okay, their common ancestor was five million years ago. Now, if we want to make this argument for human genetics and look at the least common ancestor in human genetics, we have to use DNA sequences, if we're interested in DNA sequences, that are not subject to evolution by natural selection. No question, right? Because that's going to be discontinuous. Those DNA sequences' mutations will not pile up over time. They'll be selected for, and then the rest of them will die out. Well, we don't want that so we want something that's not being selected—usually these repeated sequences in the genome where half of our genome are these repeated sequences, or sequences that are not expressed as protein. That's fine. So, we'll select some of those. Well, that's 98% of the genome, so we've got lots of places to select. Second, we want sequences that are not going to be shuffled when the gametes are formed. You'll recall when gametes are formed we go from, as Mendel described, two sets of chromosomes to one set, and some genetic shuffling can occur then. We don't want a situation that has this shuffling going on. Well, the sequences we can use in humans for looking at evolutionary clocks are sequences on the Y chromosome, which is passed through males, and on the mitochondrial DNA, I'll describe that shortly, which is passed only through females. Both of these DNA sequences are not subject to selection if we choose the sequence properly, and they are not shuffled around when gametes are formed.

First, the Y chromosome sequence. On the Y chromosome are regions that, as I mentioned, are nonselected and mutate at a constant rate. Do you remember the Y chromosome has very few functional genes, the most notable of which is the one that determines maleness? If we look at these markers, the DNA sequences, they're not necessarily genes coding for anything. They're just DNA sequences. My brothers and I probably have identical sequences. Our last common ancestor is our father. There's probably not much time to have DNA sequence changing in us. We just got it from our father. My first cousins have a common grandfather, right? So, maybe there might be a change one generation to the next. But remember it's the same grandfather, my father's father. My third cousins, a couple of generations ago, might have some slight differences because we had a common ancestor a longer time ago. My fourth, and fifth, and sixth cousins, I'm sure I have some, though I don't know who they are, and they might be more and more different. So, we could make the family tree that way.

A survey of Y chromosome sequences, these marker sequences, in different men from all over the world was conducted by Allan Wilson. And the most diversity, the group with the most diversity comparing one individual to the next, and who obviously had the common ancestor the longest time ago—they had the greatest differences between them as they exist now—were Africans. That says that the ancestor of this particular Y chromosome sequence on the humans lived in Africa. How long ago? Well, we can calculate the rate at which it changes, and the Y chromosome, Adam (we'll call this person Adam; I'll give you a caveat for that in a moment—he's not necessarily the first man), according to Wilson, lived about 80,000 years ago. There have been other calculations of other markers that show similar conclusions. So, about 80,000 years ago lived this man whose Y chromosome has been passed on uninterrupted to the current Africans. It's changed over time because every couple of generations there are mutations that happen that get passed on. They're not selected. They get passed on. So, the current Africans are different from each other.

Is that Adam the first man that ever existed? No, it's the man whose Y chromosome has passed on uninterrupted because—well, look—I have no son. My Y chromosome is not being passed on to anyone. That's it. No more evolution of my Y chromosome DNA. It stops with me in my particular case. So, you can envision lots of men have existed throughout history whose Y chromosome didn't pass, but it's an interesting calculation to make. It shows that humans probably began in Africa as far as the Y chromosome evidence is concerned. In females, there is a DNA sequence that is passed on just through women, just through the mother to the daughter. It's passed on to the sons, but the mothers pass it on. This is the sequence called the mitochondrial DNA, and this has to do with the mechanics of fertilization.

The sperm is extremely small compared to the egg. The egg is a very, very large cell. The sperm is very small, and the sperm has its DNA concentrated in a very, very small area, only the head of the sperm. That's the only part of the sperm that gets into the egg. So, it's a lunch box. It's got all of the lunch, but the sandwich is the only part that gets in. The apple and the milk don't get in. If that's a bad metaphor, I apologize. The egg has an entire lunch box. It's got all the good stuff. It's got the sandwich, but it's got everything else, and included in that lunch box is a part of the cell called the mitochondrion, which has DNA, a very small amount of DNA, and some of this DNA is not subject to natural selection. So, it's a small sequence, small chromosome that is passed on from mother to offspring, male and female offspring. But only the mother passes it on because the sperm doesn't pass it on.

So, we can do the same analysis as we did with the Y chromosome. We could look at sequences and compare Africans to Africans, and Asians to Asians, and Africans to Asians, etc., and we find mitochondrial DNA marker sequences, and we find the greatest diversity again is Africans. The mitochondrial "Eve," whose DNA is passed uninterrupted all the way to us, lived about 150,000 years ago, mitochondrial Eve. Now, wait a minute, that's not Eve. That's not the first woman, and she didn't live the same time as Y chromosome Adam, but that's just because of who passed on what, which sequences were passed on. Because if a woman dies and doesn't reproduce, her sequence doesn't get passed on.

These molecular markers can identify human populations. For example, migrations—as the human population spread over the earth from its origins, those people starting new populations have their selection of markers, and we can look at how these genetic markers, like skin color, for example, changed over time. So, these DNA markers, the Y chromosome marker and the mitochondrial marker, can be used to identify populations, and we can use the clock to find out where they diverged. There are projects such as *National Geographic*'s genographic project that is looking at groups of people from all around the world and tracing the migrations of people through ancient, ancient history by looking at the current people and saying, how different is the current person is from the original? How long a period of time has evolved since they diverged, and at what time did they arrive in this certain place? You can use these markers in very interesting ways. There's a Y chromosome sequence, for example, that's found commonly in men in East Asia where the Mongols lived centuries ago, and these men have some differences between them in this sequence. This sequence doesn't seem to be present in this form in other people, in other men. If you compare the men's sequences, you find that they're genetically different. Do the clock, and it traces back to the origin right about the time of Genghis Khan. That's kind of neat. These men can say they are descendents of Genghis Khan.

Interesting aspect of genealogy—in the Jewish tradition there is a group of priests called Cohens. You've seen people called Cohen. These are not the only Cohens, and this comes from a tradition in their Bible of Moses turning around to Aaron, his brother, saying, okay, you are the high priest and all of your sons and their sons will be these priests that have special functions in the Jewish service. Now, this event happened when Moses lived, which is about 100 generations ago—about 3300 years ago was about the time Moses is thought to have lived and gave that story. So, here is a tradition of males passing on to their sons, to their sons, to their sons, a tradition of being involved in a priestly part of the service.

But 15 years ago, a Cohen physician, his name is Karl Skorecki, was attending the synagogue services in Israel when the rabbi at the front called for, okay, now we need a Cohen up at the front to do this thing. Skorecki stood up, but some guy at the front stood up ahead of him and beat him to it. Skorecki looked at this person in the front and said, that guy has a different skin color. His eye color is different than me. His facial features, his hair is different than me. He is really different than me. How could it be that we descend from the same line of people through the Y chromosome? So, Skorecki and another scientist set up a Y chromosome data bank, and they looked at Jews who identified themselves as Cohens, and they looked at their Y chromosome in males, and they looked at all other Jews, and they looked at the overall population. They found, lo and behold, that there was a sequence in common, a genetic sequence in common with all of those Cohen men. They were different from each other somewhat, so they could do a molecular clock. The molecular cock focused in back to about 100 generations. So that's kind of neat when you think about it. It's possible confirmation of a Biblical story and a long tradition of the Y chromosome marker being passed on, and along with the Y chromosome marker, of course, is a religious tradition.

This type of approach has been spread to many other groups of using these genetic sequences that identify people. American Indians can identify what tribe they are a member of. African Americans can relate their heritage back to tribes in Africa. Asians can relate their heritage as well. The issues are personal satisfaction. The issues can be family identification. Different families have backgrounds. For example, there was a Dr. Sykes in Britain who started looking at all the Sykes over time and found lo and behold a DNA sequence that the Sykes have in common. So, you can trace your ancestry in that way.

Genome sequencing is highlighting human evolution these days. In 2005, the chimpanzee genome was sequenced. Now, the chimpanzee's genome is the same size as the human genome in base pairs. It's about 2% different from us. Now, 2% is a lot. That means there are 15 million differences in base-pair sequence, and our last common ancestor is about 6 million years ago. The physical characteristics and other characteristics that make us human—well, what are they and how are these reflected in the genome sequencing? First, there's culture—the use of tools. Well, we don't know any genes for that yet. There hasn't been any correlation yet made, but people are just as we speak analyzing the chimp genome for these kinds of things. There are a couple of others—walking upright. We walk upright. The chimps don't, as you know. Well, there's a single gene, the gene is called AHI1, and this gene appears to control placing one foot in front of the other. Humans have this gene intact. Chimps have a mutated sequence that's nonfunctional. So, the single gene might be involved in that evolutionary step in humans. A large brain—we have a larger brain than chimps. There is a chimp gene called MYH16 that humans have a mutated form that's nonfunctional. Now, this gene in chimps makes a muscle protein that makes the muscles in the jaw very strong as the jaw develops and prevents the skull from growing so the brain can't grow larger. So, over evolutionary time, if chimps got mutations to have a larger brain, they wouldn't survive because the brain just wouldn't be able to get larger. By having this gene mutated—that ends up in humans—the brain can get larger.

Another difference between humans and chimps, of course, is thought. The human genome has a number of repeated sequences for a number of genes that are expressed only in the brain, and it's been recently found that these micro-RNAs that seem to be involved in gene expression are more expressed in humans than the chimps. So, this is an ongoing comparison between the human and chimp genomes. And it's going to reveal possible evolutionary relationships. The evolution of development has been one of the big surprises of modern biology. Development is a process by which an organism goes from a fertilized egg to birth, and in humans it involves about a third of our genes. Think of it—about a third of your genes make you what you are, a newborn. You can think of the complexities involved, making all the bone, and all the tissues of the human that happens before birth. It's amazing. The incredible aspect of development is that there's a basic tool kit of genes involved in making complex organisms, and it's similar throughout biology.

A limited number of genes make a worm, or a fruit fly, or even a human. The first hint of this came from the discovery in the 1980s of genes that control which segment or part of a fruit fly develops which structure, a leg or a wing. It turns out there are genes that control that—not the leg, but control that a leg is going to come out—make that decision. These are involved with transcription factors that control which genes are transcribed, and those genes are very similar to the genes of the body plan in a mouse and in a human. It's an amazing discovery, a whole new field called evolutionary developmental biology, evo-devo, has come out of this. For instance, most animals have eyes, but they're different eyes. They're the camera eye in humans and the compound eye in insects. But the same switch can control both of them. The switch is identical in humans and in fruit flies for turning the eye on. The evolution of variations I've described in humans has led to the current human genome.

In the next lecture, I begin a description of molecular medicine by describing screening for genetic variations that cause human disease. Thank you.

Lecture Eighteen
Molecular Medicine—Genetic Screening

Scope: Genetic testing for mutant alleles in people is now possible at both the phenotype and gene levels. It can be done in newborn babies or adults, and even prenatally. Screening is done either on the whole populations (e.g., all newborns for phenylketonuria) or on populations in which an allele is prevalent (e.g., African Americans for sickle cell disease). The tissues used for screening range from blood serum to any cell for DNA testing. The tests must be both reliable (repeatable) and valid (an accurate reflection of the genetic condition). Newborn screening for disorders such as phenylketonuria and hypothyroidism has been successful in terms of optimizing human potential and economic and social benefit. DNA testing can be effective only if the mutation targeted is known. The next frontier in genetic testing is the identification of alleles for altered susceptibility to drugs and for susceptibility to complex diseases.

Outline

I. Opening story: an early diagnosis.
  A. Diagnosis of a genetic disease is now possible on early embryos.
    1. John and Mary were concerned about their infant son, who was not gaining much weight. Jimmy was listless and seemed to have a cough all the time. Searching the internet over the weekend before a Monday appointment with the pediatrician, Mary came across cystic fibrosis as fitting Jimmy's symptoms. When she licked his neck and tasted salt, she was pretty sure. The doctor confirmed it.
    2. Cystic fibrosis is due to a recessive allele and is one of the most common inherited diseases, with a carrier frequency of about 1 in 50 and a birth frequency of 1 in 2500. It is caused by a mutation of the CFTR gene, so that its product, a protein that allows chloride salt into and out of cells, does not work. As a result, mucus accumulates in the respiratory system and blocks the digestive secretions of the pancreas from reaching the intestine.

3. The disease appears during childhood, with persistent infections, digestive problems, diabetes, and later, infertility. Treatment of these symptoms has improved the lifespan for these patients: 40 years ago, few survived to their teens. Now, most survive until their mid-30s.

4. The most common mutation in the CFTR gene in Caucasians is a three-base-pair deletion of DNA at amino acid coding position 508. This results in a single amino acid missing in the large, 1480-amino-acid protein. This tiny deletion is enough to inactivate the protein. This is the mutation that Jimmy had. And because this is a recessively inherited disease, he had two mutant alleles—both John and Mary were carriers, with one normal and one mutant allele.

5. Two years later, with Jimmy's condition stable, John and Mary decided to have another child. This time they wanted a child without the disease. They knew the chances for a normal child were three in four. Fortunately, a new test is available to detect the cystic fibrosis allele.

6. First, Mary was given drugs to augment the number of eggs she would produce; instead of just one in the next monthly cycle, eight were matured. In the clinic, the eggs were removed, and John's sperm was used to fertilize them. Six eggs were successfully fertilized. Over the next three days they began to divide—the egg produced two cells, then four, then eight.

7. At this point, the thin membrane surrounding the cells of one of the embryos in the dish was punctured and a tiny straw used to suck out one of the eight cells. PCR was used to amplify the single cell's CFTR allele, and the presence of the missing three base pairs and normal CFTR allele were probed. The probe did not detect the mutant allele, only normal ones. The remaining seven cells were enough to go on to divide further, and after a week the embryo was implanted in Mary's womb. Thirty-seven weeks later, she gave birth to Susie, a child without cystic fibrosis.

B. This preimplantation genetic diagnosis, while not widespread, is the culmination of reproductive and genetic technologies.

II. Genetic tests identify alleles in people.

A. Screening involves testing people, often without symptoms, for the presence of an allele.

   1. Screening should provide information that is useful to the patient (or guardian) for decision making and/or for the physician in treatment.

   2. Screening can be done on different groups.

      a. An age group when the allele gets expressed: newborns for cystic fibrosis.

      b. Targeted populations: African Americans for sickle cell disease.

   3. Screening can be done on tissues expressing the phenotype or any cell's DNA. For example:

      a. Blood: serum for proteins, cells for DNA.

      b. Mouth: cells washed out for DNA; this was done on Saddam Hussein when he was found.

      c. Hair, semen: for forensic purposes.

      d. Fetal tissues (embryo, as above; chorionic villi at 6 weeks; amniotic fluid at 12 weeks).

   4. A test for an allele has two components.

      a. Reliability: Is it reproducible? Do two radiologists looking at a mammogram or two pathologists looking at a PCR result come to the same conclusion?

      b. Validity: Does the test actually indicate the allele? This in turn has two components.

         i. Sensitivity: The proportion of people with the allele who test positive. Failure here is a false negative.

         ii. Specificity: The proportion of people without the allele who test negative. Failure here is a false positive.

B. Phenotype screening at the molecular level involves looking for the abnormal protein.

   1. In sickle cell disease, the change in hemoglobin involves an amino acid with a neutral charge replacing the normal amino acid with a negative charge. Although this is only one amino acid in hundreds, the slight difference in overall charge of the protein (less negative in the mutant) is easily detected in a blood sample. This takes an hour.

   2. For phenylketonuria, screening is harder. As you may recall from Lecture Six, the protein missing in PKU is an enzyme present in tiny amounts. And it occurs only in the liver. Taking a piece of liver out to make the diagnosis is invasive. Instead, the test is done on a newborn's blood for the phenotypic effect of the missing enzyme.

    a. Since the liver enzyme, phenylalanine hydroxylase, catalyzes the conversion of what I will call X (it's actually phenylalanine) into Y (tyrosine), when the enzyme is missing, X piles up in the liver and spills out into the blood.

    b. A drop of blood is taken from the heel of the infant on the first day of life and put onto a blotter card. That drop is then used to the test for X (and therefore, PKU). This test, invented by Robert Guthrie in 1962, is now widely used.

    c. A number of other tests for genetic abnormalities can be done on the same drop of blotted blood.

III. Testing for alleles by DNA is possible.

    A. Sequencing DNA would be the ultimate test for a genetic abnormality. But this is very costly at present (although the costs continue to fall).

    B. For now, other rapid tests are used.

        1. DNA hybridization probe is feasible. In Lecture Fifteen, we described the use of nucleic acid hybridization, in which a single-stranded DNA probe is used to see if it binds, or does not bind, to the tested target DNA. Consider the example of cystic fibrosis in the opening story. In this case, DNA on the blotter paper of a newborn would be hybridized with DNA probes that match the known mutation in the two parents. If the probe found its match, the newborn would be considered to have cystic fibrosis. It would be important to show that a probe to the normal allele did not bind in this case; if it did, the infant would be a carrier.

        2. Polymerase chain reaction can be used to detect the presence of an allele. PCR begins with a short strand known as a primer (like what you paint on a wall). The primer must bind by base pairing to a known part of the DNA to be amplified. Now, consider the DNA on the blood blotter. To get PCR going, a primer that binds to the normal, intact allele would be used. This primer would not bind to the deleted, mutant allele. So the amplification of the CFTR gene would depend on whether it was intact or not.

IV. Screening programs are widespread.

    A. Newborn screening is medically and economically beneficial.

        1. Consider PKU: Testing was begun in 1965 and is now mandatory for all newborns in most countries and all U.S. states.

            a. Babies who test positive and are put on a special diet end up mentally normal. Untreated, a person with PKU has an IQ of about 55 and is severely retarded. The human costs are huge.

            b. The economic analysis is that the test costs about $2. The frequency of newborns with PKU is about 1 in 14,000. This means it costs $28,000 in tests for every infant with PKU detected. Add to this the costs of being PKU in terms of diet and medical care—about $3,000 per year—and for 30 years the total cost is $118,000. This is far lower than 30 years of caring for a mentally retarded person.

        2. Other diseases are screened in newborns, such as some rare genetic disorders and genetic hypothyroidism. The latter used to be hidden as a cause of mental retardation. Of 5 million infants screened a year, 1500 have it: They are treated with thyroid hormone, and retardation is prevented.

        3. Cystic fibrosis DNA testing has begun in some places, as has sickle cell DNA testing. (Many states and countries are working toward testing newborns for over 20 genetic disorders.)

    B. Screening adults and children in target populations has been successful.

        1. African Americans have set up screening for sickle cell disease, and this has led people to treatment.

        2. Jewish groups have screened for Tay-Sachs disease (most common in Jews), and the test reveals carriers. Since so many have been screened, marriages between carriers are now rare, and prenatal testing is done on the fetuses. Studies show that the mother usually chooses to terminate the pregnancy when the test is positive. It is now very rare for a Tay-Sachs child to be born of Jewish parents.

    C. Pharmacogenomics and disease susceptibility testing are the next frontier.

1. When any outside agent enters the body, it passes through the liver, where a series of proteins transforms it to more water-soluble forms for excretion in the kidney. This is evolutionarily advantageous, as it gets rid of these substances.
   a. This system is under genetic control: There are alleles coding for proteins that are more or less active.
   b. Consider smoking. The poisons in cigarette smoke are changed by the liver system. In most cases, the changes make them more water-soluble but also more harmful to cells, causing DNA damage that can lead to cancer.
   c. If a person carries a mutation in the liver system that causes less activity on the molecules from smoke, there will be fewer poisons produced. We all know long-term smokers who do not get cancer; many have the right alleles.
   d. The same goes for drugs. They are also modified by the liver. Having the right alleles may make one more or less susceptible to the actions of drugs. This is why drug companies sponsored the private human genome sequencing effort. They wanted to identify these alleles.
2. Many diseases, such as cancer and heart disease, have complex causes and many gene products interacting. So there are many disease susceptibility genes that are being identified. Tests will be developed for them.

Essential Reading:

Jack Pasternak, *An Introduction to Human Molecular Genetics*, 2nd ed. (Bethesda, MD: Fitzgerald Science Press, 2005).

David Sadava, Craig Heller, Gordon Orians, William Purves, and David Hillis, *Life: The Science of Biology,* 8th ed. (Sunderland, MA: Sinauer Associates; New York: W. H. Freeman and Co., 2008), chap. 17.

Supplemental Reading:

Thomas Devlin, *Textbook of Biochemistry with Clinical Correlations*, 6th ed. (Hoboken, NJ: Wiley-Liss, 2006).

Susan Lindee, *Moments of Truth in Genetic Medicine* (Baltimore: Johns Hopkins, 2005).

Philip Reilly, *Is it in your Genes? How Genes Influence Common Disorders and Diseases that Affect You and Your Family* (Woodbury, NY: Cold Spring Harbor Laboratory Press, 2004).

Questions to Consider:

1. Were you or your children tested for genetic diseases as newborns? If so, what is the difference between the current testing program in your area and the one that was in place when you were born?

2. Should employers or health insurers be informed of the results of a genetic test? What about a genetic test for disease susceptibility?

Lecture Eighteen—Transcript
Molecular Medicine—Genetic Screening

Welcome back. As I described in the last lecture, evolution has resulted in the current human genome. This genome contains variations—mutations—and some of these cause disease. In the next five lectures, I'm going to describe molecular medicine and how molecular biology and DNA have the potential to, and the reality of, changing the way we treat and detect human disease. I begin with screening; that is, detecting mutations. My opening story is about an early diagnosis. Diagnosis of human genetic disease is usually quite difficult. My story is about John and Mary. John and Mary were concerned about their infant son. Jimmy was six months old but not gaining much weight. He was getting listless, and he seemed to cough all the time. Searching the Internet over the weekend before a Monday appointment with the pediatrician, Mary came across cystic fibrosis as fitting Jimmy's symptoms. When she licked his neck and tasted salt, she was pretty sure, and the doctor confirmed it.

Cystic fibrosis is probably the most common inherited disease. The carrier frequency in our population is about 1 person in 50; birth frequency about 1 in 2500. It's caused by a mutation in a gene called CFTR. Because we're here in a science course, I'll tell you what CFTR is, and then I won't say what it is again. It's called the cystic fibrosis transmembrane conductance regulator. I'll call it CFTR. It's caused by a mutation in the CFTR gene so that its protein product, which is a protein that sucks chloride and allows it to go in and out of cells, doesn't work. And the result of this lack of passage of chloride salt, in and of itself, results in mucus accumulating in the respiratory, or breathing, system. In addition, the digestive secretions of the pancreas are blocked from reaching the intestine.

Cystic fibrosis appears in early childhood with persistent infections detected on X ray, and digestive problems—not surprisingly because of the pancreas problems—diabetes, and later on, infertility. Treatment of these symptoms has improved the life span of these patients quite dramatically. Forty years ago, few people with cystic fibrosis lived to their teens. Now it's pretty common for them to live into their mid-30s, and even into their 40s. The most common mutation in cystic fibrosis, in the CFTR gene, in Caucasians is a three-base-pair deletion of DNA at amino acid coding position 508. Now this is a 1480-amino-acid protein—1480 beads in the chain—and because there are three base pairs missing at number 508, we're missing one amino acid, because, remember, three base pairs code for an amino acid. So we're missing one word, and therefore we're missing one amino acid. This tiny deletion is enough to inactivate the protein. It doesn't fold right, and therefore it doesn't function as a chloride transporter. This is the particular mutation that Jimmy had. It was detected in his DNA.

Because cystic fibrosis is a disease that's inherited as a recessive trait, Jimmy had two mutant alleles, and both John and Mary, his parents, were carriers. They had a normal and a mutant, and of course there's a one in four chance of having a child with this disease. Two years later, with Jimmy's condition stable under good treatment, John and Mary decided to have another child. This time they wanted one without the disease. Now they knew the chances of a normal child are three in four; think of the genetics now. Each of them is a carrier, so the chances of having a normal child are three in four. Fortunately in this case, there was a new test to detect whether the child would be a normal child, having at least one normal allele, or a child which is homozygous for having both copies of the mutant allele and having cystic fibrosis.

Here's the way it worked. Mary was given drugs to augment the number of eggs she would produce in her monthly cycle. Instead of just one in the next monthly cycle, she matured eight eggs. In the clinic, the eggs were removed, and John's sperm was used to fertilize them. Six eggs were successfully fertilized. Over the next three days, these eggs began to divide; one to two, to four, then eight cells over the next few days. At this point, a procedure was done. The thin membrane surrounding the cells of the embryo—this thin, thin coating—was punctured by—well, I'll use the term "pipette," a fancy word for "straw," and a tiny straw was used to suck out one of the eight cells of this embryo.

At this point, PCR—we know this already from previous study; polymerase chain reaction—was used to amplify this single cell's CFTR alleles. The presence of the missing three base pairs, as well as normal gene, was probed by DNA hybridization. So, a couple of hours later, this hybridization experiment was done using probes for both the normal allele and the allele that would be mutant in cystic fibrosis, looking for the missing three base pairs. They didn't find it. They found that the probe did not detect the mutant allele; only normal ones were present. Now, the remaining seven cells of this little embryo are totipotent. When they were left to divide further, after a week the embryo was implanted in Mary's womb. Thirty-seven weeks later, she gave birth to Susie, a child without cystic fibrosis.

This preimplantation genetic diagnosis, while certainly not widespread, is the culmination of both reproductive and genetic technologies.

I want to talk about genetic testing in three ways. First, I'll describe genetic tests: what they are and how you identify alleles in people. Second, I'll talk about testing for alleles by DNA testing—and this is possible and used. Third, I'll describe genetic screening programs: how they work, what they're doing, and what the logic of them is. First, genetic tests. What is screening? Screening involves testing people, often without symptoms, for the presence of an allele. I want to repeat that. It's testing people who might not even have symptoms for the presence of an allele; for example, this eight-celled embryo, which I described testing for the parents for cystic fibrosis. The parents were concerned with having a child with cystic fibrosis. They tested an eight-celled embryo; no symptoms there. They were testing for the allele; that's screening.

Screening should provide—the objective is to provide—useful information to a patient or the guardian, if it's a parent, for decision making and/or for the physician in treatment. It's important that screening provide useful information. Now the question becomes, who should be screened? Well, we can first ask the question, what age group? Well, we could screen newborns. We could screen embryos. We could screen adults for genetic disorders, for alleles. So, for example, if an allele gets expressed at birth, we could screen for cystic fibrosis, typically in newborns, or PKU. Now who to screen also concerns which population to screen. If we're screening for hereditary breast cancer, who's the target population? All women. I doubt that you screen men for that, although it's possible for men to get breast cancer, but it's very rare. You might screen targeted populations. For example, in the last lecture I described sickle cell disease as being much more common in African Americans, so you might screen African Americans if you're doing genetic screening for sickle cell disease. It would be rare in others.

Next the question is what to screen, what tissues. Well, if we're screening for the protein phenotype, we'll screen for tissues that express that particular phenotype. You want to know who's got red hair? That's easy, right? Or you could screen any cell for DNA. We can screen blood, for example, the blood serum for proteins if we're looking for a certain protein, or we can screen the cells in blood for DNA. We can screen the mouth. Cells are washed out of the mouth for screening for DNA. I do that when I teach students about genetic screening. We actually do a genetic test on their DNA, and they take some of the cells from their mouth. We can screen hair or seminal fluid for forensic purposes to identify genes and alleles there, as I described earlier in the course. We can screen fetal tissues, embryonic tissues even. At 6 weeks, for example, the embryo sends little projections into the wall of the uterus called chorionic villi. You can stick a needle in and get little embryonic cells there and screen them for genetic abnormalities. At 12 weeks, screening can be done called amniocenteses, where the amniotic fluid in which the baby is floating can be screened, and there are cells there that come from the fetus, and we can detect abnormalities there.

What about the "how" of genetic screening? Well, any test—any medical test, for that matter—for an allele has two components. The two components are reliability and validity. Reliability asks the question, is this test reproducible? If there are two radiologists looking at a mammogram for breast cancer, do both of them agree, hey, that's breast cancer? Or do two pathologists looking at a PCR result looking for the amplification of a gene, do they agree that gene is there? They come to the same conclusion; that's called reliability. Is this test giving a consistent result? The second aspect is validity. Does it actually test for the mutant allele? I mean, the two people may agree, but they may be wrong. Just agreeing doesn't mean that they're necessarily right. Validity of a screening test has two components. The two components are called sensitivity and specificity. Sensitivity is the proportion of people who have this mutant allele who test positive for this test. We're testing for this allele. That's a positive test; they have the allele.

How are you going to find that out? You're going to have a bunch of people you already know have this genetic disease, and you test them for it; do the test for cystic fibrosis, for example, on people with cystic fibrosis. Now, if the test comes up negative in a certain number of people, that's called a false negative. False negatives are a bad thing, aren't they? Because we're going to apply this test to nonsymptomatic people, people who don't have cystic fibrosis. They'll walk in for a genetic screening, and we'll ask if they have the allele for cystic fibrosis—whether it be an embryo or a newborn child. We're testing for cystic fibrosis in a newborn child. If we certify the child as not having the disease, and the child has the disease, that's a medical disaster, right? False negatives are medical disasters. So we'd like to have 100% sensitivity of our test. We'd like to always get it. Life's not like that; neither is medicine. We go for the high. We try to get over 90%, but it's pretty hard in genetic screening. There are false negatives, which is sad.

The other aspect of screening tests is called specificity. Specificity is the proportion of people without the allele who test negative. So we take some people we know don't have cystic fibrosis, and then we apply the test to them. Now if the test comes out positive, and we say you do have cystic fibrosis, that's a burden on the medical care system and on the person because you have to bring them back into the clinic and run exhaustive sets of confirmatory tests, and that costs a lot of money and creates anxiety. That's a burden on the medical care system. It's not a disaster like a false negative, where the person walks out saying, hey, I'm okay, but they're not. It's a hassle. So specificity is a problem, and it exists in all the screening programs I will describe, as does sensitivity not being high enough. We try to be 100%, but we usually don't reach it.

Phenotype screening at the molecular level involves looking for the abnormal protein. Let's look at sickle cell disease. The change in hemoglobin in sickle cell disease—in this mutation that results in an abnormal amino acid at one position, you'll recall, in this large protein—is a change from a glutamic acid—I'll just give you the names of the amino acids in the normal—to valine; it's a different amino acid in the mutant situation, sickle cell. Glutamic acid is negatively charged. Valine has a neutral charge. So we're going, overall, from a more negative protein to a less negative protein. How about that? By placing proteins in an electric field, we can detect the difference between these. It's quite easy. So a protein that's less negative versus more negative would be different.

The more negative protein will migrate more toward the positive end of an electric field—positive and negative attract—and the less negative, less so. So it's quite easy to make this detection on the basis of the difference in charge of the protein. Blood is really easy to get. We just take a drop of blood, and we can find out the phenotype, and therefore infer the genotype of a person for sickle cell anemia. So it's easy to get carriers that way. All you need to do is take a drop of blood and find out, do they have both types of hemoglobin or just the one type, depending on whether they're negative or less negative.

Well, phenylketonuria is a little bit more difficult, PKU. Remember in Lecture Seven, I described the protein missing in phenylketonuria is an enzyme present only in teeny, tiny amounts, and it occurs only in the liver. So I want to find out where that protein's missing; we'll take a piece of liver. Not a good idea if you're doing screening. You're going to take every newborn and take a piece of liver out? That's rather invasive. Instead, the test is done on a newborn's blood for the phenotypic effect of the missing enzyme. Now recall, in the liver this enzyme, called phenylalanine hydroxylase, catalyzes the conversion of what I'm going to call X—it's actually phenylalanine—to Y; it's tyrosine. So from now on, I'll just say it converts X to Y.

The enzyme is missing in PKU. So X piles up and accumulates in the liver, and this spills out into the blood. A newborn baby who has this disease will have a lot of this X in the blood, and so you can test for it in the blood. A blood drop is used to test for X and therefore PKU. This test was invented by Robert Guthrie in 1962, and the test, and variants of it, are used worldwide. There are other tests of genetic abnormalities that can be done on the same drop of blood. So, generally, a heel stick sample is taken—a small drop of blood is taken from the heel of a newborn baby on the second day of life—and the blood is dried on a little card. Then you can detect how much of X is in the blood, as well as other chemicals that we can test for.

We can test for alleles by DNA testing as well. Now the ultimate test for alleles, of course, is by sequencing DNA for genetic abnormalities. Well, sequencing has been very costly. Now it's about $100,000, going down all the time. The objective is to get a $10,000 sequence within a couple of years. Maybe we'll have the $500 sequence. So now instead of doing sequencing, if we want to test for DNA abnormalities, we use the molecular biology that I described earlier on. There are two ways to do molecular biology testing: the DNA of these dried blood spots in a newborn or cells from another person. In Lecture Fifteen, I described the use of nucleic acid hybridization. This is a technique where, remember, a single-stranded DNA probe is used to find out if it will bind to its complement.

So this might be a bunch of As in the DNA, and we're looking for a bunch of Ts in the unknown DNA in the person to see whether they're complementary there, see if there's DNA that's missing. So, for example, this is what was done in the cystic fibrosis story that opened this lecture. DNA on the blotter paper—this dried blood spot of a newborn, for example—could be hybridized with DNA probes that matched the known mutation in the two parents. So you have to know what the mutation is in the parents so we can look for it in the offspring. That's exactly what was done on this single cell that had been amplified by PCR. It's important to show that a probe to the normal allele didn't bind if we're trying to make the diagnosis. If it did, of course, the infant would be a carrier. Because both probes bound, the normal and the mutant probe, the child would be a carrier.

A second way of doing DNA screening is by the polymerase chain reaction, PCR. Now a little bit of the chemistry of PCR. PCR begins with a short strand of DNA called a primer. You know when you paint a wall, you don't put the paint right on the wall? I've tried that; it doesn't work. You put a primer on that'll stick to the wall and stick to the paint. Well, it's the same thing with PCR. We begin with a short piece of DNA that primes the rest of the DNA as the DNA is multiplied in the polymerase chain reaction. Now if we design this short piece right, we could have this short piece actually binding to either the normal or the mutant piece of DNA. Now if the primer doesn't bind, the mutant is there, for example, and the DNA would not be amplified. The presence or absence of amplification in PCR—if we had the CFTR gene, for example—would depend on whether the gene is intact or not. So PCR is another way of detecting the presence or absence of an allele.

Screening programs are widespread; newborn screening especially. Let's consider PKU, phenylketonuria. Testing for PKU was begun in 1965 and is now mandatory for all newborns in most countries and in all U.S. states. The medical result of testing is the following. A baby who tests positive for PKU—has a lot of that X—is put on a special diet where they don't take in a lot of X. Now let me step back a moment and describe what X is. X is an amino acid; it's part of proteins. Some proteins, just by their very nature, have a lot of X in them; other proteins don't. So we just put the child on a special diet that has a low level of this particular amino acid. So you choose the proteins wisely that you eat so you don't get a lot of X accumulating in your body. This is a phenomenally successful medical intervention. It's a very simple one, a very simple dietary intervention.

Untreated, a person with PKU has an IQ of about 55 and is severely mentally retarded. Treated with the diet, their IQ is, average, 100. I've had students in my classes where I work as a professor who had IQs above 140 who are PKU people, and that's amazing. The medical and social costs, and the human costs, of a child who develops into an adult with an IQ of 55, of course, are huge. The economic analysis is, again, something we have to consider as a society when we're doing any medical intervention. Here's the economic analysis of PKU in a nutshell. A test for PKU costs $2, the screening test of a newborn. The frequency of newborns with PKU in America is about 1 in 14,000. That means we spend $28,000 as a society in testing (two times $14,000) for every one PKU patient that we detect. That's the cost that we have in the screening program. We add to that the cost of a person with PKU in terms of the diet and medical care, and that's about $3,000 a year for the first 30 years of life. So let's see; $90,000 of medical and special diet costs for 30 years, plus $28,000 for the screening costs where we didn't detect any PKU; that's $118,000. Compare this to 30 years of caring for a mentally retarded person. The economic—again, and the human—costs are huge.

Other diseases are screened for in newborns as well. Some of these others are rare genetic disorders similar to PKU, and hypothyroidism. This is a low level of thyroid hormone. The latter, this hypothyroidism, used to be a hidden cause of mental retardation until we started looking at it in these newborn blood tests. Of 5 million infants screened a year, 1500 have this hypothyroidism. We never used to know what this was, and now you simply treat them with thyroid hormone, and this mental retardation that they would get is prevented. Cystic fibrosis DNA testing has begun in some places, as has sickle cell DNA testing on newborns.

What about screening for adults and children in targeted populations? In Lecture Seventeen, I described how some diseases are more common in certain populations. The bottleneck—do you remember that?—where a small group of people begins a population and then an allele spreads in that population. Here the allele might be for a genetic disease. For example, African Americans have set up screening for sickle cell disease, and this has led people to treatment. Jewish groups have done screening for this disease, Tay-Sachs, which I described as being more common in that group. In this case, the test reveals carriers as well as the sickle cell. So, for example, since so many people in the Jewish group have been screened, marriages between carriers are now rare, and prenatal testing is done on all the fetuses of such marriages. Studies have shown that women who have an affected child will usually choose to terminate the pregnancy. It's now very rare for a Tay-Sachs child to be born of Jewish parents. That's the result of screening.

Pharmacogenomics—"*pharmaco*" means "drugs"; "*genomics*" means the "genome"—and disease susceptibility testing are the next frontier of genetic screening. Now a little bit of pharmacology, the study of drugs and the body. I always have to tell my students the study of pharmaceutical drugs and the body, but it's any kind of outside agent and the body. When any chemical that's not part of you enters your body, one of the first things that happens is it goes to the digestive system, and it passes through the liver. In the liver, a series of enzymes coded for by genes transforms this substance into something that is more soluble—able to dissolve in water. The reason for doing that is that it will be able to dissolve in water so you can excrete it or get rid of it through the kidney in the urine. So, evolutionarily, this is a protective mechanism. Outside agents are made more easy to dissolve so they don't get stored in the body. You'll get rid of them in the urine.

There are alleles for these genes that affect outside agents. You can imagine that because they are genes that code for proteins, so there'll be alleles, and there are mutant proteins that these alleles code for. So there are alleles that code for proteins that make this liver system more active, more able to convert things. There are alleles that code for proteins that make it less active. There are alleles even in the promoters of this system that cause it to be more made, and therefore more active, more expressed, or less expressed. All of these have now been described. Consider cigarette smoking. I've mentioned before that in cigarette smoke there are a number of poisons that are there. These poisons do not cause genetic damage by themselves. It's their liver product that causes damage. How did the liver product get formed? It's formed when the components of cigarette smoke get changed by this liver enzyme system, under genetic control.

In most cases, these changes make these substances more water-soluble; great. Unfortunately, on their way to the urine, they become more harmful to cells as well when they're more water-soluble. They get into cells more, and they can cause DNA damage, which can lead to cancer. If a person carries a mutation in the liver system so that they have less active changing of this poison to an active form, well, I think you can imagine. Less poisons are made by this molecule, this smoke molecule, so the people can smoke almost to their lungs' content because they don't activate the poisons when they smoke. We all know people who are smokers of many, many years who don't get cancer. Maybe these are people who have the right alleles that code for the proteins in their liver, and they don't activate the cancer-causing molecules.

Pharmaceutical drugs are also modified by this liver system, and having the right alleles there makes one more or less susceptible to the actions of the drugs. For example, there are alleles that make the drugs less active. So if you're going to metabolize the drug more, you'll need more drug to come in in the first place. This is why drug companies sponsor the private effort in sequencing the human genome. They wanted to identify, and still do, what these alleles are. Many diseases, such as cancer and heart disease, have complex causes, and many, many gene products are interacting. Genes are now being identified in the human genome for these complex diseases.

When looking at the genome and disease susceptibility, you could have alleles of those susceptibility genes as well.

The age of genomics is really upon us, and genetic testing is now going to make it possible to predict which complex diseases a person might develop later in life. An amazing and special type of genetics helps us fight invading harmful organisms. In the next lecture, we turn to the immune system. Thank you.

Lecture Nineteen
Molecular Medicine—The Immune System

Scope: The immune system identifies substances that are not part of an individual's genetic makeup and reacts to them by eliminating them. For example, this happens when a person is exposed to a virus or a blood transfusion from an unrelated donor with different genes. White blood cells first identify the substance, called an antigen, as foreign to the body and then initiate a two-pronged response. White blood cells called T cells identify and attack any body cells harboring the antigen; B cells make proteins called antibodies that bind to and eliminate the antigen if it is in the bloodstream. There is tremendous diversity in antigens, so there must be diversity in the T and B cells that attack them. This diversity is generated by an unusual recombination of genes in the cells so that a few hundred genes can be randomly selected and combined to make millions of "super-genes" that code for proteins. Vaccines are inactive antigens that provoke an immune response that stands ready to rapidly eliminate the true antigens when they infect a person. Antibodies can be used as very sensitive detectors, as in the pregnancy test, or to bind to cancer cells to get the body to attack them.

Outline

I. Opening story: George Washington and smallpox.

    A. Smallpox has played a major role in history.

        1. "Finding smallpox to be spreading much, and fearing that no precaution can prevent it from running through the whole of our army, I have determined that the troops shall be inoculated. Should the disease rage with its usual virulence, we should have more to dread from it than from the sword of the enemy."

        2. So wrote the commander in chief of the U.S. Continental army to his chief physician on January 6, 1777. During the previous year, the disease had ravaged General Horatio Gates's American Northern Army. Of his 10,000 troops, over half got smallpox, and his military campaign had to be suspended for a month.

3. Commander George Washington knew whereof he wrote in that letter. When he was a teenager, he had a mild case of smallpox.
   a. As a survivor of this often-lethal disease, Washington developed a healthy respect for it.
   b. Washington had heard about inoculation. In Boston, Cotton Mather, the famous minister, watched three of his children nearly die of smallpox. Then, a slave from Africa, Onesimus, told him that in his homeland a person would be protected if a little dried pus from an infected person was put into a cut on the skin. When some sailors inadvertently brought smallpox to Boston and the next epidemic hit in 1721, Mather convinced a physician, Zabdiel Boylston, to try inoculating some normal, undiseased people. The epidemic was stemmed.
   c. The 1777 inoculation ordered by Washington was the first known inoculation of an army, and it worked well. Casualties from smallpox were greatly reduced.
   d. Smallpox claimed 300 million lives worldwide in the 20th century. As late as 1967, there were 15 million new cases and 2 million deaths due to the disease.
   e. A massive effort at inoculation led to the eradication of smallpox from the world in 1979.

B. A series of events in the immune system is involved in this story.
   1. Smallpox is caused by a virus that infects only humans. For 30% of people exposed, lethal infections such as pneumonia soon follow, and death is the inevitable result.
   2. Fortunately, after the virus entered Washington's body, some white blood cells engulfed it, digested it into pieces, and presented some of the viral protein fragments on their cell surface. Other white blood cells recognized this "I've got a protein" flag, setting in motion an army of cells that destroyed other cells harboring the virus. Still other white blood cells made antibodies, proteins in the blood that would bind up any virus outside of Washington's tissues. This two-pronged attack—cells to kill infected tissues and antibodies to bind up free viruses—swiftly reduced the infection to a mild one.
   3. After the infection subsided, most of these two armies of white blood cells died. But a small contingent remained, ready to do battle in case a new infection occurred.

4. These "memory cells" were behind the inoculation of the Continental army: When dead smallpox viruses entered the body through a cut in the skin, they looked enough like the real, live thing that they provoked the immune system to send in the two armies. Of course, there was no real infection to fight. Most of the cells went home (died!), but once again, memory cells stayed around, at the ready for a new infection.

II. The immune system involves cells and molecules.
   A. There are two purposes of the immune system.
      1. It recognizes nonself cells, viruses, or chemicals from self ones.
      2. It destroys the nonself agents before they can do harm.
   B. Three types of cells are major players; they are all white blood cells.
      1. Phagocytes surround and engulf nonself cells or viruses. They present the products of digestion on their surface.
      2. T cells recognize the nonself products in the cell surface. Some of them signal other T cells to attack other cells harboring the invader.
      3. B cells respond to the T cell signal by making antibodies.
   C. Three types of molecules play important roles in the immune system.
      1. Antigens are the nonself substances that provoke an immune response. They are any small chemical grouping that is foreign—that is, an arrangement of atoms that the particular individual does not have. A virus may have many of these groupings and provoke many immune responses. Many groupings on the viral surface may look just like self chemicals and not provoke the immune response at all.
      2. Antibodies are proteins made by B cells that bind to antigens. Since antigens are chemical groupings, they have a specific shape (lock). Antibodies fit into this shape exactly (key). Each B cell can make one specific type of antibody that fits an antigen.
      3. T-cell receptors are the proteins on the T cell surface that bind to antigen fragments presented by the phagocytes. Like antibodies, these receptors are highly specific for each antigen fragment, and there are millions of different ones.

III. The genetic control of the immune response is unusual.

    A. There are millions of different B cells, each making a specific antibody. There are millions of different T cells, each making a different T-cell receptor. These cells are constantly being made in small numbers. If they are not used (no antigen for them), they die within days. If they are used (antigen present), they divide many times and form the cellular army to perform their roles.

    B. Genetically, one might expect there to be millions of genes, one coding for each antibody or T-cell receptor protein. This cannot be so: We humans only have a total of 24,000 protein-coding genes.

        1. The solution is to combine alleles, each of which codes for a part of the antibody molecule (or T-cell receptor).

        2. For one type of antibody, there are many alleles for four regions in one of its chains: 300, 10, 5, and 2 = 30,000 possibilities for different chains (multiply the combinations), and 300, 1, 5, and 2 for the other chain = 3000 possibilities. So when the two protein chains that make up the final antibody are considered, there are $30,000 \times 3000 = 90$ million different types of antibodies! This from only 625 genes.

        3. These genetic shuffles are going on all the time to make T and B cells to respond to any possible chemical grouping that is not self. We can make antibodies to substances we have never seen and have not even been invented yet.

IV. The immune system can be manipulated in medicine.

    A. Vaccines make use of memory cells.

        1. After an infection, the T and B cells made in response to it die off, except for about 1% of them, which stay around as memory cells.

        2. This is why people who have had the flu won't get it twice that year: Their memory cells expand rapidly to fight off any new infection.

        3. A vaccine is an inactive or dead antigen. It provokes an immune response that leaves memory cells. These cells then fight off any infection by the real agent carrying that antigen.

        4. For viruses or bacteria that have a rapid rate of mutation (due to errors in DNA replication), the mutated infectious agent might be different in its antigen, and so the vaccinated person's T and B memory cells do not recognize it. This is why there is a new flu vaccine every year.

B. Antibodies can be used for detection and therapy.
   1. Because antibodies are so specific, they will bind to their target antigen in a mixture, like a magnet. Rosalyn Yalow and Solomon Berson invented the immunoassay—a way to tag an antibody so that the antigen it binds to would be tagged. This is the way that substances in tiny amounts such as hormones can be measured.
      a. Pregnancy is indicated when a developing embryo makes a hormone called human chorionic gonadotropin, which is released into the blood and urine. This is detected rapidly.
      b. The immunoassay also led to testing newborns for hypothyroidism and to eliminating their symptoms of retardation by giving them the missing hormone.
   2. Antibodies have been developed that bind to antigens that are expressed on cancer cells. These antibodies can be injected into a patient, and the binding initiates cancer cell death. The new drugs Herceptin (for breast cancer), Erbitux (for colon cancer), and Rituxan (for lymphoma) are in this class.

Essential Reading:

Jeremy M. Berg, John Tymoczko, and Lubert Stryer, *Biochemistry*, 6th ed. (New York: W. H. Freeman, 2006), chap. 33.

Lauran Sompayrac, *How the Immune System Works* (Malden, MA: Blackwell Science, 2002).

Supplemental Reading:

Richard Goldsby, Thomas Kindt, and Barbara Osborne, *Kuby Immunology*, 6th ed. (New York: W. H. Freeman, 2006).

Benjamin Lewin, *Genes VIII* (Upper Saddle River, NJ: Pearson Prentice-Hall, 2005), chap. 26.

Questions to Consider:

1. There is concern about the development of smallpox as a biological weapon. What are the challenges in making a smallpox vaccine?

2. HIV infects the T cells that orchestrate the immune response. How does this cause the immune deficiency in AIDS?

Lecture Nineteen—Transcript
Molecular Medicine—The Immune System

Welcome back. In the last lecture, I introduced the idea of molecular medicine by talking about screening for genetic mutations in humans. Now I'd like to continue this discussion of molecular medicine by talking about the special genetics of the immune system. My opening story is about smallpox. I'm going to read to you from a letter.

> Finding smallpox to be spreading much, and fearing that no precaution can prevent it from running through the whole of our army, I have determined that the troops shall be inoculated. Should the disease rage with its usual virulence, we should have more to dread from it than from the sword of the enemy.

This letter was written by the commander in chief of the U.S. Continental army to his chief physician, dated January 6, 1777. In the previous year, smallpox had ravaged General Horatio Gates's American northern army. Of 10,000 troops, over half of them got smallpox, and the military campaign had to be suspended for a month. The commander who wrote the letter, George Washington, knew whereof he wrote in that letter. As a teenager, Washington took his half brother Lawrence to the island of Barbados, hoping it would help with Lawrence's tuberculosis. The trip didn't do much good for Lawrence, but George came back with a souvenir, a mild case of smallpox. As a survivor of this often-lethal disease, George had developed a healthy respect for it.

A century before, smallpox had decimated the native population of the colonies. Two years previously, in 1775, it had incapacitated an army that he had dispatched from Massachusetts to lay siege on Quebec—at that time a nonindependent colony—hoping to convince the Canadians to join the Union. Washington had heard about inoculation. In Boston, the famous minister Cotton Mather watched three of his children nearly die of smallpox. Then a slave of Mather's from Africa, Onesimus, told him that in his homeland a person would be protected from this disease if a little dried pus from an infected person was put on skin that had been cut—interesting idea. In 1721, some sailors inadvertently brought smallpox to Boston, and the next epidemic began.

Mather convinced a physician, Zabdiel Boylston, to try inoculating some normal, undiseased people in the way that his slave had described. Boylston did so, first on two slaves as well as his own son. When it worked—they didn't get smallpox—he did it on many others, and the result was that this particular epidemic of smallpox was greatly stemmed in Boston. The 1777 inoculation ordered by Washington in the letter that I read to you was the first known inoculation of an army, and it worked pretty well. Casualties to smallpox were greatly reduced, and history tells us that the colonists, of course, won the Revolutionary War. Smallpox claimed about 300 million lives in the 20th century. It's always, until very recently, been a serious disease. In 1967 alone, 15 million new cases of smallpox were detected, and there were two million deaths. In 1979, however, inoculation, which had gone on worldwide since the 1960s, led to the eradication of smallpox from humans. It's one of the great successes of public health.

A series of events in the immune system, the system that fights disease, is involved in this story of George Washington and smallpox. Smallpox is caused by a virus whose genome contains DNA. This virus only infects humans, and that, by the way, was the key to eliminating smallpox from the world, because if we got rid of transmission from human to human, inoculated everyone, the virus would have nowhere to go. There are very few smallpox viruses still existing. We keep stocks of the virus in case it comes back in some way, in case some other virus mutates to be smallpox. There are pox viruses that affect animals, for example, so we worry about that. The virus is kept under very close lock and key.

Back to George Washington. The teenaged George Washington who contracted smallpox probably caught it by being around a victim of smallpox on his trip to Barbados and breathing in droplets that contained the virus, the typical mode of infection. It's quite contagious. After two weeks, Washington probably got a severe rash, and the remains of it probably scarred him for life. He had little spots. You don't see these spots on pictures of George Washington. Of course, Washington was not a famous guy until he was well into his 40s, so there aren't any paintings of George Washington as a youth showing the ravages of smallpox that he had been exposed to several years previous.

About 30% of people who are exposed, as Washington was, get pneumonia. Serious infections soon follow, and death is inevitable. Now fortunately, Washington's immune system, the system that fights disease, fought off the infection in several steps. After the smallpox virus entered Washington's body, some white blood cells called phagocytes—"phago" means "eat"— engulfed the virus. They digested it to small pieces, chopped it up, and they presented some of these protein fragments of the virus on their cell surface. Then other white blood cells called T cells recognize this flag called "I've got a protein"—and this set in motion a series of events. This series of events signaled a still other group of T cells called killer T cells to come in and destroy not only the cell that had the virus sticking out, but any other cell that had the virus in it. That's called the cellular immune system, the T cell immune system.

Now still other white blood cells called B cells made antibodies. These are blood proteins that would bind up any viruses that were outside Washington's cells, that hadn't infected a cell but were in the bloodstream, for example. These antibodies would bind up to it. So these B cells made a whole army that would make antibodies that would bind them up. This two-pronged attack—cells to kill infected tissues and antibodies to bind up free viruses; that is, viruses that are out in the bloodstream—swiftly reduced the infection to a mild one in Washington's case. After the infection subsided, most of these two armies of white blood cells—the T cells attacking all the cells that harbored the virus, and the B cells making antibodies that were binding up and destroying the virus in the bloodstream—died. They went home. Well, they didn't go home; they died. That's a good way to reduce an army, isn't it? They died. These cells underwent programmed cell death.

But a small contingent of the armies remained, these armies specifically directed against smallpox. This contingent was ready to do battle in case a new infection occurred. It's a standing army of T and B cells. These are called "memory cells," and they were behind the inoculation of the Continental army. When dead smallpox viruses from the pus that was put into cut skin of the Continental army entered the body of these soldiers through the cut in the skin, they looked enough like the real live virus to provoke the immune system to send in the two armies. So the armies were sent in. They reproduced large numbers of T and B cells to fight this imaginary disease. There wasn't a real infection to fight at the time, and so once the armies fought this imaginary war, they died off as they normally would, but left memory cells. The memory cells stayed around, ready for a new infection. When these soldiers were exposed to a live virus, they had their standing army all ready to handle it before a serious infection occurred.

That's my introduction to the immune system. I'm going to talk about the immune system first of all in terms of the cells that it has—I've introduced them to you as T and B cells—and the molecules that it has. I've introduced one to you called antibodies. Then I'll describe how this system is controlled genetically. It's a highly unusual mode of genetic control. Then I'll describe how we can manipulate this immune system in molecular medicine. The purposes of the immune system are two. First, the immune system recognizes nonself things, things that aren't us—aren't me, my immune system—that are not cells of me: viruses, chemicals, anything from the outside that is not you. So it recognizes nonself from self. Second, after it recognizes, it destroys the nonself agents before they can do harm. It's a defense mechanism.

There are three types of cells that are major players, and they are all white blood cells. I've introduced them to you. First there are the phagocytes that surround and engulf the nonself cells, or viruses. They present products of digestion on their surface to signal the other two types of cells to do their thing. First, the T cells: The T cells recognize the nonself molecules on this presenting cell fragment. By the way, as a side note here, T cells are what HIV attacks, and that's why people with HIV end up susceptible to infections if they're not successfully treated. Some of these T cells signal other T cells to go and attack any other cells harboring the invader. Those are the killer T cells. Then the third type of cell is the B cells. B cells respond to the T cells signaling that there's an invasion by making antibodies that are specific proteins that bind up to the invader.

Three types of molecules play important roles in the immune system. The three types of molecules are antigens, antibodies, and what are called T cell receptors. First, antigens. Antigens are nonself substances. It's obviously something that's not in your body. We often refer to antigens as large things, like a smallpox virus is an antigen. "Anti" means it's antibodies, and "gen" means it generates, so it provokes the immune system to do something, to recognize and destroy. But really the agent that provokes the immune system is actually a small chemical grouping that has formed, this small chemical grouping that exists only in the invader and not in us. It's a particular arrangement of atoms that an individual doesn't have. A virus itself may have many of these particular groupings of atoms, so a single virus may provoke many different immune responses because it has different groupings of atoms. Some of its groupings, of course, are in common, and so they may have groupings in the viral surface that look just like self things that I have in myself, so that part of the virus doesn't provoke an immune response. But you can bet the virus has some things unique to the virus, and each one of them will provoke an immune response. That's an antigen.

Antibodies are proteins made by B cells that bind to antigens. Since antigens are chemical groupings that have a certain shape, then antibodies are proteins that have a shape that fits it, just like enzymes fitting their substrates. A three-dimensional structure of protein is designed to fit the antigenic group of atoms, lock and key. Each B cell can make only one specific type of antibody that fits a specific antigen. So when many B cells are made in an immune response to a complex substance like a virus, each one of them makes their own specific antibody. Wait a minute. Here's the problem. There are millions of potential antibodies, one for every possible chemical grouping that's not self.

Now, T cell receptors, the third molecule I want to introduce. These are proteins, like antibodies are, on the surface of a T cell. They're going to bind to (like a lock and key) to the antigenic fragment on a phagocyte. The phagocyte digests the virus to small pieces, presents these pieces that are antigenic, and now a T cell will bind to it and recognize it. Well, it's got to have a T cell receptor that recognizes that like a lock and key as well. So there's got to be millions of T cell receptors for millions of antigenic fragments in that system.

How does this specificity arise? The way that it happens is by, first of all, clonal selection of B and T cell specificity. There are millions of different T cells made, each of them with their T cell receptor to bind specifically to any antigen on the cell surface. If the antigen is present, the only cell that will be selected for division, and to make a clone or an army, will be the T cell that binds that antigen. For example, if a phagocyte digests the smallpox virus and sticks a piece of smallpox virus out, and that's antigenic, the particular T cell—now there's millions of T cells cruising around—that has its receptor that fits that one will then be signaled to make an army. You'll make a lot of T cells that fit that particular one. That's the one that will be a clone, a genetically identical cell, of that particular T cell.

By this same token, millions of different B cells exist, and each of them makes a specific antibody. The one that's selected for clonal expansion will be that B cell that makes an antibody against a particular antigen that's under consideration. The rest of them just hang around, and ultimately they will die. After the T and B cell response is over, almost all the clone dies—well over 90% of it dies—but some of them remain as immunological memory cells, so they're ready for the next invasion by that particular antigen.

So, clonal selection; how is this under genetic control? The genetic control of the immune system is highly unusual. Here is the challenge. There are millions of different B cells. Each of them makes a specific kind of antibody against a potential antigen, just like there are millions of different groups of atoms that I don't have. That particular group and arrangement of atoms presents a surface; there's got to be an antibody that'll fit that. So millions. There are millions of different T cells. Each of them makes a T cell receptor, just like there are millions of different invading virus groups, and the virus can stick out on the surface of a phagocyte that digests it, and there are millions of T cells that'll bind to it. George Washington and you constantly make T and B cells that'll respond to smallpox long before you're ever exposed to that virus. I am making antibodies, I am making T cell receptors, that will bind to HIV. I've never been exposed to it.

Here's the problem with that type of model. That type of model assumes that there are millions of genes then, each one of them coding for a specific T cell receptor or specific antibody that would then bind up that particular group of atoms. It just can't be. We know from genome sequencing that the human genome has a measly 24,000 genes. I mentioned when I talked about the human genome that we can make do with 24,000 because we can do more things with them, but it nowhere approaches millions and millions and millions of potential chemical groupings. We can't have one gene for each protein; one gene for each T cell receptor, another gene for mutant 1, another gene for allele 2, another gene for allele 3, another gene for allele 4, up to millions. We just don't have enough DNA to do that.

The solution is a very interesting one in terms of genetics and protein synthesis. We have separate subgenes that code for regions of the antibody or the T cell receptor. Consider a protein that has four different regions in it: region A, region B, region C, region D. If we want to make 16 different proteins here, we could have four subgenes and two alleles each, and then splice them together. Remember I told you about alternate splicing at the messenger RNA level to make different proteins. Now we have alternate splicing of DNA. So we could have eight alleles, and we could choose allele number one from subgene A, allele number two in subgene B, allele number one in subgene C, and allele number two in subgene D. So now the possibilities are the product of the independent, which is $2 \times 2 \times 2 \times 2$, which is 16 possibilities.

Now let me describe the reality of the number of genes we have in an actual antibody protein. Antibody proteins have four chains. The actual mature protein has four chains. They're called heavy and light chains. The two heavy chains are identical, and the two light chains are identical. So for our purposes, we'll say it's got a heavy and a light. The variable region in this Y-shaped protein is what actually binds to the antigen. This is the region at the variable end. It is the region that binds to the antigen. Now let's look at the number of genes and the number of alleles that are involved. In the heavy chain, there are four genes, four subgenes. These four genes that are actually separate genes—I'll call them subgenes—have the following number of alleles: 300 (region A), 10 (region B), 5 (region C), and 2 (region D). The total possibilities here—if we combine them, combine the DNAs, for example—I could make a protein off of subgene 17 from the 300, subgene 3 from the 10, subgene 1 from the 5, subgene 2 from the 2. So I multiply them out: $300 \times 10 \times 5 \times 2$ is 30,000 possibilities. The total number of alleles, however, is 317—not much DNA to make 30,000 different proteins; very clever.

For the light chain, the second chain of the antibody, there are 4 genes, and once again you have 300 in the subgene regions, 1—and only 1—, 5, and 2. Here we have 3000 different chains possible. So now we combine the possibilities of the light chains and the possibilities of the heavy chains, $3000 \times 30,000$: so 90 million different possible proteins can be made from a total of 625 alleles in DNA. That's a little bit of DNA, but we cut the splice and we can make lots of different possible antibodies. The same thing happens in making T cell receptors in cellular immunity. So this is a DNA shuffle. The rest of the alleles are lost. This amazing process, these genetic shuffles, are going on all the time to make T and B cells to respond to any possible chemical grouping that is not self. You and I are all making antibodies and T cell receptors to things we have never seen, or that have not been even invented yet.

This knowledge of the immune system I've described can be manipulated in medicine, and I'm going to describe a couple of examples of that, namely vaccines and antibodies, and then talk a little bit about monoclonal antibodies in terms of the antibodies for therapy. First, vaccines. Vaccines make use of memory cells. After infection, the T and B cells made in response to it, as I mentioned, die off, except for a couple of percent that are used and stay around as memory cells. That's why, as you recall with George Washington, and now we know from the flu, people who had the flu won't get it again in the same year. You already have built up memory cells against that strain of flu, so if it tries to invade you again, your army will knock it out before it can do much harm.

A vaccine is defined as an inactive or dead antigen; it's dead in terms of a virus or bacteria. It provokes an immune response and leaves the memory cells, and these cells will then fight off any infection when the real agent comes in. The infectious agent must carry the same antigen as the vaccine. I've made an army that recognizes a certain antigen. My T and B cell army is there. The memory cells stand ready to fight that antigen. But if the antigen now has mutated, like viruses do because they don't do very good repair of their genome when they replicate it, then there's a new variant of the virus coming in, and my memory cells don't recognize it anymore. That's why we need a new flu vaccine every year, because the flu virus is constantly mutating, and it presents a new shape, and the serum immunity doesn't recognize it anymore.

Antibodies can be used for detection and therapy. Because antibodies are so specific, they'll bind tightly to their target antigen in any kind of complex chemical soup. So we can have 5000 different chemicals in a solution, and if I take an antibody—it's like a magnet—it'll zero in on its specific antigen if it's there, and it'll only bind to it. The binding is extraordinarily tight, like a lock and a key. Rosalyn Yalow and Solomon Berson used this property of specificity to invent what's called an immunoassay. In this system, an antibody against a target antigen is tagged with color or some other way for detection. After the antibody binds to its target, the complex—that is the antibody or antigen—is separated. And if the antibody is attached to some paper or something like this, the complex would be on that paper and colored. The result is the antibody-antigen complex can be quantitated; we can measure how much is there, how much of the antigen is there, by how much binds to the antibodies.

This is extremely sensitive. You can measure tiny amounts of things like hormones, which we never used to be able to measure before. For instance, pregnancy is indicated when a developing embryo makes a unique hormone called the human chorionic gonadotropin. That's a hormone only made, essentially, by a developing embryo very early on, human chorionic gonadotropin. This hormone is released in the blood and the urine, so that's how you detect pregnancy. It's made by the embryo. In the old days, urine was injected into a female rabbit to find out whether it had this hormone. There was no way of finding out how much of the hormone was there. We couldn't detect it, the amounts are so small. So the urine would be injected into a female rabbit to see if the bunny developed large ovaries in response to the hormone. Sometimes the animal had to be killed to confirm the ovarian response to this hormone. Now we can do this by immunoassay in a minute, and there are home pregnancy kits that will do it.

Immunoassay is also used to test newborns for hypothyroidism, eliminating their symptoms of mental retardation, so it's no wonder that Rosalyn Yalow and Solomon Berson won the Nobel Prize for developing this technology. These antibodies can also be used to bind to antigens that are expressed on cancer cells. If an antibody against an antigen expressed in the cancer cell is injected into a patient, the antibody will zero in on the cancer cell, and this initiates cancer cell death. A number of drugs—Herceptin, for example, for breast cancer; Erbitux for colon cancer; Rituxan for lymphoma—are in this class of newly-developed drugs for treating cancer. They are antibodies that bind to antigens unique to tumor cells, and the binding initiates cell death.

In the next lecture, we'll continue with cancer, which is a major challenge to molecular medicine. Thank you.

Lecture Twenty
Molecular Medicine—Cancer

Scope: Rapidly increasing knowledge of the details of cancer at the molecular level has led to the development of new drugs like Gleevec, which is used to treat a form of leukemia. Tumors form because of inappropriate cell division. Cells normally have finely tuned genetically inherited internal and external controls of cell division. In addition, cells stick together in tissues. In cancer, these controls break down, and tumor cells divide, spread to other tissues, and even recruit their own blood supply. In some cases, an activated oncogene that stimulates cell division is brought into cells by a virus, and in other cases a person inherits a mutation in a tumor suppressor gene that cripples this gene that normally blocks cell division. In most cases, cancer is caused by a series of mutations in these genes. While some cancer-causing agents such as those in cigarette smoke are known, most are not. Cancer is treated by surgery, radiation, and chemotherapy.

Outline

I. Opening story: Molecular medicine treats cancer.

    A. A new treatment is targeted for a leukemia.

        1. Alan noticed that he tired easily and had shortness of breath, so he decided to see his physician.

        2. Tests showed that Alan had over 200,000 white blood cells per milliliter (one-fifth of a teaspoon): 40 times higher than normal. In the next few days, a hematologist took a sample from Alan's bone marrow and looked at the immature white blood cells. She saw an abnormality in the chromosomes called the Philadelphia chromosome, and the diagnosis was made: chronic myelogenous leukemia.

        3. In this type of leukemia, the DNA in two different chromosomes in an immature white blood cell is cut and spliced. Parts of two genes, ordinarily on separate chromosomes, come to be right beside one another. The cells carrying it are stimulated to divide rapidly.

        4. Alan, now under the care of an oncologist, was given drugs designed to kill any reproducing cells. One drug bound to

DNA, another interfered with making the nucleotide building blocks that make up new DNA, and a third inhibited the mechanism that partitions chromosomes to new cells during cell division. These drugs had bad side effects, but Alan stayed the course for six months. His white blood cell count went down to 80,000 cells per milliliter and then stalled. This was still 16 times higher than normal.

   5. Alan's oncologist now tried a new approach—a specific drug. During the 1990s, the molecular biology of this leukemia was described in detail. The new gene made by chromosome shuffling was sequenced and its protein product studied. Chemists went into the lab and designed a drug that would specifically bind to and inactivate the new gene product in the tumor cells.

   a. At the University of Oregon, Dr. Brian Druker coordinated a clinical trial, in which patients like Alan who were stalling in conventional treatment were given the drug.

   b. It worked: Alan's white blood cell count went down to 5400. There were no white blood cells with the abnormal chromosomes in his bone marrow. He was cured.

B. The development of this drug, Gleevec, is the prototype of the molecular approach to cancer treatment.

C. The aim is to find out precisely what is going wrong in a tumor cell and design rational treatments on this basis.

II. Cancer develops in stages.

A. Cancer cells are different from normal cells.

   1. Cancer cells lose control over cell division. Normally, cells have two strategies to control when and where they will divide.

   a. Internal controls: Normally, an internal "clock" triggers events in the cell division cycle. Each event is under separate control, and this determines whether and how fast the cell divides. Most mature, specialized cells don't divide (like the white blood cells in the bloodstream). Immature cells divide rapidly (like the ones in bone marrow). What keeps cells from dividing is a set of proteins called tumor suppressors that act as "brakes." These act at the control points, for instance to block DNA from replicating. Cancer cells have defective tumor suppressors ("bad brakes").

   b. External controls: Hormone-like proteins called growth factors stimulate cells to divide by acting like a "gas pedal" on the cell cycle control points. Genes whose protein products stimulate cell division are called oncogenes. Cancer cells often make their own growth factors (self-stimulate) or have changes that make them hypersensitive to even tiny amounts of growth factors. They turn on the "gas pedal."

2. Cancer cells can spread to other organs. This is the most feared aspect of cancer, called metastasis. It makes cancer hard to treat (you can't operate to remove tumors that are all over the place) and leads to multiple organ failure.

   a. Normal cells have a "glue" that is adherent and specific. Cancer cells lose this adhesion.

   b. Cancer cells can detach from a growing tumor, chew up adjacent cells until they reach the bloodstream or lymph system, enter these vessels, travel to a new organ, and then stop there, growing a "satellite tumor" or metastasis. They even recruit nearby blood vessels to make branches to the tumor, ensuring it oxygen and nutrients from the blood. This is called angiogenesis.

B. These events—inactivation of tumor suppressors, activation of oncogenes, metastasis, and angiogenesis—occur in sequence. Cancer is a multistep disease.

III. Cancer is a genetic disease, but not usually inherited.

A. The major events in the development of cancer all involve the expression of genes: oncogenes, tumor suppressor genes, metastasis genes, and angiogenesis genes.

   1. Viruses can bring active oncogenes into cells.

      a. Tumor viruses were first discovered by Peyton Rous in 1910, when he showed that a muscle (meat) tumor in chicken could be passed from bird to bird in the hen house, and that this passage was virus induced.

      b. Tumor viruses have active oncogenes (e.g., for growth factors), so when they get into cells they stimulate cell division.

       c. Only about 10% of human cancer is caused by viruses. The most important ones are hepatitis B virus, which causes liver cancer, and a papillomavirus (warts), which causes cervical cancer. In both cases, antiviral vaccines are being used to prevent infection and cancer.

   2. Inherited mutations in tumor suppressor genes can allow cells to divide inappropriately.

       a. About 10% of cancers are inherited. These include 10% of breast cancer and colon cancer, as well as some childhood tumors.

       b. Compared to sporadic (noninherited) cancers, inherited tumors occur earlier in life (e.g., in breast cancer, in the 20s and 30s instead of after their 50s) and in numerous places (e.g., in breast cancer, in multiple locations and/or both breasts, instead of one tumor in one breast).

       c. Arthur Knudson proposed a "two-hit" hypothesis for inherited cancer. For tumor suppressor genes, both copies must be mutated to make inactive proteins so that cell division is no longer blocked. People with inherited cancer have one bad allele already through inheritance; they just need a mutation in a cell with the "good" allele to have no good tumor suppressor protein made.

B. Most cancers are sporadic and need many mutations in their cells to form. This means that carcinogens (which cause cancer) are usually mutagens (they damage DNA).

   1. Spontaneous mutations can lead to cancer. Many people get cancer with no risk factors for carcinogen exposure. Recall that errors in DNA replication can lead to mutations.

   2. There are some known carcinogens. These include cigarette smoke (which damages specific tumor suppressor genes in lung cells) and ultraviolet light from the sun (damages skin cell DNA in many genes).

   3. Most carcinogens are natural substances in the diet, and in most cases we now know what they are.

IV. There are three ways to treat cancer.

  A. Surgery is the most common treatment.

   1. Removal of a localized tumor can be curative.

2. Much of cancer surgery has become conservative of surrounding tissue, as another treatment is used to get rid of any surrounding tumor in the area.
B. Radiation is used on localized regions that cannot be removed in surgery.
   1. This might be in a diffuse area, or if a tumor is right against a vital organ.
   2. Radiation damages DNA. The amounts used are very large and focused on the tumor. Lifetime exposure of a person to radiation from all sources is 0.12 gray [a physical unit]; during the course of radiation treatment, the tumor gets 50 gray in a month. This is 400 times the lifetime dose!
C. Chemotherapy is used when tumors have spread over the body.
   1. Typical chemotherapy drugs kill all dividing cells, including the tumor. So there are side effects where there are dividing cells in normal tissues (bone marrow, intestines, skin, etc.).
   2. There is a wide array of drugs that block cell division. Some are natural products, others are synthetic.
   3. Precise molecular descriptions of the chemical biology of cancer are leading to targeted chemotherapies in molecular medicine.

Essential Reading:

Vincent DeVita Jr., Samuel Hellman, and Steven Rosenberg, *Cancer: Principles and Practice of Oncology* (Philadelphia: Lippincott Williams and Wilkins, 2005).

Lauren Sompayrac, *How Cancer Works* (Sudbury, MA: Jones and Bartlett, 2004).

Robert Weinberg, *The Biology of Cancer* (New York: Garland Science, 2007).

Supplemental Reading:

Ricki Lewis, *Human Genetics*, 7th ed. (New York: McGraw-Hill, 2006), chap. 18.

Gerald Litwack, *Human Biochemistry and Disease* (New York: Academic Press, 2007).

Questions to Consider:

1. A vaccine was developed against human papillomavirus, which causes genital warts and cervical cancer. Since this is a sexually transmitted disease, who should get the vaccine? Why is there some controversy about its widespread use?

2. What is the difference between the molecular medicine approach to cancer treatment and the conventional approaches now used?

Lecture Twenty—Transcript
Molecular Medicine—Cancer

Welcome back. In the previous two lectures, I've introduced you to molecular medicine. First, I introduced genetic screening, where we looked for mutations in humans that are connected to human disease. In the last lecture, I described the unique genetics that controls fighting diseases in the immune system. Now I'd like to turn to cancer. My opening story is about Alan. Alan first noticed it when he was at the gym. He tired easily, and it got worse over several weeks. When he began to have shortness of breath even when he walked from room to room at home, he decided to see his physician. When his doctor looked at a drop of blood under the microscope, he saw many white blood cells. This was unusual because white blood cells are usually dwarfed in numbers compared to red blood cells.

A blood sample of Alan's was sent to the laboratory, and the lab confirmed that he had over 200,000 white blood cells per milliliter; a milliliter is about 1/5 of a teaspoon. This is 40 times normal. In the next few days, a hematologist—that is, a specialist who looks at blood—looked at bone marrow as well as the blood of Alan and found a lot of immature white blood cells. In addition, she saw an abnormality. This was a funny-looking chromosome called the Philadelphia chromosome. The diagnosis was made at this time of chronic myelogenous leukemia. No one knows how, but in this disease, chronic myelogenous leukemia, a type of white blood cell cancer, the DNA in two chromosomes inside an immature white blood cell is cut and spliced.

Two chromosomes exchange material so that parts of two genes that are ordinarily on separate chromosomes come to be right beside one another. Think of it this way. Supposing we have two sentences: "This course is good," and the other sentence is, "Politicians are boring." Now we can cut and splice; then we can get totally different meanings, can't we, if we take the last words and change them. The shuffled chromosome that was seen in Alan's white blood cells was first noticed by scientists in Philadelphia in 1960, so that's where it got its name. White blood cells carrying this strange chromosome are stimulated to divide very rapidly, and so you had this huge number of cells in Alan.

Now, first Alan was treated with standard chemotherapy. He was under the treatment of an oncologist, who is a specialist in cancer, and was given drugs designed to kill any reproducing cells; not just the reproducing cells of his cancer, but these drugs will kill other cells as well. It's a side effect. One of the drugs bound to DNA. A second drug blocked the assembly of the building blocks of DNA. A third drug blocked the mechanism that partitions chromosomes to new cells during cell division. As I mentioned, these drugs had bad side effects on other dividing cells, but Alan stayed the course for six months. His white blood cell count went down from 200,000/ml to 80,000/ml and then stalled. This is still 16 times normal.

The drugs that Alan took blocked cell division all over the body, as I mentioned. They were nonspecific. They weren't specific for his tumor. Alan's oncologist now tried a new approach, a specific drug. In the 1990s, the molecular biology of this leukemia was described in detail. You'll remember that molecular biology is the study of the large molecules in the cell, of DNA, the genetic material, and of protein, which is the expression of genes. The new gene made by this genetic shuffling for the Philadelphia chromosome was sequenced, and its protein product was studied—an example, by the way, of reverse genetics. We got the DNA sequence first, and then we found out what the protein was. And indeed, the protein turned out to be a terrific cell division stimulant. It causes cells to divide without control.

The next step was that chemists at a drug company went into the laboratory and designed a brand-new substance, a chemical that would specifically bind to and inactivate this new gene product in the tumor cells—unique to this unique target. At the University of Oregon, Dr. Brian Druker coordinated a clinical trial with this drug, in which patients with CML, chromic myelogenous leukemia, were given this drug, first to test for its safety and then to test for its effectiveness. Patients like Alan who were stalling in conventional treatment, whose blood concentration of white blood cells was still high, were given the new drug, and the result was spectacular. In Alan's case, his white blood cell count went down to a normal 5400/ml. In fact, when the hematologist looked at Alan's white blood cells, she found no cells with abnormal chromosomes in his blood or in his bone marrow. He was cured. The development of this drug, which is called Gleevec, is the prototype, is the great example, of a new molecular approach to cancer treatment. The aim is to find out precisely what's going wrong in a tumor cell and design rational treatments on this basis.

For the remaining time in the lecture, I want to describe cancer. First, I'll talk about cancer developing in stages. Then I'll describe how cancer is a genetic disease, but it's not usually inherited. And finally, I'll describe the ways that we treat cancer. First, the development of cancer. Well, we all know that cancer cells are different from normal cells, and one of the hallmarks of cancer cells, and there are many, is that cancer cells lose control over cell reproduction. They just reproduce without control. Normally, cells control when and where they reproduce, and they do it, really, in two ways. First, there are internal controls. Normally, there is an internal clock inside a cell—and actually, biologists use this term, "clock"— that triggers events in the cell division cycle.

Now, from Lectures Three, Four, and Five, you can envision what some of these events to reproduce a cell should be. The first one is going to be duplicating DNA. The second will be packaging DNA into compact chromosomes, structures we can actually manipulate. The third will be separating the chromosomes from one another so that each new cell gets a complete set of chromosomes; and finally will be dividing that big cell that has these two nuclei, both with the entire chromosome set, into two smaller cells. Each of these four processes I've just described is under separate control, and each control determines whether, and how fast, cell division will occur. Now, most mature—and I tell my students that is in older people like me—no, no, mature is a specialized cell, if we're describing a cell. A mature cell is a white blood cell, not an immature white blood cell in the bone marrow. A mature cell doesn't divide, like a white blood cell. It's out there; it does its function. It's not dividing. And it's almost a mathematical axiom, like a statement of fact, in biology that cells that are specialized do not divide.

Immature cells, on the other hand, divide rapidly. Think of an embryo, or think of the bone marrow where there are cells constantly dividing to replace cells that die. What keeps cells dividing is a group of proteins that stimulates them, and what prevents them from dividing is a set of proteins that blocks them from cell division. And because they block tumors from forming, we call them tumor suppressors. Think of them as the brakes in an automobile. These proteins in the cell that are under the control of genes, DNA, act at these control points—DNA duplication, separating chromosomes, et cetera—for cell division. Cancer cells have defective tumor suppressors. They have mutations in their DNA that cause the protein that normally functions to block cell division to not function. It's like having bad brakes in the car. Cars will move really well if you don't have the brakes on.

Now, those are the internal controls in cell division. There are also external controls in cell division. The external controls are hormone-like substances called growth factors; it's a very apt term. They stimulate cells to divide by acting like a gas pedal in a car at the cell cycle control points. So, at every one of these control points, there is a gas pedal that makes it go forward, and there's a brake that keeps it from going forward. Let me give you an example of what we mean by a growth factor. I talked in a previous lecture about blood clots and getting rid of blood clots. Remember we talked about biotechnology. We had a brand-new drug that would dissolve away blood clots. Well, now I want to talk about clot formation. So a blood clot forms, and then the wound heals. The skin around the blood clot heals, and the clot, as we would say, goes away. The going away was the subject of the previous lecture.

These cells that surround the blood clot have to be stimulated in some way to do so. Those cells have to surround the blood clot and close the wound. Now, closing the wound is not a biological term. There must be a lot of cell division going on there. It turns out, just as these are the cells that close the wound, that stimulate the clot to dissolve, the cells that form the clot stimulate the cells above it to heal. So the clot cells, the cells that form the blood clot, make a growth factor that stimulates the skin cells to divide, reproduce, and then heal the wound. It's a very good example of a growth factor. Genes whose protein products stimulate cell division in this way are called oncogenes. "Onco" means "mass"; "genes" obviously are genes. An oncologist deals with a mass, which is a tumor. Cancer cells often make their own growth factors; they stimulate. So they will have an oncogene that has either been mutated or its promoter has been mutated, so it's making a constant stimulation for cell division. Other cancer cells may have genetic changes that make them hypersensitive to even tiny amounts of growth factors. So these are the genes, the oncogenes, that turn on the gas pedals of cell reproduction.

The most fearsome aspect of cancer is that cancer cells can spread to other organs. This is called metastasis, and it makes cancer hard to treat. You can't do surgery if a tumor is all over the place. This leads to multiple organ failures, and it's really what very often causes people to die of cancer. Think of metastasis in the following way. Normal cells have a glue that causes the cells to stick to one another, and this glue is specific. The skin cells—and if you're driving your car, please don't do this. If you pinch your skin, you will notice that the cells of the skin stick together and are separate from the bone.

They don't stick to the bone at all. The cells can stick to each other, but not to the bone, so they must have a specific skin cell surface molecule that allows them to stick. Well, these are proteins; they're cell recognition and adhesion proteins. Cancer cells lose this adhesion.

There are several steps in metastasis, in a tumor spreading. First, cancer cells have to lose their adhesion and detach from a growing tumor at one place in the body. Then the cells make a beeline for the blood system or lymphatic system, which is a different, but related, system in the body where cells can move. So they chew up, as they're making this beeline for the blood, the adjacent cells and tissues to get to the bloodstream. Then these tumor cells have to enter the blood vessels, and in the blood, they'll go through the blood as a red blood cell would, and they travel to an organ. Then they stop at the new organ. They weasel their way out of the blood and into the new organ, and now they grow a satellite tumor, or metastasis. We know all of these steps in great detail at this point.

During the process of growth of a metastasis, or even of a normal tumor, the metastasis must recruit nearby blood vessels to make branches to the tumor. All cells, all tissues of the body, need oxygen to survive, and they need the blood to take away things they don't want, like carbon dioxide and waste products. If you don't have blood, you're going to die as a tissue. Well, the tumor needs that. It's a bunch of cells, and it literally sends signals out to the nearby blood vessels and says, hey, come here; make a branch and send blood over to here. This process is called angiogenesis. You hear of angiograms, which visualize the blood vessels. Angiogenesis means starting new blood vessels. These four events—inactivation of tumor suppressors, activation of oncogenes (turn on), metastasis (spreading), angiogenesis (getting blood vessels)—occur in sequence. So, we can define cancer as a multistep disease.

Now I want to turn to cancer as a genetic disease and talk about the genes involved in these four processes. These four events I've just described are obviously controlled by genes, which we all have, and these genes are getting changed or turned on in some way. Oncogenes, tumor suppressor genes, metastasis genes, angiogenesis genes are all getting inappropriately expressed. Now there's a couple of ways we can get these genes inappropriately expressed. One of them is to bring an active oncogene into a cell. If a cell has an oncogene that is not being expressed, a virus can actually bring it into the cell. Tumor viruses were discovered in a very interesting way in 1910 by Peyton Rous, working at what was then called the Rockefeller Institute in New York City and is now the Rockefeller University.

He got a call from chicken farmers on Long Island that the chickens were all getting these weird horrible tumors on their meat, and it was spreading throughout the chicken coops, and so he thought this is maybe a communicable disease. He went out to Long Island, and to make a long story short, he showed that there was a virus that was spreading from chicken to chicken and causing this muscle tumor, which is called a sarcoma. It would be passed from bird to bird in the house. He did this by using Koch's postulates, where he isolated the virus and then infected a naive animal who didn't have the tumor, and showed that the animal got the tumor. Then from the tumor in that animal, he re-isolated the virus and repeated.

Rous was awarded the Nobel Prize in 1966, 56 years later. Why did it take that long to recognize him? It took a long time because people thought this is kind of specialized. No one really wanted to believe that cancer could be a communicable disease. People started looking at proteins and DNA after 1910, 1920, as we know, and sort of attention in biochemistry shifted and kind of put this on the back burner. In the 1950s and '60s, it got back on the front burner. It's good for all scientists to know that you can still win a Nobel Prize 56 years after you do your work. There's hope for all of us. Now tumor viruses, it turns out, have actively expressed oncogenes. So, there's a tumor virus that has an actively expressed oncogene for that growth factor that comes from the blood platelets that go to the wound-healing cells. When these active oncogenes get into a cell, brought in by the tumor virus, they stimulate cell division.

Approximately 10% of human cancer is caused by viruses. In our society, there are two major ones that are important. First, hepatitis B virus is associated with liver cancer; and second, a papillomavirus, or genital warts, is associated with cervical cancer. In both cases, the good news is antiviral vaccines are being used and developed so that people will be able to take a vaccine and prevent getting this cancer, which is essentially communicable. Inherited mutations in tumor suppressor genes can allow cells to divide inappropriately. It turns out about 10% of cancers are inherited. I said 10% are caused by viruses, and 10% are inherited. This includes about 10% of breast cancer, 5% of colorectal cancer, a larger percentage of some solid tumors of childhood. Compared to noninherited cancers—these are also called sporadic—inherited tumors typically occur earlier in life—for instance, inherited breast cancer will be in women in their 20s up to the 30s, instead of usually after their 50s—and in numerous places. For instance, you won't have an isolated breast cancer in one breast. You might have multiple locations in one breast or in both breasts.

After looking at the data comparing inherited and sporadic cancers in the two ways we've described, early onset and multiple tumors for heredity, Arthur Knudson proposed what he called the "two-hit" hypothesis involving tumor suppressor genes and inheritance. The tumor suppressor genes normally block cell division. Recall from Mendelian genetics, most cells have two copies of every gene. Knudson proposed that for tumor suppressor genes, both copies have to be mutated so that the only proteins made are inactive ones, so cell division can no longer be blocked. It's like taking your foot off the brakes and releasing the parking brake to let your car move forward. You need both types of brakes. Both alleles of the tumor suppressor gene must be off.

People with inherited cancer have already inherited in all of their cells one bad allele. And so if later on they get a mutation in that cell of the second allele, they'll get a tumor. That can happen reasonably soon; whereas people who inherit two normal alleles need two mutations, and that's going to happen later on. Most cancers turn out to be sporadic, so they need many mutations in order for the tumor to form. What do I mean by many mutations? Not only in the tumor suppressor genes, but remember oncogenes are turned on, metastasis genes are turned on, angiogenesis genes are turned on. So you need all these events to occur in a sequence. These mutations have to occur in all of these four processes in order for a tumor to finally happen.

A doctor at Johns Hopkins University, Bert Vogelstein, and his colleagues spent a lot of time during the 1990s looking at the sequence of genetic changes of these four types that I have described. Specifically, he looked at colorectal cancer, which develops first as a small group of cells called a polyp in the colon, and then that group of cells gets larger and larger and larger over time. You can actually follow these. In a colonoscopy, the objective, of course, is to remove the polyp before it becomes a tumor. But if you remove the polyp, you obviously have a sample of an early, very early, cancer. So what Vogelstein did was make a survey of all of the genes involved in cancer in these polyps as they went through the stages developing to colorectal cancer.

What he found was a very dramatic series of events. That is, first there were mutations in tumor suppressor genes, and then there were mutations in oncogenes in the cells, and then there were mutations in metastasis genes, so they would detach. And finally, when they detached and became antistatic, there were mutations in angiogenesis genes to turn them on. Describing cancer in this amount of molecular detail is an amazing achievement of modern biology and medicine, and it will lead to treatments, as we have seen in the case of Gleevec.

Now, if we're talking about genetic changes, of course, we're talking about the fact that anything that causes cancer must be causing these genetic changes. So I've described two ways that DNA can change in this course. First, there are spontaneous mutations. Spontaneous mutations are ones that we get just by the fact that we're made of DNA. Many people get cancer with no risk factors of any kind of bad stuff that they're being exposed to. This is because of errors in the duplication of DNA or other chemical reasons. This is a rare event, but think of the fact that the body has trillions of cells and that cancer can come from one cell that goes bad in a number of ways. The second type of mutations are induced mutations: mutations that are caused by something else, something from the outside. Most cancer mutations are caused by the environment; no question about that.

We know one environmental factor quite well from an earlier lecture: cigarette smoke. You'll remember that damages a specific tumor suppressor gene. You'll remember the molecule, benzpyrene, that bound to DNA in a specific gene in the lung called p53, and it's a tumor suppressor gene. Now we can understand a little more of what that does. Benzpyrene causes DNA of p53 to get mutated, and so this no longer acts as an active tumor suppressor gene. Ultraviolet light from the sun causes skin cancer, DNA damage. However, these things are obvious—cigarette smoke, ultraviolet light. For the case of most cancer-causing things, we really don't know what's going on. In fact, many carcinogens—things that cause cancer—are natural substances in the diet. In most cases, we just haven't identified them yet.

Let me repeat that. Many carcinogens are dietary, and we haven't identified them. They're not the things that you might think of, the preservatives and other things in foods. They're natural molecules that plants make to defend themselves that are there in small amounts. How do we know this? We know it—that diet is important—because of country differences in cancer incidence, and the fact that when someone moves from one country to another, they, and then their offspring—who are the same genetically; haven't changed much genetically—will adopt the cancer rate of their new country. When you look very carefully, you find that it's probably diet.

There are three ways to treat cancer, and those three ways are surgery, radiation, and chemotherapy. First, surgery. Surgery is by far the most common treatment of cancer. Removal of a tumor that is localized, that is in one place, can be curative. That's how you cure cancer; you get rid of all the tumor. The surgeon says, we got it all. Much of cancer surgery in recent years has become conservative of the surrounding tissue. That is, any treatment used—and other treatments might be used to get rid of any surrounding tumor cells ... For example, the breast might be conserved by what is called a lumpectomy, and only the tumor can be removed, and then some other treatment will be used again to clean up any cells that remain.

Radiation is used in cancer treatment on localized regions that can't be removed in surgery. This might be in a very diffuse area, or it might be useful if there's a diffuse area around the tumor that's been removed, or it might be useful to shrink a tumor if it's up against a vital organ and the surgeon is afraid of damaging that vital organ. Radiation damages DNA. It causes both strands of DNA to be broken. It breaks the bonds between the beads on the chain of DNA. The amounts of radiation used are small from the military viewpoint, but quite large, and they're focused on the tumor. I'll give you an example. The lifetime exposure of radiation of a typical person on the earth from all sources is about 0.12, or 1/8 of a gray. Now don't worry about what the gray is as a unit; it's a physical unit. Just remember 1/8. During the course of radiation treatment, the tumor itself gets 50 gray over five weeks. That's 400 times the lifetime dose going to, we hope, a localized area. So radiation therapy is a highly scientific, highly focused procedure.

The third method of treatment is called chemotherapy, and that's general therapy for cancer. It's used when tumors have spread over the body because when you put a drug in the blood system, it'll be distributed everywhere in the body. Typical chemotherapy uses, as we saw with Alan, our patient in the opening story, drugs that kill all dividing cells, including the tumor. So there are side effects to chemotherapy anywhere where there are dividing cells in normal tissues, such as bone marrow, and the intestines, and skin, etc. A wide array of drugs that block cell division have been isolated and are used. Some are natural products we get from plants; others are synthetic—we build in the laboratory—as was the case of Gleevec.

Precise molecular descriptions of the chemical biology of cancer are leading to targeted chemotherapies and molecular medicine, such as our opening story.

In the next lecture, we turn to perhaps the most daring of all therapies based on genetics, and that is gene therapy. Thank you.

Lecture Twenty-One
Molecular Medicine—Gene Therapy

Scope: Gene therapy is the addition to humans for medical benefit of protein-coding DNA along with a promoter sequence for its expression. There have been many successful pilot experiments on animals, including the production of "marathon mice" with altered muscle composition and improved endurance. In humans, gene therapy can be done by removing cells from the body, adding the new gene, and reintroducing the cells (ex vivo). Or the gene can be given directly to the patient (in vivo). Approaches include adding a new gene to correct the effects of a defective one and adding a gene that enhances cell killing by the immune system or drugs. Disabled viruses are used as vectors. There have been some modest initial successes at gene therapy for genetic diseases and for cancer.

Outline

I. Opening story: Gene therapy for athletic performance?

    A. Gene therapy produces a marathon mouse.

        1. Sprinters are different from long-distance runners, and a lot of the reason is, not surprisingly, in their muscles. The skeletal muscles that move bones in your arms and legs have two types of fibers.

            a. Slow-twitch fibers need abundant oxygen from the blood to work well. They contain a lot of mitochondria, which are the energy-producing factories of cells and generate a long-lasting supply of energy for muscle contraction. They don't get tired.

            b. Fast-twitch fibers, on the other hand, don't need as much oxygen. They have fewer mitochondria and generate quick bursts of energy but fatigue easily.

            c. Not surprisingly, sprinters have more fast- than slow-twitch fibers, and in distance runners the situation is reversed.

            d. Training improves the blood supply and even changes the ratio of fibers somewhat. But a lot of the ratio appears to be genetically determined. You don't hear of a person winning both the marathon and the 100-meter dash.

  e. Distance runners also seem to burn fat effectively; they eat a lot and don't get fat.

2. Enter the marathon mouse. No, this isn't a video game or cartoon character. It's a mouse that has been treated with gene therapy to change the ratio of its slow- to fast-twitch fibers.

  a. Dr. Ron Evans, who created this mouse in his lab, found that a protein called PPAR-delta (if you need to know, the "PPAR" stands for "peroxisome proliferator-activated receptor") got fat tissue to break down stored fat for energy.

  b. Evans then wondered what would happen if mice were genetically modified to express a high level of PPAR-delta in muscles, which also need energy. He predicted that they would burn fat for energy. So he did gene therapy: He put the gene for PPAR-delta beside a promoter that would be expressed in skeletal muscle. This recombinant DNA was put into a vector, and the vector injected into fertilized mouse eggs.

  c. As expected, the genetically modified mice that grew up did not gain extra weight on a high-fat diet, as the PPAR-delta stimulated fat breakdown. What was unexpected was that the composition of the skeletal muscles changed from an even ratio of slow- to fast-twitch, to a marked increase in slow-twitch fibers. There were more mitochondria to burn the fat.

  d. The performance of the mice on an exercise wheel reflected the muscle fiber changes. The genetically altered mice ran almost twice as long and twice as far on a wheel as normal mice.

B. This serves as a good example of gene therapy, the addition of genes to humans or animals for medical purposes.

II. There are several strategies for gene therapy.

A. Gene therapy is based on several assumptions.

  1. We know the gene involved in a disorder.
  2. We have a normal copy of that gene.
  3. We know where and when the gene is normally expressed.

      4. We are pretty sure what will happen when the normal gene is expressed appropriately.

      5. Molecular medicine is giving us much of this knowledge.

B. Gene therapy must do the following:

      1. Get the gene to the appropriate cells.

      2. Get the gene expressed in the cells.

      3. Get the gene integrated into the genome of the target cells.

      4. Have no bad side effects.

C. The strategies for gene therapy are:

      1. Gene augmentation is used for diseases in which a functional gene product is lost. The idea is to introduce extra copies of the normal allele so that the protein product is made and function is restored. An example might be muscular dystrophy, in which the muscles lack dystrophin, an organizing protein.

      2. Targeted cell killing uses a gene that either produces a toxin that kills certain cells or stimulates the immune system to do so. This is useful in cancer, where it is called "suicide gene therapy."

      3. Targeted mutation correction attempts to replace a bad allele with a good one. This is needed if the harmful allele makes a harmful gene product. This might be useful in cancer where a mutation in an oncogene has occurred in which the gene product, a growth factor, is always made. This stimulatory allele must be destroyed.

D. Method 3 above has been used successfully on animals but not humans. The human clinical experiments (trials) have used methods 1 and 2. No one has suggested germ line gene therapy on eggs or sperm. All of the potential uses are on nonsex (somatic) cells.

III. There are several methods for human gene therapy.

A. In ex vivo therapy, cells are removed from the patient, the new gene added in the lab, and the cells put back into the patient.

B. In in vivo therapy, the DNA is actually added directly into tissues, by injection or some other way.

C. There are several DNA vectors for human gene therapy.

      1. These must be expression vectors with active promoters to express the gene of interest. They have the same requirements as vectors in recombinant DNA experiments on cells, plants, and animals: small size, a marker gene to show the vector got into the targeted tissue (harmless and easily detected gene product), and restriction enzyme sites for insertion of the DNA of interest. Most gene therapy vectors are viruses that are infective but have been genetically modified to not produce more viruses (they just get in and deliver their DNA).

2. Adenovirus: This is a large DNA virus that causes colds. The DNA remains outside of the cell's chromosomes, and so it will only affect the cell that gets the virus.

3. Adeno-associated virus: This small virus inserts its DNA into the host chromosome at a specific site (chromosome 19). It is not pathogenic (an advantage) but small in DNA carrying capacity (a disadvantage).

4. Retroviruses: These viruses use RNA as genetic material and reproduce in an unusual way. They incorporate their DNA into the host cells, but at any location, and so there is a chance they will get into the wrong place.

IV. Some gene therapy looks promising.

A. Very few successes have been reported in humans. The reasons are:

1. Therapy does not last long. Target cells often divide rapidly, and if the new gene does not get into most of them, the treated cells will be outnumbered.

2. Patients may mount an immune response to the vector. This has occurred unexpectedly, and all gene therapy was stopped for a time in 1999 when an 18-year-old boy died in this way.

3. Many diseases cannot be cured with a single gene therapy. Heart disease, diabetes, Alzheimer's, and arthritis are caused by defects in many genes interacting with the environment.

B. Here are some examples of gene therapy.

1. Severe combined immunodeficiency: A patient has neither cell-mediated nor humoral immunity due to a gene mutation for adenosine deaminase (ADA), which is normally expressed in white blood cells.

a. Prior treatment for this disease was to totally shield the patient from any germs in the environment (the "bubble boy") and give blood transfusions. Unfortunately, the bubble boy died of viral infection in a blood transfusion

from his sister. Recall that there must be a genetic match in transfusions.
   b. Then physicians tried giving the patients the missing protein, ADA, isolated from cows. This was moderately successful.
   c. Finally, they tried ex vivo gene therapy, using gene augmentation to supplement the ADA injections: The patient's white blood cells were removed and the good ADA gene inserted into them via a retroviral vector. The cells were put back into the patient and made ADA, lowering the dose of external ADA necessary. But these blood cells were T cells, and they died after a few months. Now the doctors do this gene therapy on bone marrow cells that live for years. Still, the gene therapy is only a partial treatment.

2. Familial hypercholesterolemia: A patient cannot remove cholesterol from the blood because of a gene mutation for the receptor expressed in the liver.
   a. Physicians tried gene therapy ex vivo, using gene augmentation to add the good gene for the receptor. A piece of liver was removed and the cells disaggregated in the lab. Then the gene was added by a vector and the cells grown to a larger number.
   b. Upon reinfusion to the patient, the therapy cells fused with the liver, continued to divide, and made enough receptor to restore most function.

3. Ornithine transcarbamoylase deficiency: A patient cannot break down ammonia released by amino acids in the liver; the ammonia is very toxic. Most die within a year of birth, but milder cases can live for years by taking a special diet and ammonia-reducing drugs. Gene therapy was done in vivo by adenoviral vector with the good gene injected into an artery leading to the liver. The virus infected liver cells, and they expressed the enzyme, lowering ammonia. This was done in milder cases, but has not yet been done on the severe cases in infants.

4. Cancer is the subject of most gene therapy trials. There have been two approaches:
   a. In vivo: gene augmentation by introduction of a virus expressing a tumor suppressor gene that is mutated in the

tumor. This has been done in lung cancer for the tumor suppressor gene p53 that is mutated so that its protein is nonfunctional in the tumor. Generally, recipients have been very sick patients who failed other therapies. Scientists have shown that the vector gets into the tumor, is expressed, and the patients generally live longer.

   b. Ex vivo: targeted cell killing by the removal of white blood T cells and addition of a T-cell receptor that binds to a tumor. The cells can home in on the tumor expressing the antigen to that receptor and stimulate an immune response to eliminate the tumor. This has been done for melanoma.

5. Muscle buildup is not just for athletes: In muscular dystrophy there is a lack of muscle repair and replacement by fat/fibrous tissue. Also, most older people have muscle wasting: Strength and mass decrease by up to one-third from ages 30 to 80. Finally, in some disabilities there is muscle wasting due to underuse: If we don't use it, the body does not repair it, and muscle cell death ensues.

   a. At the University of Pennsylvania, Lee Sweeney is finding what controls muscle repair. He has found two genes involved and the proteins they code for: IGF-1, which stimulates nearby cells to promote muscle buildup; and myostatin, which stimulates muscle breakdown.

   b. If the IGF-1 gene is added to mice, using an AAV vector for muscle expression, treated mice get bigger muscles.

   c. If gene therapy adds a protein that inhibits myostatin, muscles get bigger as well.

   d. Clinical trials are planned on patients with muscle disorders. There is concern that this may be abused by competitive athletes.

6. There have just been a handful of successes in gene therapy, which is proceeding with caution but promise.

Essential Reading:

Ricki Lewis, *Human Genetics*, 7th ed. (New York: McGraw-Hill, 2006), chap. 20.

Joseph Panno, *Gene Therapy: Treating Disease by Repairing Genes* (New York: Facts on File, 2005).

Supplemental Reading:

Susan Barnum, *Biotechnology: An Introduction* (Belmont, CA: Thomson Brooks-Cole, 2005), chap. 10.

Gavin Brooks, *Gene Therapy: Using DNA as a Drug* (London: Pharmaceutical Press, 2003).

Questions to Consider:

1. Do you think gene therapy to change the germ line, such as giving new genes to eggs, should be banned?

2. There have been many news stories of successful gene therapy in animal experiments but few in humans. Why?

Lecture Twenty-One—Transcript
Molecular Medicine—Gene Therapy

Welcome back. In the last three lectures, I've been describing molecular medicine. I talked about screening. I talked about the molecular biology and genetics of the immune system, and I talked about cancer. With few exceptions, most of this molecular biology discussion has been involved with describing things. We now have pretty good molecular descriptions of what's going on in cancer, and we're beginning to scratch the surface on treatment, using molecular genetics to treat. Now let's talk about gene therapy, which is really a dramatic way of improving a genetically caused disorder.

The skeletal muscles that move the bones in your arms and legs come with two types of muscle fibers. The first type are the slow-twitch fibers, and the other type are the fast-twitch fibers. First, slow-twitch fibers. Slow-twitch fibers need a lot of oxygen from the blood to work well. They contain a lot of these powerhouses of the cell I referred to earlier in the course, called mitochondria. Remember we talked about the mitochondrial DNA. The mitochondria happen to be these powerhouses of the cell that produce energy, so these are factories in the cell that produce energy. The mitochondria generate a long-lasting supply of energy from oxygen for muscle contraction. Slow-twitch fibers don't get tired. Fast-twitch fibers are different. They don't need as much oxygen as the slow-twitch fibers. They have far fewer mitochondria, and they generate quick bursts of energy, but they get tired easily.

Now it's not surprising that when you look at sprinters in the Olympics or in other athletic competitions, sprinters have more fast-twitch fibers than slow-twitch fibers. They get tired fairly easily, but they finish the race by the time they get tired. For distance runners, the situation is reversed. They have more slow-twitch fibers than fast-twitch fibers. Training improves the blood supply to muscles, and even changes the ratio of fibers somewhat, but a lot of this ratio of fast- to slow-twitch seems to be genetically determined. You don't hear of the same person winning both the marathon and the 100-meter dash in the Olympics. Distance runners also seem to burn fat effectively. My friends who run marathons seem to be able to eat a lot, and they just don't get fat.

Enter the "marathon mouse." Now this is not a video game or a cartoon character. No, it's a mouse that has been treated with gene therapy to change the ratio of its slow- to fast-twitch fibers. Ron Evans, a scientist at the Salk Institute in California, who produced this mouse in his laboratory, was not looking for a super athlete mouse. He was interested in the control of the breakdown of fat. He's an anti-obesity researcher. Evans had found in his laboratory, with his colleagues, a protein called PPAR-delta. Now if you need to know, "PPAR" stands for "peroxisome proliferator-activated receptor." We'll call it PPAR-delta. This protein seemed to be able to get fat tissue to break down stored fat in the fat stores of what is called adipose tissue, which is the tissue that stores fat. To put it mildly, the drug companies got very interested in what Evans was doing.

PPAR-delta is a transcription factor. It binds to the promoter for genes that produce the proteins that are involved in fat breakdown. Now let me review a little bit about promoters and transcription from earlier on in the course. Genes are expressed as proteins, and the intermediary between genes being expressed and the protein expression is messenger RNA, a copy of the gene, as you recall, that is sent out to the ribosome to then be translated into protein. The determination of which genes will get turned on and expressed in which tissue is a property of the promoter, the region adjacent to the gene. The promoter is a place where these proteins called transcription factors do their magic. They either turn genes on or turn genes off. In the case of PPAR-delta, it's a transcription factor that binds to promoters for a number of enzymes involved in the breakdown of fat.

Now, Evans had already done experiments to show that PPAR-delta, if you turn it on in fat tissue, will cause the fat tissue to shrink. No wonder the drug companies were involved. Now he wondered, what would happen if mice were genetically modified to express a high level of PPAR-delta in muscles? You know, muscles need energy just as any other tissue does, and fat breaks down to energy. So he predicted from his experiment that the mice would burn fat that's stored around the muscle for energy and that they might get leaner, as well, if this gene was also expressed in fat tissue. So Evans did gene therapy on the mouse. He put the gene for PPAR-delta, which is a protein, beside a promoter that would be expressed in skeletal muscle. This is recombinant DNA time. So he took this recombinant DNA, put it into a vector, and the vector was injected into fertilized mouse eggs. We've seen this technology before. Animals with the recombinant DNA were selected. He had a selectable genetic marker, as you would always do in recombinant

DNA work. And then these animals were tested for weight gain, composition of muscle, and performance.

Now the results. As he had hypothesized, the genetically modified mice did not gain extra weight on a high-fat diet. This PPAR-delta protein was being expressed in large amounts, and it stimulated fat breakdown in the fat stores and in the muscle. An unexpected result was that the composition of the skeletal muscles had changed from an even ratio of 50/50 slow- to fast-twitch to a marked increase in slow-twitch fibers. There were more mitochondria burning the fat. When he put the mice on an exercise wheel, the performance of the mice reflected these muscle fiber changes to more slow-twitch fibers. Normal mice can run about 90 minutes or 900 meters, about a half mile, before getting exhausted on a wheel. The genetically altered mice ran almost twice as long and twice as far. It was as if they were trained as elite athletes. Can gene therapy be used on muscle tissues to help produce long-distance human runners? Well, the answer is unclear, but athletic competition authorities are concerned. I'll come back to this later on in the lecture.

For now, this serves as a good example of gene therapy, which I define as the addition of genes to humans for medical purposes. In this case, we were doing it on mice, but it's the addition of genes for medical purposes to humans if we're talking about human therapy. There are several strategies for gene therapy. Gene therapy is based on a couple of assumptions. We have to know the following. First, we have to know the gene that is involved in the thing that we're doing therapy for. Second, we have to have a normal copy of that gene in our hands in the laboratory to put in for therapy. Third, we have to know when and where this particular gene is normally expressed. Fourth, we have to be pretty sure what's going to happen when the normal gene is expressed at its appropriate time and place.

The knowledge I just described is coming to us fairly rapidly by molecular medicine. The more molecular biology we describe of human tissues, the more we know which gene is turned on where and how. Gene therapy must do the following. First, gene therapy must get the gene into the appropriate cells. Second, gene therapy must get the gene expressed in those cells. Third, we have to get the gene hopefully integrated into the genome of the target cells so it'll be there permanently. Fourth, you better not have any bad side effects to gene therapy, like any therapy in medicine. Gene therapy has been the subject of numerous what are called clinical trials, experiments in humans with various disorders.

There are a couple of major strategies for actually doing the gene therapy. I've gone from the general to the particular. These three strategies are gene augmentation, targeted cell killing, and targeted mutation. First, what do I mean by gene augmentation? Gene augmentation is used for diseases where a functional gene product, the protein we need for function, has been lost, is no longer there. The idea of gene augmentation is to introduce extra copies of the normal allele for this gene that obviously has been mutated in a person. So this protein product will be made, and function is restored. I'll give you an example. We could hypothetically think of muscular dystrophy as a good target for gene therapy. We know that muscles lack the protein dystrophin. It's an organizing protein, so we'll put in the good gene for good dystrophin.

The second type of gene therapy is called targeted cell killing. Targeted cell killing uses a gene that either produces a poison that kills certain cells or stimulates the immune system to kill the cells. So targeted gene therapy is useful in cancer, where it's called "suicide gene therapy": suicide for the cancer cells. A gene is put into cancer cells that allows them to produce a protein that will make a toxic drug from a harmless chemical. So the idea is we inject a harmless chemical into the body. It goes all over the body, and when it enters a tumor cell, it's converted into a poison by the gene product of the gene that we've put in for gene therapy. Now the way to do this would be putting a gene into cells to enhance the immune system's reaction against the tumor. We might put in a gene that will cause a protein to be made that attracts killer T cells. So the tumor will stick up its hand and say, come kill me now. Good idea for cancer therapy.

Targeted mutation correction is the third method of gene therapy, and here we're pretty ambitious. We want to take the bad allele and replace it with a good one. We're not just going to add a good allele where the bad allele is already there; that's gene augmentation. We're going to take the bad one out, and we're going to replace it with a good one: genetic shuffling, if you will, gene replacement. This is needed if the harmful allele that is in the disease is making a harmful gene product, and no matter what we add, we can't overcome the effects of that harmful allele. It's called a very interesting term—this is called a "dominant negative gene product." It's negative, it's bad, and it's dominant. No matter what you do, it's going to be made. This is a gene we have to get rid of. Now this might be useful in cancer where, as I mentioned in the last lecture, a mutated oncogene—remember the oncogene turns on cell division—is making a growth factor that's saying, turn on cell division, turn on cell division. It's the gas pedal, right, continuously being made. Well, you can't do anything about that. The only thing you can do is to destroy that gene, and that's going to be hard to do.

This is targeted mutation correction. It's been used successfully in animal experiments, but not in humans at all. Human clinical trials, experiments, have been done using the other two methods, gene augmentation and targeted cell killing. No serious suggestion for looking at the germ line— that is, the cells that produce egg and sperm—for inherited characteristics by gene therapy has been made. No gene therapy on eggs and sperm. All potential uses of gene therapy now being proposed are on nonsex, or somatic, cells. We're in the dark here in a lot of instances, and so to play with the whole human genome and add new genes to a whole human genome and the sex cells is a little bit ambitious at this point.

There are a couple of ways to do gene therapy, and now I'm zeroing in even more. In ex vivo gene therapy, outside of life—"ex," outside; "vivo," life— cells are removed from the patient, the new gene is added in the laboratory dish, and then the cells are put back in the patient. So remove the cells, then put them back. Now this will be done on diseases that affect the blood, or cells that we can easily remove, treat and put back in the patient. It's hard to do with a bone or a brain. You can't remove the brain; take the brain out and correct it and put it back. The other type of gene therapy is in vivo gene therapy; "in life," inside life. This is Latin. The DNA is actually added directly to the tissues by injection or some other way. So you could do this on the skin. If you wanted to do gene therapy of the cells in the skin, you could put a cream and have some DNA there. Or on muscle, as I've just described; you might take a gene therapy on muscle. On a solid tumor, you could actually use a CT scanner and guide a needle to squirt gene therapy right on the tumor.

There are several vectors for gene therapy. It's like any recombinant DNA experiment. We're going to need a vector: a chromosome or a piece of DNA that is recognized and can get into the cell and will carry our gene that we're interested in into the cell using that vector. Now there are four requirements for these vectors. First of all, they must be expression vectors with active promoters. We want our gene to be expressed in our therapeutic setting. Second, they've got to be small in size so we can handle them in the laboratory. A single human chromosome has 100 million base pairs of DNA. It's hard to cut and splice and do things with something that big. We want something smaller. Third, we need, as I mentioned before, a marker gene, a gene whose phenotype will show that the vector got into the targeted issue but is harmless. So we might use a green fluorescent protein or some other thing like that—antibiotic resistance, harmless, easily detected, hopefully. And fourth, our gene therapy vector better have restriction enzyme sites. Do you remember that? That's the way we can cut DNA open in our genetic engineering. So we'll be able to cut DNA open by the restriction enzyme site for insertion of the DNA of interest.

As it turns out, most gene therapy vectors for humans are viruses. It's a piece of DNA. It's got a code on it. It can get injected into a cell. So what we do with a gene therapy vector that's going to be a virus is that we take a virus that's infected, that's got the genes for infecting the cell, but we remove the genes for reproducing inside the cell. So the virus will shoot its DNA in but won't kill the cell and turn the cell into a virus factory. The knowledge of this, of course, comes from our knowledge of all of the molecular biology details of viral infection. There are three gene therapy viral vectors that are commonly used in human clinical work. The three are called adenovirus, adeno-associated virus, and retrovirus. A couple of remarks about each one of these before we proceed with actual clinical trials.

First, adenovirus. Adenovirus is a large DNA virus. Sometimes it causes colds. Now, of course, we're going to disabled the virus, and it won't cause a cold. We'll just have it infect. The DNA of this virus remains outside of the cell's chromosomes after infection, and that's a negative in the sense that it won't be carried to the daughter cells when the cells divide in our target. So we're going to have to give adenovirus repeatedly if we're doing gene therapy. It's an easy to isolate and easy to work with virus; it's a DNA virus.

The second virus is called the adeno-associated virus. It looks kind of like adenovirus, but it's smaller. It doesn't cause a disease in humans. In this case, however, the viral DNA is spliced into the host chromosome at a specific site on chromosome 19. This adenovirus injects the DNA and puts it in at chromosome 19 along with, we hope, our gene therapeutic DNA. It's small in its capacity. It can't put in many, many genes, but it's a very widely used virus in gene therapy.

The third type of viruses are called retroviruses. Retroviruses are unusual. They have RNA as their genetic material, but they reproduce by making a DNA copy. Remember DNA makes RNA. Here, RNA makes DNA, and they splice this DNA into the host cell. The problem with retroviruses—we know a lot about them, but they splice in their DNA in any location on the genome. Well, since for 98% of the genome, it's not going to be harmful, I guess that's okay. On the other hand, what if you go to that 2%, and you splice a random piece of DNA and disrupt a functional gene in the cells? That's not a good thing at all. So we run a risk sometimes when we use retroviruses for gene therapy.

Some DNA viruses and RNA viruses have led to successes in gene therapy. Some gene therapy looks promising, but there have been very few successes. It looks good on paper. It works well in mice, and when you go to humans, things seem to get a little more complicated. Some of the reasons for these failures in humans are the following. First, the gene therapy very often doesn't last long. The target cells often divide rapidly, and if our gene therapy gene doesn't get into all of the cells in this target tissue, then all the new cells won't have it, and they'll be far outnumbered pretty soon. So we'll have a very small minority of the cells that have the gene therapy DNA. The second problem is that patients may mount an immune response against the gene therapy vector.

Now, these three viruses I've mentioned are viruses that normally infect people, so you would expect that we wouldn't necessarily mount an immune response against them because the virus has evolved a way to avoid our system because it naturally infects us, and our immune system normally doesn't react to it in the extreme way. All gene therapy trials were stopped for a time in 1999 when an 18-year-old boy who was given a gene therapy vector died unexpectedly by a massive immune response against the virus. It was totally unexpected and has never been fully explained. So that's a tough part of gene therapy.

Third, there are a lot of diseases that you can't cure by a single gene therapy. You'll remember one of my criteria for doing gene therapy is we've got to know what the gene is that causes the problem. Heart disease—not a single gene causing heart disease. Multiple genes are involved with heart disease, as well as environment. Diabetes—multiple genes, especially in the non–type I diabetes, the diabetes called type II, where it's not the problem of not making insulin, but it's other things. Alzheimer's disease, arthritis, cancer—as I've just described in the previous lecture, many genes involved. If there are many genes involved interacting with the environment, it becomes quite difficult to use just one gene for gene therapy, and no one is yet proposing giving seven genes at once in a massive gene therapy trial.

Here are some examples of gene therapy. First, severe combined immunodeficiency. In severe combined immunodeficiency, well, it's what it says, immunodeficiency. They don't have a good immune system. The patients have neither cell-mediated nor antibody immunity. They have a gene mutation for an enzyme coding for a protein called adenosine deaminase; let's call it ADA. They have a gene mutation in a gene coding for ADA normally expressed in white blood cells, both T and B cells. So the T and B cells don't develop, and these people cannot be around any infective agent; otherwise they'll die. They'll die of any normal infection. They have no immune system. The treatment used to be just totally shielding them from any germs—you remember films and pictures of the "bubble boy"—and you give massive blood transfusions as well. Unfortunately, the bubble boy died of a viral infection in a blood transfusion from his sister. We didn't know the virus was there when he was given the blood, and he died of a massive infection that a normal person could fight off.

Now, physicians then tried giving patients with this disease the protein itself, the missing protein. They isolated it from cows, and later on they cloned it and got it by biotechnology. The result was moderately successful. Some of the white blood cells would take up this protein and develop into immune system cells. Then they tried some ex vivo gene therapy in the early 1990s using gene augmentation to supplement the ADA injections. So here's what happened. The patient's white blood cells, ex vivo, were removed. The normal ADA gene was put in using a gene therapy vector, retroviral vector. Then the cells are put back in the patient, under the hope that they would continue to divide and form good white blood cells, and they did. The patient's need for ADA was reduced, and the gene therapy was moderately successful. This has been repeated on a number of patients since.

The second disease treated by gene therapy, with very few cases, is familial hypercholesterolemia. "Familial," that's the family; it's inherited. "Hyper," high; "cholesterol," you know what that is, the cholesterol in the blood; "emia," blood. So familial hypercholesterolemia, high amounts of cholesterol in the blood. In this case, the reason is the patient cannot remove cholesterol from the blood when the patient eats. There is a gene mutation in a gene that normally codes for a protein that's a receptor for cholesterol that's expressed in the liver. So this receptor grabs the cholesterol from the blood and puts it in the liver where it breaks down to something else, harmless things. Instead, this protein is not there, and so the cholesterol just stays in the blood.

So here's how that was done. First, a piece of liver was removed. The liver cells were disaggregated, or separated from one another, in the laboratory. The gene for this receptor protein was added by a vector, normal vector, and the cells were grown to a larger number of liver cells, then were put back in the patient. What's nice about the liver is it's fairly plastic in its genetic capacity, and so these cells actually fused with the liver and continued to divide. The result was the liver now made enough of the receptor protein to remove cholesterol from the blood, and the patient's blood cholesterol went down—moderately successful.

Another disease, ornithine transcarbamylase deficiency. Okay, I'll call it OTC deficiency. Here the patients cannot break down ammonia, amine groups, that are released by amino acids when they are digested. Well, ammonia turns out to be very, very toxic to humans, and most patients with the disease die within a year of birth, but milder cases can live for years by taking a special diet with ammonia-reducing drugs. In this case, in vivo gene therapy was done by an adenoviral vector, and the normal gene was actually injected into an artery leading to the liver in this vector. The virus infected the liver cells, and the result was the liver did express the enzyme, lowering ammonia levels. So this was moderately successful in these patients. This was done in the milder cases of this disease. It has not yet been done on the severe cases in infants, which can be lethal.

Cancer is my fourth example of a disease treated by gene therapy. Cancer actually accounts for most gene therapy trials, and there have been two approaches. First, in vivo, gene augmentation by the introduction of a virus expressing the normal tumor suppressor gene when it's mutated. Remember p53, that gene in lung cancer that gets mutated by the component of cigarette smoke: p53 is no longer functional as a tumor suppressor, so gene therapy has been done by introducing, in vivo by a catheter squirting, the good p53 in a vector onto the lung cancer cells. Generally this has been done on very sick patients who failed other therapies, and the result so far has been that the vector does get into the tumor. The gene is expressed, the good p53, and the patients have generally been living longer. A second approach to cancer by gene therapy has been ex vivo targeted cell killing by removal of white blood cells. The T cells were removed from the patient, and the addition was made of a T cell receptor that essentially binds to the tumor and causes cells to home in and kill the tumor. This was reported recently successfully for melanoma. The melanoma was wiped out by this new immune stimulant added by gene therapy.

Back to our opening story with muscle. Muscle buildup is not just for athletes. In muscular dystrophy, for example, there's lack of repair of muscles, and it gets replaced by fibrous tissue, fat. In most older people, muscle wasting occurs. The strength and mass of muscles decreases by up to a third from age 30 to 80, no matter what we try to do. Disability—if a person is disabled, the muscles are going to waste. They're going to be wasted away because of underuse. If you don't use it, the body doesn't repair it, and cell death of muscle occurs. At the University of Pennsylvania, Lee Sweeney is finding out what controls muscle repair when muscles need to be repaired, which they do all the time after their being used. Well, it turns out he's found two genes involved, and the proteins coded for them. The first is called IGF-1, which stimulates nearby cells to promote muscle buildup; and the other is called myostatin, which stimulates muscle breakdown.

So he has been doing gene therapy, and he's doing it on mice first, by adding the gene for IGF-1, the buildup protein, that's targeted to muscles in mice by either making them genetically modified or by gene therapy, using an adeno-associated virus vector. The gene gets expressed in muscle, and lo and behold, muscles get bigger. Then you could add another gene therapy vector that makes a protein that blocks myostatin. If it blocks myostatin, the same thing's going to happen. You'll prevent muscle breakdown, and you'll get bigger muscles as well. Clinical trials of both of these approaches are planned on patients who have muscle wasting. The question now is, will athletes get to it first?

While gene therapy may hold some promise for repairing damaged tissues, cloning and stem cells also have great potential. We turn to them in the next lecture. Thank you.

323

Lecture Twenty-Two
Molecular Medicine—Cloning and Stem Cells

Scope: Cloning is the production of an organism genetically identical to another organism of that species or cell. Plants can be cloned easily from specialized cells. This shows that these cells have all the genes for all other cell types; that is, they are totipotent. Showing this is harder in complex animals. The nucleus of a specialized cell can be transplanted into an egg whose nucleus was removed, and the resulting egg can be induced to form a new organism, or clone. This was first done on frogs, then sheep (Dolly), and now many other animals. Reasons for animal reproductive cloning include preservation of valuable genotypes, preserving endangered species, and preservation of the genes of a pet. This technology makes human reproductive cloning feasible. Stem cells are constantly dividing cells that make a pool for specialized cell formation to replace cells that are lost or damaged. Stem cells can be pluripotent, such as those in bone marrow that form several kinds of blood cells, or totipotent, as in embryonic stem cells that can form all the kinds of cells in the body. There is potential in using specialized cells derived in the laboratory from stem cells to repair damaged tissues, ranging from heart to brain. Stem cell technology can be combined with cloning in the process of therapeutic cloning. This may make stem cells and tissues that will not be rejected by the recipient.

Outline

I. Opening story: stem cells from fat.

    A. Many tissues have stem cells.

        1. As a plastic surgeon in Los Angeles, Dr. Marc Hedrick's practice included liposuction, in which unwanted fat is removed from the body.

        2. When he looked at some of the fat under the microscope, he saw not just fat cells, but some other types as well. He proposed that these specialized cells got there because fat tissue harbors some stem cells—unspecialized cells that constantly divide to form a pool of cells that then specialize when needed. He thought that the fat stem cells might form a population for cells whose origin in the embryo related to fat cells: muscle, bone, cartilage, blood vessel, and of course fat.

   3. Hedrick and some colleagues set out to find these stem cells in discarded fat, and indeed found them. When implanted into animals, these cells will specialize into the tissue where they are located: So stem cells from fat can be put into damaged blood vessels and will take a hint from that environment and specialize into blood vessel cells, repairing the damage.

   a. Fat stem cells are reaching the clinic. An advantage of using them is that a person's own fat can be used to get them so they will not be rejected as nonself when implanted into an organ. Hedrick has invented a way to get fat stem cells in about an hour in the operating room while a patient is there waiting for the implant. About 450 grams (a pound) of fat is enough to obtain 200 million stem cells, sufficient for therapy.

   b. Recently, some women in Japan received fat stem cells to help repair breast tissue after mastectomy for cancer, and a child in Germany got them to help repair the skull after damage in an accident.

B. The biology behind this has come from studies on the molecular genetics of cells, focusing on a key biological question: How does an unspecialized cell become specialized? Put another way, how does a fertilized egg form the entire organism? The biological basis for the answer is that every somatic cell in the body has all of the genes necessary for the entire organism. That is, all cells are totipotent.

II. Cloning in plants confirmed totipotency.

A. In 1958, Frederick Steward, a plant biologist, showed directly that a specialized cell is totipotent.

   1. Steward took specialized cells from a carrot (a certain cell type in the root that we eat) and put them into a chemical environment that mimicked the embryo. This provided signals for the root cells to first despecialize, then form a carrot embryo, and then form an entire carrot plant. The plant was a clone, genetically identical to the initial root cell.

   2. This can be done for many different plant cells and organs. Specific chemical signals can turn one cell type into another.

III. Animals can be reproductively cloned.

    A. Cloning animals cannot be done the same way as plants.

        1. Some simple animals can regenerate organs from other cells (worms, hydra, starfish). This means that their specialized cells are easily manipulated and "plastic" in their genetic program.

        2. For most complex animals, such as mammals, this kind of cloning cannot be done.

        3. The proof of totipotency in animals came from studies not on the whole cell but the cell nucleus.

            a. The idea was to surround a specialized cell's nucleus with the chemical environment of the fertilized egg. Scientists did it by replacing the egg nucleus with the specialized cell nucleus, thereby giving the latter an "egg" environment, with its proper signals to go on and become an embryo.

            b. The first experiments were done on frogs: Their egg cells are large and easy to get from the water. The egg nucleus was removed and replaced with another nucleus, and then the egg was coaxed to try to form a tadpole and then a new frog. Donor nuclei from the embryo always worked; later stage embryo and tadpole nuclei sometimes worked; adult cell nuclei worked—but rarely.

            c. The frog experiments showed that there is totipotency (all of the genes) in a specialized cell nucleus. But something prevents consistent cloning as the cell gets more specialized.

            d. For 30 years, scientists tried to figure out what made an animal specialized cell nucleus largely unsuitable for cloning. In 1996, Ian Wilmut and colleagues found out. By starving the donor cells in the laboratory, they found that their nuclei would be much better for transplant into an enucleated egg and then cloning: Dolly the sheep was the result.

            e. Dolly was cloned not just to give evidence for totipotency. The company Wilmut worked for was trying to produce transgenic animals that would make a human protein in their milk that treats cystic fibrosis. Cloning was the best way to propagate such an animal. This has now been done for human growth hormone made by cows, for example, as described in Lecture Twelve.

4. There are several reasons for reproductive cloning in animals.
   a. Propagation of valuable animals (see above).
   b. Preservation of endangered species that won't breed in zoos.
   c. Preservation of a pet; the company doing this has done cats and dogs but is no longer in business because of lack of demand.

B. Human reproductive cloning is possible.
   1. Human clones are born all the time: identical twins. The cloning of animals makes deliberate human reproductive cloning possible.
   2. There are some reasons why human cloning might become available.
      a. Many people have problems with normal reproductive mechanisms but want a child genetically related to them.
      b. There may be a desire to perpetuate valuable genotypes. What if there was an old woman who never got cancer because she has certain mutations? These will die out with her, unless she is cloned. A person with unique characteristics (Einstein) might be cloned to preserve the genes that made him unique (whatever they are).
      c. Perpetuation of a dying child.
   3. But there are several concerns.
      a. The process is not efficient. Dolly was 1 of 277 nuclear transplants; the others failed. The technology has improved, but it is not as good as test-tube baby technology.
      b. In some species, clones have some problems. Defects in the immune system and disease susceptibility have been noted.

IV. Stem cell technologies are developing rapidly.

A. There is a need for new cells in medicine, for example:
   1. In a heart attack, there is often permanent damage to the heart muscle.
   2. In the brain, Parkinson's and other diseases result from a lack of functional cells.

3. In diabetes, the pancreas is damaged and its product (insulin) must be replaced.
4. In the musculoskeletal system, breaks and tears are often hard to repair.
5. Two problems in getting new cells are:
    a. A source for these specialized cells. Organ transplants are hard to get.
    b. The immune system ultimately rejects transplants as nonself.

B. Stem cell transplants are already performed.
1. Bone marrow gets damaged in cancer radiation therapy and chemotherapy as the dividing cells are killed. This makes the patient severely anemic and immunocompromised.
    a. If the patient's bone marrow is removed before therapy and stored, it has enough pluripotent stem cells to form the new blood cells when returned to the patient after therapy.
    b. If there is a blood cancer, the patient's bone marrow cannot be used. So a genetically related donor is sought.
    c. There have been instances of parents conceiving a child to provide genetically appropriate bone marrow for transplant.
2. Bone marrow also contains stem cells that do not form blood but form the tissues around blood: blood vessels, muscle, and bone. These have been used as well and are pluripotent.
3. Pluripotent fat stem cells are just starting to be used (see opening story).

C. Embryonic stem cells are totipotent.
1. In the early embryo, cells are totipotent. The preimplantation genetic diagnosis described in Lecture Seventeen shows this. One cell could be removed from an eight-celled embryo, and the rest of the cells took over.
2. At about the 10-day stage in a human embryo, there are several dozen of these undifferentiated, totipotent cells. These cells can be removed from the embryo. In 1998, James Thomson showed that they could be put into a lab dish and grown indefinitely.
    a. In laboratory experiments, these stem cells can be induced to form many different cell types. In animals, these cells have cured brain, heart, muscle, and pancreas damage.

This had led to great excitement about potential for humans.

    b. It is proposed to use lab-grown stem cells as a supply. Not a lot of embryos would be needed. But these cells might be rejected, as they are nonself.

3. A solution to this rejection problem combined cloning and stem cells: therapeutic cloning.

4. Here is the scenario: I have a damaged heart because of a heart attack. Some of my skin cells are removed and grown for a few days in the lab, then sent to a cloning lab. There, a woman donates an egg cell after being induced to ovulate. Her egg cell nucleus is removed and replaced by mine. The egg is stimulated to divide and forms an early embryo. After 10 days, the embryonic stem cells (genetically mine) are removed, placed in a lab dish, and induced to form heart cells. These heart cells are then sent to me and implanted in my heart, where they repair it.

5. Another method produces embryonic stem cells without the embryo. Shinya Yamanaka at Kyoto University has found that mouse skin cells can be reprogrammed to act like embryonic stem cells if four genes are added by vectors for high expression. All four genes code for transcription factors. Their gene products cause cells to divide, prevent cell death, and cause them to be totipotent embryonic stem cells. Indeed, in mice these cells can be coaxed to form true embryos that develop into newborn mice. So a possible scenario might be for skin cells to be reprogrammed to make stem cells, which would then be reprogrammed to make heart cells in the example above.

6. In any case, like fat stem cells, this is a way to get around concerns about using cells from embryos: These cells never get to be part of an embryo.

Essential Reading:

Susan Barnum, *Biotechnology: An Introduction* (Belmont, CA: Thomson Brooks-Cole, 2005), chaps. 7 and 10.

David Sadava, Craig Heller, Gordon Orians, William Purves, and David Hillis, *Life: The Science of Biology,* 8th ed. (Sunderland, MA: Sinauer Associates; New York: W. H. Freeman and Co., 2008), chap. 19.

Supplemental Reading:

Michael Bellomo, *The Stem Cell Divide* (New York: AOMCOM Press, 2005).

Jay Gralla and Preston Gralla, *The Complete Idiot's Guide to Understanding Cloning* (New York: Penguin, 2004).

Christopher Thomas Scott, *Stem Cell Now: From the Experiment That Shook the World to the New Politics of Life* (New York: Penguin, 2005).

Questions to Consider:

1. Do you think that there are suitable alternatives to embryonic stem cells?

2. What are the moral and ethical arguments against reproductive cloning in humans?

Lecture Twenty-Two—Transcript
Molecular Medicine—Cloning and Stem Cells

Welcome back. In the previous lecture on molecular medicine, I ended by describing how gene therapy might be useful to help alleviate symptoms of muscle wasting. Now I want to talk about a different way of treating tissues that are damaged—that is, cloning and its associated stem cells. As a plastic surgeon in Los Angeles, Dr. Marc Hedrick's practice included liposuction, where unwanted fat is removed from the body. Rather than throw the goo away, he asked if there was something useful in it. When he looked at the fat under the microscope, he saw not just gooey fat cells but some other cell types as well, including what appeared to be bone and cartilage. Hedrick proposed that these specialized cells, these extra specialized cells of bone and cartilage got there because fat tissue must have some stem cells.

Stem cells are unspecialized cells in the body that constantly divide to form a pool of cells, a group of cells, that can then specialize when they are needed. Hedrick knew about stem cells and bone marrow from his medical training, and these are the stem cells that form a constantly replenished population from which red blood cells and white blood cells get formed. You'll recall that red and white blood cells have a limited lifetime in the bloodstream and have to be replaced. Hedrick thought that fat stem cells might form a population for cells whose origin in the embryo related to fat cells. For example, muscle and bone and cartilage and blood vessel, and of course fat, all come from the same group of cells in the embryo.

Hedrick found these stem cells in the discarded fat from liposuction. And when he took these stem cells and implanted them in animals, the cells would specialize into the tissue where they were located, kind of like "when in Rome, do as the Romans do" if you're a stem cell and can change your options in life. If you're a specialized cell already and you're put into another environment of a different specialized tissue, well, good luck. You're going to stay the way you were. Stem cells from fat can be put into damaged blood vessels in animal studies and will take a hint from their environment and specialize into blood vessel cells, repairing the damage. Fat stem cells are reaching the clinic.

The advantage of using fat stem cells is that a person's own fat can be used to get these cells, so they won't be rejected as nonself cells by the cellular immune system. You'll recall from a previous lecture that T cells in the immune system recognize things that are not self, that have genetic flags on them, proteins on them, that say, I'm not from you, and so you should reject me. Well, a fat stem cell from you will not be rejected by you when implanted into an organ. Hedrick and his colleagues have invented a way to get fat stem cells in about an hour in the operating room while a patient is there waiting for the implant of stem cells. He can get about 450 grams, which is about a pound, of fat, and that's enough to get 200 million stem cells. This is enough for therapy.

A couple of examples: Recently some women in Japan received some fat stem cells to help repair breast tissue after they had breast surgery for breast cancer. In Germany, a child got his own fat stem cells to help repair his skull after damage in an accident. The biology behind all of this has come from studies on the genetics and molecular biology of cells. A biological question is, how does an unspecialized cell like a stem cell become specialized into bone or blood vessel, or fat for that matter? Put another way, how does a fertilized egg form the entire organism? The key biological basis to all of this is that every somatic, non-sex-forming, cell in the body has all the genes necessary for the entire organism. That is, all cells except for the sex cells are totipotent. They can give rise to all other cells in the body.

I want to talk about cloning first in plants and then in animals, and then we'll get back to stem cell technology. In Lecture Three, I described cloning in plants. You'll recall what was done by Frederick Steward at Cornell University in 1958. He took specialized cells from the root of a carrot plant, put them into a growth medium that was proper, that would signal these cells to become embryo cells. The cells indeed formed a carrot embryo, and then that grew up into a functional carrot that had roots, stems, leaves, and flowers—all the organs of a plant. If he did five cells from the carrot, he got five identical carrots. They were clones. The plants were all clones, genetically identical to each initial root cell.

Cloning in plants, which proved totipotency, can be done for many different plant cells and organs. There are specific chemical signals that we know of that can turn one cell type into another, so plants are pretty easy to work with in this way. In Lecture Twenty-Four when I talk about agriculture and biotechnology, you'll see how this process has been very important. Animals can also be reproductively cloned because remember, in the plant we are producing a reproductive organism, a full organism with all the organs and systems for reproduction. The straightforward experiment from plants that I described, where I could take a cell of my finger and put it into a growth medium that has the right signals and it would all of a sudden become a fertilized egg and give rise to a brand new me, which can't be done. My students are very thankful for that. Some simple animals can regenerate organs from other cells. For example, worms, the little hydras that live in fresh water, and starfish can regenerate organs. Largely, we can't.

So, in these animals that can, their specialized cells are easily manipulated by injury or some other purpose, and they're plastic in their genetic program. They have the genes, and the genes can be turned on at will. But most complex animals such as mammals, like us, can't do this. Proof of totipotency of the animal cell came from studies on the cell nucleus. You'll recall from many lines of experimental evidence that the cell's nucleus is the location of the genetic material. The idea was, let's surround not the whole cell with some chemical signals, but let's surround the cell nucleus with the chemical environment that says, you're in a fertilized egg now. You're not in a skin cell; you're in a fertilized egg. This can be done by a little bit of surgery here. We can replace the nucleus of the egg with the nucleus of a specialized cell, and thereby we'll give that nucleus of the specialized cell the eggy environment. This is done by pipettes, little straws, and you can suck out the nucleus of an egg cell, and you can insert the nucleus of a specialized cell. It's technically absolutely feasible to do.

Of course, this nucleus that's in the egg cell—it's from a differentiated specialized cell—now has signals around it that say, you're no longer in skin. Start acting like a fertilized egg because that's your environment. The nucleus might start doing that. The first experiments in this regard were done on frogs. Why would scientists do it on frogs? Again, model organism time. Scientists use organisms they can manipulate to show what they need to show experimentally. The frog lays its eggs in the water. The eggs are very large, and they're easy to obtain, so the experiments were done on frogs. Here's what was done. This was done first in the 1950s. The egg nucleus was removed, as I just described, and it was replaced with another nucleus. Then the egg was coaxed—and there's ways to do this—to try to form this tadpole that a frog forms, as you'll recall, and then an adult frog. Would it happen?

Here are the results from different nuclei. If the donor nucleus that went into this empty egg was from an early embryo, it always worked. You always got a tadpole, and you got a brand-new frog. Ten nuclei from an embryo would give 10 frogs. Later in the embryo, if you were a later embryo that was a little bit before the tadpole time—before tadpole, but still an embryo—they would usually work. If the nucleus donor was from a tadpole, it sometimes worked. Now we're into the 1960s. These experiments are continuing. John Gurdon at Oxford University took the nucleus from adult cells—first an intestine cell, then skin cells—and it worked, but it worked rarely. It was pretty hard to get it to work well. Gurdon's experiment was historic because it showed that even though it worked rarely, it worked. It meant that the nucleus of a specialized animal cell hasn't lost any genes at all. It's got all the genes that are present in the nucleus of a fertilized egg because it can replace the nucleus of a fertilized egg.

But something was not working well here. Something was preventing consistent cloning as the cells seemed to get more specialized, as the organism got older, as the frog was born and had specialized organs, rather than a tadpole or an early embryo. For the next almost 30 years, scientists tried to figure out what it was that made an animal specialized cell nucleus largely unsuitable for cloning. In 1996, Ian Wilmut and his colleagues found out the answer. What they did was they starved the donor cells in the laboratory before they took the nucleus out of the donor cell. Why this worked, no one kind of knew. No one really knew that it would work; it was just an experiment. So they kind of didn't give them much food for a week, and somehow an eager nucleus of a cell, which at that point is not dividing because it's starving, was very good for transplantation. They could transplant it into an enucleated egg, and then it would give rise to a brand-new organism.

Now wait a minute. If we take 10 nuclei from that same organism, no matter what it is, vertebrate animal, and we take it into 10 eggs that are enucleated, the nucleus will program the formation of all 10 new organisms, and all of those 10 are genetically identical because their nuclei came from the same organism, and so they are clones. This is cloning, and Dolly the sheep was the result of Wilmut's experiment. History was made. Dolly was born in 1996 and announced in 1997. When Dolly was announced, by the way, as a clone, it was important for Wilmut and his colleagues to show that indeed Dolly was identical genetically to the source of the nucleus in this enucleated egg experiment. So they showed short tandem repeat data, just like the forensic identification I talked about earlier in the course. They proved by DNA analysis that this was indeed a clone.

Dolly was cloned not just to give evidence for totipotency. This was not done as some trick. We kind of knew by then that nuclei were totipotent.

Cloning just hadn't been successful for technical reasons. The company that Wilmut worked for was trying to produce transgenic—that is, animals that have been genetically transformed analogous to gene therapy—animals that would make human protein in their milk. This particular protein was a human protein that treats cystic fibrosis. Once you made the animal, the best way to propagate the animal, to get more, is not normal reproduction because this transgenic technology really is not too stable. The best way is to clone the animal and get multiple copies. So that's why they invented cloning, to get multiple copies of an animal that might be used to get a drug to treat cystic fibrosis. This has now been done for human growth hormone made in cows, as I described in an earlier lecture, in Lecture Twelve. A single cow that had the gene for human growth hormone has been cloned, and now there's a bunch of them that will give all the growth hormone we will ever need.

There are several reasons for doing reproductive cloning in animals. I alluded to one of them, and that is propagation of valuable animals. A second reason is preservation of endangered species that won't breed in zoos. A friend of mine, Dr. Oliver Ryder, has had a dream job for about 25 years. He is a geneticist at the San Diego Zoo, and he works with endangered species. About 20 years ago, he took cells from a bunch of species that were having a lot of trouble reproducing in captivity and froze them so they would remain alive, but they're in a suspended state until the time that cloning might be possible.

He figured that if we can't reproduce the animals to get a decent-sized herd of these animals—if they're horses, for example—in a zoo, and they're not out in nature, and they won't reproduce in nature, let's get a large enough herd by cloning, maybe, once the technology is developed. So he froze these—he calls it a Noah's Ark of frozen cells—until Dolly was cloned, and now the technology is available. They've begun to do some cloning of endangered species. It's more or less a semi-farfetched idea. That's probably not the way we're going to preserve endangered species, but it's a potential use of cloning animals.

A third use of cloning animals might be preservation of a pet. The company that was doing this for cats—you may have heard of this. This was done for cats in the late 1990s to early 2000s, and dogs as well. The company is no longer in business, maybe because of the lack of demand. They charged about $30,000 to clone a pet. Now why would someone want to clone a pet? Well, because they love the pet that just died. "Are the characteristics of the pet genetically determined?" is a good question. The lady who had the cloned cat said with delight, the cat behaves just like my dead kitty, who was the nuclear donor in this case. One can be skeptical of that. Maybe there's wishful thinking. At any rate, as I speak, this company has been out of business for a year, and there's no plan to bring it back. So three reasons for doing cloning in animals: one, propagation of valuable animals, pretty likely; the second, preservation of endangered species, a little less likely; and the third, preservation of a pet, not a viable business proposition so far.

Human reproductive cloning. Is it possible? Well, human clones are born every day, identical twins. An identical twin is the product of an egg that divided into two, and each one of those fertilized eggs then formed an embryo. They're genetically identical. Since cloning has been done on a number of animals, it makes it possible to deliberately do human reproductive cloning. Why would anyone want to do this? A couple of reasons: First of all, cloning might be useful in people who have problems with normal reproductive mechanisms. Many people have these problems, but they want a child genetically related to them. For example, a woman might not be able to make eggs, but wants a child related to her. Well, she could be a nuclear donor to make a clone carried by another woman, of course, or even by her if the egg donor might be another woman. It's just another reproductive technology like in vitro fertilization. You may recall that in vitro fertilization—"test tube babies," which have been around now for 30 years—was greeted with horror when it first happened, and now it's more or less a routine procedure.

A second reason for doing human reproductive cloning might be that there is a desire to perpetuate valuable genotypes. We might have an old woman who all of a sudden we discover never gets cancer. Well, she's beyond reproductive age, and she might be carrying certain mutations, and you want to study these mutations in a real person, so it might be better to study if the person is cloned. Or we could clone a unique individual, like an Einstein, to study the genes that made this person unique, whatever those genes are. A third reason for doing human reproductive cloning is a sad one, perpetuation of a dying child. There have been movies made of this possibility, where a child is dying and the parents want the child back.

Well, there are several concerns about doing human reproductive cloning. First, the process is not a very good and efficient one. Dolly was one of 277 nuclear transplants into sheep that Wilmut tried. All the others failed. Things have improved somewhat, but it sure isn't as good as test tube baby technology now is, in vitro fertilization. Second, in some species, clones have medical problems. Dolly the sheep died young, and the claim is Dolly did not die of anything to do with the cloning, but other animals have also died young. There have been defects in the immune system, disease susceptibility in clones. There are a lot of unknowns, and no scientific group is seriously proposing doing human reproductive cloning at this time.

Now I turn to stem cell technologies, and I will come back in a loop to cloning as the lecture goes on. There is a need for new cells in medicine to replace cells that are damaged. In the last lecture, I alluded to that when I talked about muscle. For example, in a heart attack, the heart muscle is damaged, and there's often permanent damage to the heart muscle. How are you going to replace that tissue? In the brain, Parkinson's disease and other diseases result from a lack of functional cells. In diabetes, especially type 1 diabetes, where there's a lack of insulin, the pancreas is damaged, and its product must be replaced; insulin must be replaced. Of course, I described last time the musculoskeletal system and the muscles that break, and the tears, and they're often hard to repair. Well, let's get some new cells to repair these.

The problem of getting the new cells, of course, is where are we going to get them? Well, if you have a bad heart, you get a heart transplant, etc., and other transplants as well. Organ transplants are hard to get. There are many, many more people waiting for kidney transplants, as you know, in our society than we have kidneys available. The second problem relating to transplanting organs is that the immune system ultimately will reject the transplant as nonself. So a person who gets an organ transplant has to take immunosuppressive drugs to keep that organ there as long as possible. Well, how about using stem cells? Stem cell transplants are already performed every day. Bone marrow gets damaged when cancer is treated with radiation therapy and chemotherapy because all the dividing cells, including the stem cells inside the bone marrow, are damaged. And so a person who is treated with radiation and chemotherapy for cancer is going to be severely anemic because their red blood cells are not being produced, and immunocompromised because their immune system will not be working because their white blood cells are not being produced in sufficient numbers. We don't wipe it out completely, but we make it really bad.

Well, the strategy is the following. If the patient's bone marrow is removed before therapy and stored, literally, in a refrigerator, this bone marrow has enough stem cells to form the new blood cells when they are returned after therapy. So we give the patient a large dose of therapy and give the bone marrow back. Now these stem cells are called "pluripotent." They're not totipotent. They can give rise to all of the blood cells, the red and white blood cells. What if a patient has a blood cancer, leukemia or lymphoma? If they have a blood cancer, the patient's bone marrow can't be used, so you need a genetically matched donor. You've probably seen advertisements in your community for becoming a member of a bone marrow registry. It's not a hard test to take, and it's a wonderful thing if you do it.

Every year at the institution where I work, which does a lot of bone marrow transplants, there's a reunion between the donor and the recipient. Imagine being able to save a life with a very simple procedure of donating some stem cells. There are even instances of parents conceiving a child to provide genetically appropriate bone marrow. Bone marrow contains other stem cells as well. These don't form blood, but they form the tissues around the blood, such as blood vessels, muscle, and bone. These are also pluripotent stem cells. I gave you the example in the opening story of fat stem cells, and these are starting to be used. So stem cells are used in medicine.

The ultimate stem cells are embryonic stem cells because they are totipotent. The early embryo cells are totipotent. You'll recall in Lecture Eighteen I described preimplantation genetic diagnosis, where we had an eight-celled embryo and took one cell out for diagnosis, and the other seven cells were allowed to take over and form a perfectly good embryo in a human. At about the 10-day stage after fertilization, there are several dozen of these undifferentiated totipotent cells in a human embryo. These cells can be removed from the embryo and grown in a laboratory dish and reproduced. In 1998, James Thompson at the University of Wisconsin showed that indeed this is possible to do. Put them in a lab dish and they will grow indefinitely as a laboratory culture of human embryonic stem cells.

In laboratory experiments on animals, not humans, these embryonic stem cells can be induced to form many different cell types. In animals, these cell types coming from embryonic stem cells, because they are totipotent, have cured brain damage, heart damage, muscle damage, pancreas damage—all of those things for which I described earlier the need exists for replacement cells. This has generated great excitement about their potential in human medicine. The proposal is to use laboratory-grown stem cells as a supply. You don't need a lot of embryos to do this. The problem, of course, then is, if I get some stem cells from someone else, they're not mine. Those cells going into my heart will replace the heart, but then my immune system will say, wait a minute. That's not genetically me. Ultimately, they might be rejected just like any transplant organ will be rejected—ultimately, if we don't watch it.

This has led to the proposal of therapeutic cloning by nuclear transplant. Here is the scenario. I have a damaged heart because of a heart attack. Second, some of my skin cells are removed and grown for a few days in the laboratory, and then sent to a cloning laboratory. In the cloning laboratory, a woman has donated an egg cell after being induced to ovulate. So the woman ovulates many eggs, and one of those egg cells is donated. Her egg cell nucleus is removed and replaced by my skin cell nucleus. The egg is then stimulated to divide and forms an early embryo. This is actually possible to do so far in human medicine. After 10 days, the embryonic stem cells of this embryo, which are genetically mine—it's my nucleus—are removed, placed in a laboratory dish and induced to form heart cells. These heart cells are then Federal Expressed to me and implanted in my heart, where they repair my heart; an interesting scenario.

There's another way we might produce embryonic stem cells, and that's by genetic engineering. At Kyoto University, Dr. Shinya Yamanaka recently showed that mouse skin cells, a fully differentiated cell, can be reprogrammed to act like embryonic stem cells if four genes are added by vectors for high expression. So we do four separate vectors, each of which has a promoter for high gene expression. All four of these genes code for transcription factors involving transcribing certain genes, and their gene products stimulate the cells to divide. They prevent cells from dying, and they cause those skin cells to become just like embryonic stem cells. They become totipotent, so Yamanaka has unlocked the key to totipotency of any cell. The cells that form after this procedure are true embryonic stem cells. They will form embryos, and these will grow up to be mature mice in the mouse experiments.

So let's repeat the scenario. I have a damaged heart because of a heart attack. Some of my skin cells are removed and grown in the laboratory for a few days and sent to a cloning laboratory that does genetic cloning. Now we add the new genes, turn them into embryonic stem cells, and send them back to me. Now the problems with this procedure are numerous. It's brand new, and we're adding new genes in humans. For example, the embryonic stem cells that come to me are cells that have several new genes in them, and two of these four happen to be oncogenes that could be involved with cancer. We really don't know, but experts feel that these are soluble problems. In any case, like the fat stem cells in the opening story, this is a way to get around concerns that some have about using cells from embryos. These cells never get to be part of an embryo, even though they form embryonic stem cells.

Totipotency and cloning have been especially useful in the genetic engineering of useful plants. We will turn to these processes now in the genetics of agriculture in the next lecture. Thank you.

Lecture Twenty-Three
Genetics and Agriculture

Scope: Agriculture is the earliest example of biotechnology. The development of agriculture was an important event in human history, as it allowed for a settled lifestyle. The challenge of agriculture is to feed a growing human population. Three crops—rice, wheat, and corn—directly provide about two-thirds of the human diet. While previously, people increased crop production by expanding the land under cultivation, now the best land is already taken. So the yield or production of crops on a given piece of land must be improved. This is done by intensively managing the soil, water, and pest ecosystems, as well as by altering the genetic capacities of the crops. The methods of crop plant genetics use the principles of Mendelian genetics and evolution by natural selection. These methods include pure line selection, hybridization, and deliberate crosses. They have been very successful but have some limitations.

Outline

I. Opening story: the green revolution in genetics.
  A. The genetics of wheat breeding culminated in Japan.
    1. An article in a newspaper in Connecticut in 1794 described a new genetic variety of wheat that grew quickly, was resistant to a major mold disease, produced more grain, and was 25% shorter and stronger than other varieties.
    2. For reasons unknown, farmers did not use this wheat when the U.S. Midwest was settled in the decades to come. But the Japanese developed a semi-dwarf variety, which obviously had the same height genes as the U.S. variety. By the 20th century, their semi-dwarf variety gave high yields.
    3. Height and grain yield are complex phenotypes determined by numerous genes.
    4. After World War II, the U.S. sent an occupation army into Japan, and among the first officers was an agricultural attaché. He was sent to find out how the Japanese had produced enough food, and once he went into the countryside and saw the short, high-yielding crops, he had his answer.

      5. The Americans sent some of the unusual wheat seeds to colleagues in the Pacific Northwest, where they were crossed with local varieties and record yields were reported.

B. Wheat breeding in Mexico benefited the poor.
      1. In 1944, a wheat research program had been set up in Mexico under the sponsorship of the Rockefeller Foundation. It was a joint U.S.-Mexico venture, with the goal of improving wheat production in Mexico as an aid to economic development. A young scientist from Iowa, Norman Borlaug, headed the plant-breeding effort.
      2. In 1953, Borlaug received some of the semi-dwarf wheat. He set out to introduce genes that would adapt the wheat plants to the climates of Mexico in particular and the poor regions of the world in general.
         a. Borlaug made his crosses and planted at two locations: One is on a cool, wet plateau near Mexico City; the other is in the hotter and drier state of Sonora.
         b. Having two sites was deliberate: Borlaug wanted two crops a year; this would speed up experimentation. And the two sites with different climates would provide a wide adaptation to climates around the world.
      3. By 1961, the crosses resulted in new wheat strains that were fast maturing so they could grow two crops a year. The crops were naturally resistant to a wide variety of pests, very high yielding, semi-dwarf, and adaptable to warm and cool climates.
         a. In Mexico, wheat yields took off and had tripled within the next 12 years. Mexico no longer had to import wheat.
         b. In 1964, Borlaug visited India, and upon returning to Mexico sent 100 kg (60 lb.) of seeds of the new wheat to his Indian colleagues. They were successful there and in Pakistan. Wheat yields skyrocketed. In 1968, an aid official described the astonishing events as a "Green Revolution."
      4. In 1970, Borlaug was awarded the Nobel Peace Prize. There is no Nobel Prize for agriculture, but it was appropriate that he be honored, because his work prevented massive starvation and the political instability that would have followed. By human impact, it was the most important genetics experiment of the 20th century.

II. Plants are humanity's major source of food.

    A. The race between population and food production is a human challenge.

        1. Agriculture is the oldest example of biotechnology. It began about 8000 years ago when hunter-gatherers found plants that they could eat, possibly growing near their garbage dumps. They ate the seeds and sowed some of them nearby for the next year. This allowed settlement.

        2. In 1999, the world population reached 6 billion, adding 75 million a year. The UN estimates that one person in seven is underfed. It could be much worse: The 20th century saw great increases in food production.

        3. Demography is the study of human populations. Population growth equals birth rate (additions) minus death rate (subtractions).

            a. When agriculture began, there was increase in the birth rate. But the death rate was high because of infectious diseases, so overall population growth was low.

            b. When education and knowledge improved, so did medicine and sanitation. The death rate was reduced and the growth rate went up: There was a population explosion.

            c. Then the birth rate went down and overall growth stabilized.

            d. The U.S. and Europe have gone through this "demographic transition"; less developed areas are at stages b and c above.

        4. Current projections are that world population will level off at about 10 billion in about 2050. This places pressure on food production.

    B. Crop plants are the major source of food.

        1. Food is any substance that provides energy (fuels conscious and automatic actions) and nutrients (substances we cannot make by our genetic limitations).

        2. Worldwide, direct consumption of plant materials accounts for 75% of the food humans eat. The rest is caught and farmed fish, and farmed animal products.

        3. Three plants provide two-thirds of the human diet: rice, wheat, and corn. These plants are called staple foods, as they grow in certain areas and the cultures have used them as their primary food.

    4. We are dependent on the genetic capacities of these plants for growth and seed production.

        a. Growth: The plants have specific environmental requirements. Modifying the environment to fit these requirements is called farming!

        b. Seeds: The seeds are "lunch boxes" for the plant embryo and contain stored carbohydrates, proteins, and vitamins. Unfortunately, the storage proteins have low contents of two of the eight amino acids that we humans cannot make. And the contents of certain vitamins of the grain are not adequate.

        c. Both a and b above are under genetic control, and a major effort in crop plant breeding has been made to improve them for our needs.

III. Agriculture maximizes the genetic potential of crop plants.

    A. Expanding the land under cultivation drove human history.

        1. This was a reason for the rise of empires.

        2. But the "easy" land (U.S. Midwest, etc.) is gone, and lands remaining are very dry ones or tropical forests.

        3. Sometimes land is not farmed, but kept bare to keep prices up.

    B. Increased crop yields is now the way to increase food production.

        1. Example: Japan in early 20th century faced a rising population but not much more land available for rice crops. To be independent of outside sources, they made a big push to increase yields on the land they had, and yields increased threefold. This was done by ecological management of the land and genetic crossing to improve the potential of the plants.

        2. The management of the crop environment takes several forms.

            a. Soil: Plowing fields and conserving the soil from runoff are important. Improving the nutrients (for plants) in the soil is essential. This is why soil is fertilized.

            b. Water: This is needed to dissolve soil nutrients and cool the plant. The problem has always been that there is too much or too little water at the wrong times. So huge dams and canals make water available and deep wells bring water to fields.

      c.   Pests: Crops are eaten by insects, molds, bacteria, viruses, animals, etc. These can be controlled by hand (e.g., weeding) or pesticides (e.g., fungicides). Pesticides must be used with care, lest they damage beneficial organisms or even humans.

IV. Plant breeding uses genetics to improve crop plants.

    A.   There are three methods of conventional plant breeding that seek to improve plants genetically so they will grow better and give better food.

    B.   Pure-line selection: This was the way that crops were domesticated.

        1.   Example: Wheat relatives that grow in the wild (the original wheat) have alleles for seed germination (sprouting) that provide for dormancy. Seeds shed by the plant will germinate at staggered intervals. Dormancy is advantageous to plants, but not to farmers. So when farmers were the selective agent, they planted seeds and harvested only the ones that grew right away. These plants were used for the next generation. After about 20 generations of selection for this multigene-determined phenotype, the plants were homozygous for lack of dormancy.

        2.   There are many such varieties selected for one genetic characteristic. Seed banks have tens of thousands of varieties stored so farmers can use them where and when they are needed.

        3.   Some varieties have been selected for nutritional characteristics.

            a.   For example, in the 1960s a group at Purdue University found a corn variety that made a seed protein that was higher than normal in lysine. Usually, corn proteins do not contain much of this amino acid, and so people who eat it are malnourished.

            b.   Lysine is one of the eight amino acids that humans cannot make because we lack the gene for the enzyme involved. So we get our lysine supply in our diet. People who eat mostly corn protein do not get enough lysine for their own protein synthesis and are malnourished.

            c.   The Purdue scientists found a high-lysine variety of corn. It was bred (see C, below) with other varieties by a team led by Surinder Vasal to give quality-protein maize, a strain that has higher yields, more protein, and better balanced protein than traditional varieties.

C. Hybridization: Crosses between pure lines give more than the individuals.

   1. Example: In 1910, George Shull crossed two pure lines of corn. Line number one had a yield of 20 bushels per acre, and line 2, with different ecological characteristics, also had 20. The offspring had 80.

   2. Hybrid corn is heterozygous for many genes.

   3. Wheat and rice do not produce good hybrids; it is not clear why.

   4. All corn in the U.S. is now hybrid. Farmers must buy the hybrid seeds from seed companies.

D. Deliberate crosses: The principles of Mendelian genetics and its successors are used to cross plants with desirable characteristics and get single ones into a recipient plant.

   1. Example: Borlaug wanted to add a gene for resistance to the wheat rust mold into the high-yielding, semi-dwarf plants.

   2. He took a variety that was genetically resistant but had none of the other desirable characteristics, and crossed it with the semi-dwarf variety that had all the desirable characteristics except resistance.

   3. The offspring were a mix. He chose those that had all the good semi-dwarf characteristics and also were moderately resistant and crossed them to the very resistant plants.

   4. After six generations he had "fixed" resistance alleles in the semi-dwarf plants.

E. These methods are widely used in a huge, worldwide effort to improve plants. But:

   1. They are using many genes in selection and crosses, and other, hidden genes that are not desirable may be also transferred.

   2. There are many genes in nature that cannot be crossed into plants because they are in different species. For example, soybeans make a more balanced protein than corn, but these genes could never mix naturally because beans do not mate with corn.

   3. It is slow. Many generations of selection or crosses are needed to get new characteristics in crop plants.

4. The ecological thrust of agriculture remains to use genetics and technology to adapt the environment to the plant.

Essential Reading:

Maarten Chrispeels and David Sadava, *Plants, Genes and Crop Biotechnology* (Sudbury, MA: Jones and Bartlett, 2003), chaps. 13 and 14.

Nina Federoff and Nancy Brown, *Mendel in the Kitchen* (Washington, DC: National Academies Press, 2004).

Supplemental Reading:

Anthony Griffiths, Susan Wessler, Richard Lewontin, William Gelbart, and David Suzuki, *An Introduction to Genetic Analysis*, 8th ed. (New York: W. H. Freeman and Co., 2007).

Benjamin Pierce, *Genetics: A Conceptual Approach* (New York: W. H. Freeman, 2005), chap. 22.

Questions to Consider:

1. Seed dormancy, a useful characteristic of plants, has been lost from crops through genetic selection. What other characteristics do you think have been changed by domestication of crops?

2. Organic foods are defined as crops that are grown in a certain way, without pesticides or chemical fertilizers. What are the benefits of the organic process for the farmer? What are the differences between organic produce and nonorganic produce? Why don't all farmers use organic practices?

Lecture Twenty-Three—Transcript
Genetics and Agriculture

Welcome back. At the start of this course, I described how genetics and DNA have made great impact on two applications of biology to human welfare. The last five lectures have dealt with medicine; my next two deal with agriculture. A newspaper article in Connecticut described a new genetic variety of wheat that had remarkable characteristics. It grew quickly. It resisted infections by a mold disease that would cause the wheat to give less seeds. It produced more grain. It was shorter and stronger because when it gave a lot of grain, it wouldn't fall over because the stem was very strong, and it was squat. So in comparison to other varieties, this wheat was much better. By the end of the century, a fair amount of this wheat was widespread in the United States at that time. The date of this article was June 30, 1794.

For reasons unknown, farmers did not use this genetic variety of wheat when the U.S. Midwest was settled in the decades to come. But unbeknownst to the Americans, the Japanese were using semi-dwarf wheat, this short, strong wheat that gave a lot of seeds and obviously had the same height genes as the U.S. variety; an example of random mutation. There could be a mutation in wheat in this country, and it could be the same mutation of wheat in Japan. The Japanese wanted to get an even higher grain yield, so by the 20th century, they were performing genetic crosses, telling which plants to mate with which, between the semi-dwarf variety, the short ones, and the U.S. variety that gave very high yields. Yield means how much wheat or food are you producing per acre per year.

Things like height and grain yield are usually complex phenotypes, sometimes determined by numerous genes, so it took years of repeated crossings until, in 1935, the Japanese were satisfied that they had a semi-dwarf wheat variety that, it turns out, was only somewhat improved over the one that had appeared in Connecticut 140 years before; remarkable story. After World War II, the United States sent in an occupation army to Japan. Among the first officers to go with the occupation army was an agricultural attaché. This agricultural attaché was sent to find out how in the world the Japanese produced enough food to survive the war. The Allies had blockaded Japan. They couldn't get food from anywhere else. How in the world could they have grown enough food to feed their population?

Well, once the agricultural attaché traveled into the countryside outside of Tokyo and saw the short, high-yielding crops, he had his answer. Never hesitant to adopt technologies by others, the Americans sent some of these unusual wheat seeds. Now remember, the wheat that had been developed 150 years before no longer was being grown to any extent. We kind of just supplanted it by other wheats. So he sent some of these unusual wheat seeds to colleagues in the Pacific Northwest. After doing genetic crosses with local varieties, farmers there got record high yields of wheat, bumper crops. This is by now the late 1940s. A couple of years previously, in 1944, a wheat research program had been set up in Mexico under the sponsorship of the Rockefeller Foundation of New York. This was a joint U.S.-Mexico venture. Its goal was to improve wheat production in Mexico to help economic development. Mexico was a desperately poor country.

A young scientist from Iowa by the name of Norman Borlaug headed the plant breeding effort in Mexico. In 1953, Borlaug received some of this American and Japanese semi-dwarf wheat that had been discovered after the Second World War by the Americans, and Borlaug set out, at this point in the '50s, to introduce genes to that wheat that would adapt these plants to the climates of Mexico in particular and of poor regions of the world in general. Borlaug made his genetic crosses and planted his wheat at two locations in Mexico, and I've visited both of these. One is in a cool, wet plateau near Mexico City. It's high; it's cool. The other is in northern Mexico, in the hotter and drier area of the Sonoran Desert. It's not quite the desert, but it's hot and dry.

Borlaug used these two places to do his wheat crosses deliberately. First, he wanted to get two crops a year, so by speeding up the experiments, these sites would provide two crops rather than one. Second, the diversity of climates would reflect the climates where poor people in the world are living, as well as in Mexico. And so wheats that would grow well in those two climates might be ones that would be adaptable to other places in the world. By 1961, Borlaug's repeated crosses hit pay dirt with some brand-new genetic strains of wheat. These genetic strains were fast maturing. Two crops a year could be grown, terrific, doubling the amount of food you can get per acre per year. Second, they were resistant to a wide variety of pests, of insects and of molds, and of viruses and of bacteria that reduced the growth of wheat. Third, they were high yielding, very high yielding; more so than any other wheats had been. And they were also semi-dwarf, so the high-yielding stem wouldn't be broken and fall over. The plants, moreover, were adaptable to both warm and cool climates.

This new wheat was a hit in Mexico. Wheat yields took off in the late 1950s and '60s, and within the next 12 years, wheat yields in Mexico tripled. Mexico no longer had to import wheat. They were growing enough to feed their expanding population. In 1964, Borlaug visited India. When he got back to Mexico, in response to requests by his Indian colleagues, he sent them 100 kilograms, about 60 pounds, of seeds of this new wheat for them to plant in some demonstration plots. These new wheats in India were so successful that he sent, the next year, 250 tons of wheat—he started with 60 pounds—and the year after, 18,000 tons of wheat seeds, in 1966. The same thing happened in Pakistan, and over the next two decades, there were wheat yield records in these countries.

Countries that had faced famine now were, in some cases, exporting food to other countries. In 1968, an aid official described this astonishing turn of events as a "Green Revolution." In 1970, Norman Borlaug was given the Nobel Peace Prize. There is no Nobel Prize for agriculture; it's just in certain areas that Alfred Nobel put in his will. But this Nobel Prize was appropriate for peace. It's appropriate that Borlaug be honored in this way because his work had prevented massive starvation and the political instability that would have followed. Estimates are that Borlaug's work saved a billion human lives. By human impact, his work was the most important genetics experiment of the 20th century. I'll repeat that—the most important genetics experiment of the 20th century.

I want to turn now to agriculture and agricultural genetics. First I'll describe how plants and plant agriculture is our major hope for feeding humanity because plants are humanity's major source of food. Then I'll describe what agriculture is, and the job of agriculture is to maximize the genetic potential of plants that we grow as crops. Then I'll describe plant breeding, the actual ways that we improve plants, improve crop plants, by using genetics.

First, plants as humanity's major source of food. The race between an expanding human population and food production has always been, and still is, a major human challenge. Agriculture, as you know, is the oldest example of biotechnology and began thousands of years ago. I've described this before when I described the domestication of barley. Hunter-gatherers found plants that they could eat, and they ate the seeds and sowed some of them for next year. This allowed human settlements. Some of the oldest sites are in the Middle East where wars have been going on, and some of those sites of early agriculture have been damaged in recent wars.

In 1999, the world population reached 6 billion, and we're adding about 75 million a people a year to the world population. The United Nations estimates that about one person in seven is chronically underfed. It could be much worse. The 20th century saw great increases in agricultural production. I want to talk about population a little bit because it has to do with food supply. Demography is the study of human populations. Now when we look at population growth, we can really simplify it if we eliminate immigration and emigration. We can simplify it as the population growth of a given year is equal to the birth rate (the additions) minus the death rate (the subtractions).

When agriculture began as a human practice, there was a great increase in the birth rate because more kids were being fed and surviving. But at that time, the death rate was also high because people were dying of infectious diseases. So birth rate high/death rate high: Overall population growth was low in human history for a long time. Well, as people started settling down, there was better education, scientific research; knowledge improved. Medicine and sanitation were the result. The death rate was reduced. Now wait a minute. The birth rate was high; the death rate is low, and so now the population explodes. There was a population explosion because the population growth rate rose.

After the population growth rate was rising for a period of time, the birth rate gradually went down for a complex of reasons, but mostly because medicine had improved to the point where people started believing in it and saying, we don't have to have so many children as insurance. And so the overall growth rate then stabilized because now the birth rate was low and the death rate was low. This process—high birth/high death, high birth/low death, low birth/low death—is called the "demographic transition." It happens over a period of decades, usually, in a society. The United States and Europe went through this transition in the last century, century and a half. Less developed areas, less rich areas of the world, are now at the later stages of this transition as birth rates are declining.

By current projections from the United Nations and other organizations, the world population will level off at about 10 billion people in the middle of this century. Even at that, this growth of the human population will place enormous pressure on food production because if we're going to have about one-third more people, we have to feed one-third more people; and even now the overall human diet is just barely adequate. The major sources of food for humans are crop plants. Now let me step back a minute and define food. Food is any substance that provides two things: energy—we can break it down for energy to fuel conscious things, like you're doing now if you're driving your car or listening to me; or automatic actions—your heart is beating, your lungs are working in the body. So food provides fuel. It provides energy for those things. And food provides nutrients, substances that we cannot make because of our genetic limitations. We can't make steak; we have to eat it. We can't make all of the amino acids; we have to eat them. We can't make vitamins; we have to eat them.

Worldwide, the direct consumption of plants as food accounts for 75% of the food we eat. The rest of the foods we eat are fish that are either caught in the wild or farmed, or animal products that are farmed. Farmed animal products also come from feeding them plants. For example, until corn, recently, in the last year or two, was grown for ethanol, almost all the corn grown in the United States was used to feed pigs. A little bit of popcorn in the theater, but that's about it. Three plants provide two-thirds of the human diet. Those three plants are rice, wheat, and corn. These are called the staple foods. A staple food grows in a certain area and grows well and produces food, and the cultures have used it as their primary food over a period of time—corn in Latin America, wheat in our country, rice in Asia, for example. We are dependent on the genetic capacities for growth and seed production of these three plants.

Now, growth of a plant requires specific things to go on in the environment. It needs soil, it needs air, and it needs water, etc. Modifying the environment to fit these growth requirements of plants is called farming. The seeds of plants that we eat—the grains, the rice, wheat, and corn—are essentially lunch boxes for the plant embryo. The plant embryo is below the ground in the seed, and it's going to sprout, as you know, and it's going to grow up a plant. But the issue is, what's it going to get for energy and nutrients in the meantime? It can't make its own food—it's not above the ground—and so it needs some stored molecules. What it uses are polymers of carbohydrates—remember, sugars linked together. That's a polymer to make a carbohydrate, starch. It uses proteins in this lunch box, so it has storage proteins, amino acids hooked together, that are used there for storage, and of course, some vitamins.

Now, what the plant will do when the seed germinates is it will break these proteins to amino acids and refashion them for its own use, and break the carbohydrates down and use them for energy. I want to focus in on proteins. The storage proteins of plants—well, the wheat—have unfortunately low contents of 2 of the 8 amino acids that we cannot synthesize. Remember we humans are mutant. We can't make all 20 amino acids. We must take in 8 of them whole in our food. It just so happens that plants' storage of proteins in rice, wheat, and corn have low amounts of 2 of these; just the way the protein is constructed. So the plant doesn't make any difference. Plants can make their own amino acids. They can make all 20; we can't. In addition, some vitamins of the grain are not adequate for human nutrition; fine for the plant, but not good for human nutrition. So we may not have made the wisest possible choice of staple foods, but there you are. These characteristics of the protein, the vitamins, etc., are under genetic control, and a major effort in crop plant breeding and genetics has been to improve them for human needs.

I mentioned that the job of farming and agriculture is to maximize the genetic potential of crop plants. There's two ways to do agriculture, to increase the amount of agricultural food production. The first is to expand the amount of land that you're growing the food on. If you need more food, just plow some more land and grow food there. The second is to expand the amount of food that is grown and produced on a give piece of land. Expanding area is the first; expanding yield is the second. Expanding area, of course, is the driving force of a lot of human history. This is the reason for the rise of many empires, including Western cultures. Unfortunately, the bad news is the easy land, like the U.S. Midwest, has been taken. It's farmed already for food. The land that is remaining in the world where crops could now be grown is either very dry or it's tropical forest, where you have to do a lot of manipulation of the environment.

Increased crop yields is now the way to increase food production. The classic example of this is Japan in the early 20th century. Japan had a rising population but not much more land for rice to grow on, so they tried to get more land, for example, by invading China. That was a great idea. Let's invade China, get more land to grow food for us. That's the way many empires have done it. The Chinese were not cooperative, and the Japanese were rebuffed when they tried that. Next, they relied on trade, just like we are doing for oil, for example. So they relied on trade. We'll trade with our enemies, and we'll depend on them for our rice for our expanding population. Bad idea. They came to the idea that they better be self-sufficient, so they made a huge effort to increase the yield, the food per acre per year, that their rice would produce. The result was the yields increased threefold, the result for wheat and rice. And there was a parallel development of semi-dwarf rice, the same as semi-dwarf wheat. The result for both of these was a terrific achievement in improvement of food production.

Farming is done by ecological management. We are adapting the land for the plants that grow on it. The management of the environment around crops takes several forms. First, we manage the soil. We'll plow the field to allow the seeds to sprout. We'll conserve the soil—there's a whole branch of the U.S. government called Soil Conservation Service—so prevent the soil from running off into the river when it rains. We'll improve the nutrients that are dissolved in the water in the soil. I've just given you an entire course in plant physiology. That's called adding fertilizer. We're improving the nutrients for the plants. A second environmental thing we manipulate around the crop plants is water. Water dissolves soil nutrients; it also cools the plant. The problem is, of course, there's either too much or too little water, and it comes at the wrong times. So this has been the story of huge dams and canals making water available, and deep wells in many areas of the world bring water up to where the fields are.

Pests. Remember my saying, "Big things have little things upon their backs to bite 'em; and lesser things, still lesser things, and so ad infinitum." Well, crops get eaten by insects and molds, and by bacteria and viruses and animals. Lots of things besides humans like to eat rice, wheat, corn, and every other crop that we grow. We can control this by hand, swatting the flies or pulling out weeds, hoeing. We can control them by pesticides. We can add herbicides or fungicides to fields to kill the invading things that way. But we have to use pesticides with great care, lest they damage beneficial organisms, or even humans. Plant breeding is the other way to improve crop plants because you can feed me all you want, as my mother would say, I'll grow big and tall; but no matter if she feeds me twice as much, I still won't grow much bigger and taller than I am. I might grow wider, but I might not grow bigger and taller because that's my genetic capacity. So let's improve the genetic capacity of plants.

There are three methods of conventional plant breeding that seek to improve plants genetically so they will grow better and give more food. The three methods are called pure line selection, hybridization, and deliberate crosses.

First, pure line selection. Pure line selection is the way that food crops were domesticated. I described this in an earlier lecture when I described the evolution of barley, and the seeds shattering, and the threshing floor. Let me give you another example now. If you look at the relatives of wheat that grow out in the wild, out in nature, what you find is that the original wheat and the wheat out in nature have alleles, genes, that code for seed germination that will happen over a staggered period of time, depending on the seed. This is called seed dormancy. When seeds are shed by a plant, they germinate at staggered intervals.

Now, for the plant, this is a terrific property, genetic property, because if one seed germinates and the environment isn't perfect, the plant might die. It might get frozen, for example. Another seed will sprout months later when the environment is good. So for the plant, this is great. For a farmer, bad idea. I want to put my seeds in the ground, and then they'll sprout. So I think you can see that early farmers selected for plant strains that would not have seed dormancy. That's what happened; dormancy was selected by humans not to be in our crop plants. It usually takes about 20 generations of selection until you've got all the genes, the alleles, being the ones that you want for a given characteristic. Now there are many, many of these varieties of plants all selected for a given characteristic. There's corn that's good for popping; Orville Redenbacher was a plant geneticist. There's corn that's colored in certain ways. There's corn that sprouts. There's corn that's high as an elephant's eye. There's many, many thousands of varieties.

In Fort Collins, Colorado, is one of my favorite buildings in the United States, on the campus of Colorado State University. It's called the National Seed Storage Laboratory, and in there are a half a million pure lines of crops from all around the world; 40,000 wheat varieties are stored there, and they're constantly testing for their potency to make sure that they can be used. So a farmer can say, I want corn of this characteristic, and then write in to the Seed Storage Laboratory for that particular strain. Some varieties have even been selected for nutritional characteristics. I mentioned the problem of low levels of essential amino acids in some of our staple foods.

In the 1960s at Purdue University, scientists screened thousands of corn varieties in their seed bank for a genetic mutant that made a seed protein that's high enough in all eight essential amino acids, and they found one. They found a corn variety that would do this, and this variety was bred with other varieties that are more adaptable to different climates by a team led in the 1980s by Surinder Vasal, and it gave what is called quality-protein maize. Maize is the term everyone else in the world uses for corn. This quality-protein maize is a genetic variety that has higher yields, more protein, and amino acid balanced protein as well. So that's our first method, pure line selection.

The second method is called hybridization, and hybridization involves crossing pure lines. The first person that did this scientifically really was Charles Darwin, who reported it in a book in the 1870s to 1880s. In 1910, George Shull, a plant geneticist, did this systematically with two lines of corn. Line number one gave 20 bushes per acre per year and had certain characteristics; line number two had different characteristics and 20 bushels per acre per year. When he crossed them, he didn't get 20; he got 80. The whole was greater than the sum of the parts. This is called hybrid vigor. Almost all corn grown in the United States now is hybrid corn, and you buy the seed from a seed company. Corn hybridization worked for corn. Wheat hybridization doesn't seem to work well, nor does rice, so we're not there yet, making wheat and rice as hybrids.

The third method of doing plant genetics is deliberate crosses, which is what Borlaug did in the 1950s and '60s. So you cross one plant with another. This is using the principles of Mendelian genetics and its successors to cross plants with desirable characteristics and get single ones into a recipient plant. This is hard when you've got phenotypes controlled by many genes. Borlaug, for instance, wanted to add a gene for resistance to a mold called wheat rust into the high-yielding semi-dwarf plant. So what he did was he took a variety that was genetically resistant but had none of the other good characteristics—he got it from the seed bank—and he crossed it with his semi-dwarf variety that had lots of good characteristics. The offspring were a mix. They had all types of genes and phenotypes. From the offspring, he chose those that have all the good semi-dwarf ones, the things that he wanted, and were moderately resistant. Then he crossed again this variety to the very resistant plants. After he did about six generations, he fixed, essentially, the resistance alleles into the semi-dwarf plants.

These methods of traditional plant breeding are widely used in a huge worldwide effort to improve crop plants, but they have four limitations. First, the limitation of hidden genes. Scientists use some genes to select for the characteristics they're interested in, in their crosses, or by pure line selection. But when you're doing a cross, you don't know what other hidden genes, which might be recessive, you're crossing into this new plant. So you might have undesirable genes that are transferred. Many pure lines in the seed bank have low yields because, in addition to disease resistance, for instance, farmers were unconsciously selecting for other alleles that the plant has that are not so good. So it might be corn that's high as an elephant's eye, but it's got lots of bad characteristics as well.

The second problem with traditional genetics is species limitation. There are many genes out there in nature that cannot be crossed into crop plants because they're in a different species. For instance, soybeans make a really well-balanced protein. Corn makes a protein that's unbalanced. But by conventional genetics, corn and soybeans don't mate. You can't do a cross between two different species; so problem number two. Third, it's slow. It takes many generations of selecting and crossing to get what you want if you're doing traditional plant genetics. And fourth, the ecological thrust of agriculture has been, and remains, to use genetics and technology to adapt the environment to the plant. In the next lecture, we'll see how molecular biology and biotechnology have been applied to these four challenges. Thank you.

Lecture Twenty-Four
Biotechnology and Agriculture

Scope: Plant biotechnology seeks to genetically modify plants for human use in agriculture. Totipotency of plant somatic cells is important because it allows any cell to be manipulated in the lab and then grown quickly to produce a plant. Specific plant expression vectors can introduce new genes into plant cells. Gene guns can shoot DNA-coated pellets into the cells. Genetic manipulation can overcome some of the drawbacks of traditional plant genetics: It transfers only single genes, any gene from any organism can be transferred, it is fast, and it can result in plants tailored to their environment. Several examples of genetically modified plants are in use, ranging from plants that make an insecticide, to herbicide-resistant plants, to rice with improved composition for human nutrition, to salt-tolerant crops. While there is great potential for this technology, some people are concerned. These concerns relate to a human aversion to manipulating nature, the safety of foods from genetically altered plants, and the danger of ecological accidents.

Outline

I. Opening story: the salt-tolerant tomato.

    A. Most plants cannot grow in salty soils.

        1. Normally, the small amounts of salts that are dissolved in soil water get removed from it by rainfall washing it down to lower levels in the ground. But in dry climates there isn't much rain, and as time goes on, salt builds up.

        2. Salt is toxic to plants in two ways. First, it impairs the roots from taking up water, and second, it inhibits some of the enzymes involved in making proteins and in photosynthesis—the process by which the plant converts solar energy into stored energy in sugars.

            a. Few plants can thrive in very salty soils, and certainly the major crops cannot.

            b. Salt buildup is a global problem. An estimated 1% of farmland a year (65,000 acres a day!) is made unusable because of saltiness.

B. Biotechnology can make plants salt tolerant.

    1. In Lecture Nine, we described the tiny mustard-like plant *Arabidopsis* and how it is a model for the genomes of major crops. In the 1990s, Eduardo Blumwald found that this plant has a gene that is expressed as a protein that takes salt from the soil and puts it in cell storage depots, called vacuoles, in leaves. This hides the harmful salt from doing damage to the plant.

        a. The problem comes when the salt buildup in the soil is high. It simply takes too much energy for the plant to keep pumping the salt into the vacuoles, so the excess salt gets into the rest of the cells, and the plants wither and die.

        b. Using genetic engineering, Blumwald added a very active promoter beside the salt pump gene so that its expression would be enhanced. Sure enough, the genetically modified *Arabidopsis* was able to not just withstand salty soil, but to thrive in it.

    2. As we saw in Lectures Ten through Fourteen, biotechnology allows scientists to transfer DNA from one organism to another. When the active salt tolerance gene was put into a tomato plant, the transgenic plant became salt tolerant. What is more, the salt was in the leaves; the tomato fruits were fine.

    3. While they are important, tomatoes are not nearly as important as the major grain crops. So Blumwald and others are busily transferring the salt-tolerance gene from *Arabidopsis* to these plants. This may make salty soils usable for farming. Salinity ruined the soils where farming began, in the Fertile Crescent of the Near East. Salt-tolerant transgenic plants may make this desert bloom again.

    4. There are several lessons in this story.

        a. Biotechnology is a powerful, specific, and rapid way to transfer genes from one organism to another.

        b. Biotechnology can lead to a fundamental change in the relationship between people, their crop plants, and the environment. Until now, we have made enormous efforts to adapt the environment to the plant. Now, we may be able to adapt the plant to the environment.

II. The methods of agricultural biotechnology are similar to those for other organisms.

A. Totipotency and recombinant DNA are essential to plant biotechnology.

1. As described in Lecture Twenty-Two, plant cells are totipotent and can be cloned to make new plants.

   a. Cloning is valuable when uniformity is necessary. For example, in forestry, trees are cloned and plantlets put in the soil so they grow to the same size for harvesting.

   b. Single plant cells can be transformed, selected, and cloned. This allows rapid screening of the phenotype.

2. There are two ways to get plant DNA into cells for transformation.

   a. Vector: A bacterial infection causes crown gall tumors in plants. The bacterium has a small chromosome that is injected into the plant cells. This chromosome DNA was isolated and its genes for plant cell alteration (but not infection) removed. It has single restriction enzyme sites for gene splicing. In addition, there are numerous plant promoters that have been described in terms of organ and time (e.g., seed formation).

   b. Gene gun: An inert pellet can be coated with DNA and literally shot into the plant cell nucleus. This is needed at times because plant cells are surrounded by a thick cell wall.

B. Plant biotechnology overcomes some of the limitations of traditional plant genetics that were listed in Lecture Twenty-Three.

1. When traditional plant genetics uses many genes in selections and crosses, other, hidden genes that are not desirable may be transferred also. In biotechnology, only single genes are transferred.

2. Many genes in nature cannot be crossed into plants by traditional genetics because they are of different species. In biotechnology, genes from any organism can be transferred.

3. Traditional plant genetics methods are slow. Biotechnology is rapid; results appear in weeks.

4. In traditional genetics, the ecological thrust of agriculture is to use genetics and technology to adapt the environment to the plant. In biotechnology, the plant can be genetically adapted to the environment.

III. Genetically modified plants are in widespread use.

A. Plants can make their own insecticides.

   1. Many insecticides are not specific. They target many insects, not just the pest. And some are toxic to the environment in other ways.

   2. Insect larvae (the grub or worm immature life stage) eat bacteria. *Bacillus thuringiensis* (Bt) bacteria solve their insect problem by making a protein that binds to the insect larva (grub, worm) intestine to make it lose fluid. The insect dies.

   3. The gene coding for this protein has now been introduced to corn, cotton, soybeans, and tomato cells, which were cloned to plants that expressed the toxin in leaves. The larvae eat the leaves and die, and their population goes down. This reduced insecticide use by 90%.

B. Plants can be made resistant to herbicides.

   1. Weeds are killed by herbicides, but a problem is that these chemicals also kill beneficial plants, and even the crops themselves. So, great care is needed in their use. Genes have been identified from bacteria and other sources that code for proteins that break down herbicides or make protein targets that are functional but unaffected by the herbicides. Such genes have been inserted into cotton, corn, soybeans, and rice.

   2. The transgenic crops are now resistant to the herbicide, and it can be applied without risk of damaging the crop.

C. Golden rice has improved nutritional characteristics.

   1. People require in their diet beta-carotene, which gets converted to vitamin A. Rice plants do not have the genes to make beta-carotene. As a result, about 250,000 children go partially blind each year because they are rice eaters and do not get enough beta carotene.

   2. Other organisms have genes coding for enzymes that can complete the biochemical pathway in rice for beta-carotene. Ingo Potrykus isolated DNA for one of these enzymes from a bacterium and two other genes from a daffodil plant. One by one, these genes were introduced to rice plants along with a promoter that would stimulate gene expression in the developing rice grain.

   3. The resulting rice plant made grains with beta-carotene that were golden and contain adequate amounts of beta-carotene, thanks to the transgenic biochemical pathway.

      4. These plants are being crossed with local varieties to make the beta-carotene phenotype part of rice that is used in different regions.

IV. There is public concern about plant biotechnology.

    A. At the start in the 1970s, there was concern about biotechnology in general. When it was shown to be safe, these concerns abated. Plant biotechnology and genetically modified foods (they are not necessarily the same—most cotton plants are now genetically engineered) have raised serious concerns, especially in Europe.

    B. The objections to biotechnology in agriculture fall into three categories.

       1. Genetic manipulation is an unnatural interference with nature.

          a. This is what a philosopher calls the "yuck factor." Eating food from a plant that has genes from bacteria is just going too far.

          b. There is no real scientific response to this emotional argument.

          c. All major crops have been genetically manipulated, but not to the extent of biotechnology.

       2. Genetically modified foods are unsafe to eat.

          a. Some modifications may create allergic proteins.

          b. Most genetically modified plants are not altered phenotypically in the food part of the plant, except for some extra DNA sequences.

       3. Genetically modified plants are dangerous to the environment. Although a single gene has been transferred to the crop plant, it may be inadvertently transferred to neighboring plants, such as weeds, in the field.

V. Overview.

    A. In this course, we have come from describing heredity to understanding its mechanism to controlling it.

       1. In the first lectures, I described what genetics is and how a monk, Gregor Mendel, and others described the rules of inheritance. Then came the identification of what a gene is (DNA) and how it works (expressed as protein).

       2. With these basics of descriptive genetics in hand, I described how this knowledge has been applied to human use in the biotechnology industry. From making products to solving crimes and cleaning up the environment, biotechnology is growing in importance.

3. Modern genetics is rewriting the "book of life" as explained by Charles Darwin's theory of evolution by natural selection. We are finding out more about how the amazing array of organisms on Earth are related, and even how we as humans may have evolved.

4. Genetics and DNA are having growing impact on medicine. With precise descriptions of genetic causes of diseases in hand, we are now able to diagnose and screen for people with the diseases, and we are beginning to design specific treatments. The areas of gene therapy, cloning, and stem cells are at the leading edge of modern medicine and hold great promise for the future.

5. I ended the course with agriculture, that other application of biology to human welfare, not just because it is important (we have to eat!) but also because so many of us in the rich world take it for granted. The applications of modern genetics and DNA to the problem of feeding the world are already profound, and an exciting future is in store.

B. The genetic genie is out of the bottle.

Essential Reading:

Maarten Chrispeels and David Sadava, *Plants, Genes and Crop Biotechnology* (Sudbury, MA: Jones and Bartlett, 2003), chaps. 6, 17, and 18.

Nina Federoff and Nancy Brown, *Mendel in the Kitchen* (Washington, DC: National Academies Press, 2004).

Supplemental Reading:

Miguel Altieri, *Genetic Engineering in Agriculture: The Myths, Environmental Risks and Alternatives* (Oakland, CA: Food First, 2005).

Jon Entine, *Let them Eat Precaution: How Politics is Undermining a Genetic Revolution in Agriculture* (Washington, DC: AEI Press, 2006).

Questions to Consider:

1. Besides the applications described in this lecture, can you suggest other genetic characteristics that you would like to see in crop plants?

2. Much of the concern about plant biotechnology boils down to the "precautionary principle." This states that if any action *might* cause harm, don't do it. The onus is on the proponents to show that it *does not* cause harm. Predictions are not enough. Can you think of other technologies where we as a society use the precautionary principle? Do you feel it is justified for plant biotechnology?

Lecture Twenty-Four—Transcript
Biotechnology and Agriculture

Welcome back. In the last lecture, I described how genetics and environmental manipulation of crop plants, also known as farming, have done incredible things with food production over the last century. These achievements have been impressive, but as I pointed out, they have their limitations; and we are faced with a challenge over the next 50 years of feeding an ever-expanding human population, which, according to UN estimates, will level off at about 10 billion people. Can biotechnology and DNA manipulation help in this process? That's the subject of this lecture.

I want to begin by talking about a real problem in agriculture that has existed for millennia. Most plants cannot grow in salty soils. When soil is irrigated, when people bring water to dry soils in order to grow crops, the water comes in, but also salts that are dissolved in the water come along with it. This temporarily allows plants to grow, and normally the small amounts of salts that are dissolved in the soil water get removed from the soil by rainfall washing it down to lower levels in the ground; it's called percolation. The salts percolate down to lower levels, so they won't harm the plants. But in dry climates, there isn't much rain, and as time goes on, salt builds up. Salt buildup has always been a major problem in agriculture. It led to civilizations falling. For example, the Mesopotamians fell as a civilization largely because of salt buildup in their soil. Today it's estimated up to 65,000 acres of farmland a day are lost to excess salt buildup, and the soils are essentially rendered unusable because of saltiness.

Salt is toxic to plants in two ways. First, salt impairs the roots from taking up water; and second, salt blocks several of the enzymes involved in important cellular processes. How does salt do that? It alters the way that these proteins fold, and if an enzyme folds incorrectly, it won't be able to do its function. The particular enzymes I'm talking about are, in the plant, involved in making proteins—well, that's bad; if you can't make proteins, you can't express the phenotype—and also certain proteins involved in photosynthesis. Photosynthesis is the process by which a plant converts solar energy into stored energy in the form of sugars, carbohydrates. Few plants in the world can thrive in very salty soil, and certainly not the major crops—you recall what they are; rice, wheat, and corn—so finding a gene for salt tolerance in these three crop plants is kind of unlikely. If you go to the crop seed bank, it's unlikely you're going to find a variety of rice, wheat, or corn that has a mutation such that it can tolerate salt. The wild relatives of these plants, which are weeds, don't grow in salty soils.

I mentioned earlier on in the course the idea of model organisms, and the model plant is a tiny mustard-like plant, a couple of inches high, called *Arabidopsis*. That's the name of it. It's a model for the genomes of the major crops, and in fact, the genome of *Arabidopsis* was sequenced first before rice was sequenced, and then other crops. *Arabidopsis* is a model plant; it does all the things that the major plants do. It has roots and stems, and leaves and flowers, and seeds and fruits, and all of those things. So it's useful to study because we can grow it quite readily in a greenhouse or a warm room near a laboratory. We have mutations of *Arabidopsis*, and needless to say, we know its entire genome sequence.

In the 1990s, Eduardo Blumwald found that this model plant, *Arabidopsis*, has a gene that is expressed as a protein, and the job of this protein is to suck up salt from the soil and take that salt and put it into storage depots inside of cells called vacuoles. These particular cells where it puts it are in the leaves of the plant. It's a pretty good way to tolerate salt. The salt will never get into the rest of the cell. In fact, it won't even surround the root because this protein will suck it up and deposit it in the leaves in these storage depots. This hides the harmful salt from doing any damage to these plants. Now a problem comes when the salt buildup in the soil is very high, as happens in soils that have been rendered unsuitable for agriculture. There's just not enough of this protein expressed, and so the excess salt then leaks out of these vacuoles, storage depots, gets into the rest of the cells, and well, the proteins that are going to be blocked will be blocked, and the plants wither and die.

Using genetic engineering, Blumwald has added a vector with a very active promoter beside the salt pump gene, beside this gene that allows the salt to be stored in the vacuoles, and so the expression of this gene will be enhanced. When he made transgenic plants using this vector for high expression of the salt tolerance gene, sure enough, the genetically modified *Arabidopsis* was able not just to withstand salty soil but to thrive in it; an amazing thing when you think about it. But Blumwald really didn't want to grow *Arabidopsis* on salty soils; that was not his objective. His objective was to get this gene into crop plants. So what he did was the following.

In Lectures Ten through Fourteen, I described how biotechnology allows scientists to transfer DNA from one organism to another. So when the active salt tolerance gene from *Arabidopsis* was put into a tomato plant, and the transgenic plant then was grown up, it became very salt tolerant. The tomato plant that was normal and didn't have this salt tolerance gene from *Arabidopsis* would wither and die in a salty soil, whereas the tomato plants that were in the salty soil and had this salt tolerance gene would be just fine. What's more, the salt, as I mentioned before, was in the leaves. The tomato fruit, which is the part we eat, was just fine. Now while tomatoes are important, they're not nearly as important as the major grain crops, so Blumwald and others are busily trying to transfer this salt tolerance gene from *Arabidopsis* and tomato to these plants, and they're going to use the same methods of biotechnology that were used in the tomato. This may make salty soils in the world usable for farming. As I mentioned, excess salt ruined the soils where farming began, in the so-called fertile crescent of the Near East. Salt-tolerant transgenic plants may make this desert bloom again.

Now there are several lessons in this story. First, biotechnology is a powerful, specific, and rapid way to transfer genes from one organism to another—and from one plant to another in particular. Second, biotechnology can lead to a fundamental change in the relationship between people, crop plants, and the environment. Until now, as I mentioned in the last lecture, we have spent enormous efforts to adapt the environment to the plant. That's what a farm is; adapting the environment to maximize the growth of a plant. Now we have the possibility of being able to adapt the plant to fit the environment. I want to talk about agricultural biotechnology. First, I'll describe the methods by which agricultural technology has been developed; and second, I'll describe some examples of genetically modified plants. As I will discuss later, there is public concern about plant biotechnology, and I'll discuss what some of those concerns are.

First, the methods of agricultural biotechnology. The best summary I can give is that the methods of agricultural biotechnology are similar to those of biotechnology in other organisms, starting with bacteria, to animals, only we add for plants the nice property of totipotency. You'll recall what that means. It means that every cell of a complex organism—and now we're talking about a plant—has the entire complement of genes for the entire organism. So every cell can be manipulated to giving an entire new plant in this case. You'll recall the experiment on carrots that I mentioned in Lectures Three and Twenty-Two. You'll recall that you can take a single carrot cell, a specialized cell from the root, put it into a growth medium that is suitably composed, and this growth medium will tell that cell to become an embryo, and then the cell will divide, and then form a little plantlet, and then grow up to be a mature reproducing plant that'll give roots, stems, leaves, flowers, etc.

Cloning is valuable in situations in agriculture—especially in forestry—where uniformity is desirable. In forestry, for example, in many instances now, trees are cloned. The little plantlets—I love that word; that's the immature little plant—are grown in greenhouses to be of uniform size, and then they're transplanted into the forest where they grow to the same size for harvesting. This actually turns out to be a very good way of conserving this resource. We know from totipotency that single plant cells can be transformed by vectors. They can be selected for containing the vectors, and then of course, they can be cloned. This allows rapid screening of the phenotype and the underlying genotype of these single cells.

There are two ways to get plant DNA into plant cells for genetic transformation, and they're a little bit different than the ways I've described for animal cells and for bacteria. The principle is the same. We're going to use a chromosome as a vector, a piece of DNA, as a carrier for our foreign DNA, but there's one other way that's physical that we get it in also. The two ways are vectors and gene guns. First, the vector. There is a disease in many plants called "crown gall tumors." Yes, plants get cancer. What's a tumor? A tumor is a bunch of cells, as I mentioned in a previous lecture, that are reproducing without any control, so they're just dividing and dividing. It turns out crown gall tumors are caused by an outside agent, and this outside agent is a bacterium.

When this bacterium infects the bud, the terminal region of the plant, this bacterium injects a small chromosome into the plant cells. This small chromosome has DNA coding for two types of phenotypic proteins. One of them is so that the DNA will get incorporated into the plant genome and expressed, and the other set of genes stimulates the plant cells to divide, so they're kind of the tumor-forming genes. Now for the bacterium, this is a good deal because this bacterium, the host bacterium that has injected this DNA, wants sugars and stuff to eat, and the plant is going to provide that. The expanding plant cells will provide even more of it. So for the bacterium, it's exactly what they want.

For the biotechnologist, this is a good idea as long as we get rid of those genes in this small piece of DNA that cause the plant cells to grow and to reproduce. So this vector can be removed from the bacterium. The genes for infection are allowed to remain, and then the genes for causing the plant cells to grow are removed and replaced by your favorite gene, by any gene we want to make the plant transgenic. It turns out this small piece of DNA, this small chromosome, has a single restriction site for gene insertion, and in addition, numerous plant promoters have been described in terms of organ and time of gene expression. So we know a lot about the promoters for seed formation, the promoters for fruit formation, etc.

I mentioned the second way of getting DNA into plants; it's called the gene gun. It's a rather interesting name, but it's true. You take an inert pellet that's not biologically active, and you coat it with DNA, coat it with the DNA you want to get into the cell, and you literally shoot it into the cell. It doesn't go through the cell because it gets slowed down. The reason for using the gene gun to get plant DNA into a cell, and into its nucleus, is that very often the plant cell is surrounded by cellulose and complex polymers called the cell wall. This makes getting foreign DNA as a vector in quite difficult, so we kind of hasten it by using this gun to get the stuff in.

Plant biotechnology overcomes some of the limitations of traditional plant genetics that I listed in Lecture Twenty-Three. Limitation number one: They are using specific genes for selection and crosses (in traditional genetics), but at the same time, other hidden genes that are not desirable may also be transferred (in traditional genetics). In biotechnology, single genes are transferred. Number two: There are many genes in nature that can't be crossed into crop plants of interest (rice, wheat, and corn) because they're in different species. Remember the idea of a soybean protein being expressed in a corn. Soybeans and corns don't mate. In biotechnology, as we know, genes from any organism can be transferred. Third problem: It's slow. Response: Biotechnology is rapid. You can see results using cells in a laboratory dish that are totipotent in weeks. Fourth objection or concern with traditional plant genetics is that the ecological thrust of agriculture has remained to use genetics and technology to adapt the environment to the plant. In biotechnology, as I gave you the example of the salt-tolerant plant, the plant can be genetically adapted to the environment.

Genetically modified plants are in widespread use. I'm going to give you three examples of this biotechnology. The first are plants that can make their own insecticides. Insecticides are chemicals that kill insect pests, but the problem with insecticides is many of them are not specific. These insecticides target many insects, not just the pests. In addition, some insecticides are toxic to the environment in other ways. We owe a debt to

Rachel Carson, the great environmentalist, who showed us that DDT, for example, can lead to the thinning of eggshells in birds. Insect larvae—that is, the immature stage of an insect; the caterpillar, the worm or the grub, they call it—eat, among other things, bacteria. They go and they chew up plants, and they chew up bacteria as well.

There's a bacterium called *Bacillus thuringiensis*—I'm just going to call it Bt—and this bacterium has a gene that defends itself against insect larvae. This gene codes for a protein that binds to the insect larvae intestine, to the gut of the insect, and makes it lose all of its fluid. It essentially gets the insect version of chronic diarrhea, and the insect dies. Well, that's a great idea for the bacterium because the bacterium can then survive. The gene coding for this toxin protein has now been introduced to corn, cotton, soybeans, and tomato cells in the laboratory. Then these cells were cloned up to make plants, by totipotency, that express the toxin in the leaf, because the leaf is where this caterpillar does its damage. As a result, the insect caterpillars land on the leaf, begin to eat, and die very quickly, and the population of this pest goes ways down. This technology in these crops has reduced insecticide use by 90%; very impressive.

My second example of crop plant biotechnology: Plants can be made resistant to herbicides. Weeds can be killed by repeated applications of herbicides; these are chemicals that kill weeds. But a problem with these chemicals is they very often kill beneficial plants as well, and sometimes even some crops themselves, so these are nonspecific toxins. Great care is needed to use herbicides properly. Well, genes have been identified from bacteria and other sources that code for proteins that break down herbicides or make altered protein targets for the herbicides. That's how the bacteria survive. So these genes have been isolated from the bacteria and put into cotton, corn, soybeans, rice, and sugar beets. And as a result, these transgenic, genetically modified, crops are now resistant to the herbicide, and the herbicide can be applied without any risk of damaging the crop. That's my second example of plant biotechnology. I will say that these first two examples are in widespread use all over the world.

My third example involves rice. I mentioned when I discussed the rice plant that rice grains are deficient in their protein in terms of the amino acid balance. You'll recall there was an effort in corn to improve that, and there is an ongoing effort in rice to improve the amino acid balance of the protein in rice. But in addition, rice does not make a required vitamin-related substance called beta-carotene. People require beta-carotene in their diet, and beta-carotene is reddish-orange in color. It's what gives the carrot its orange color. This gets converted to vitamin A in the body. Rice plants do not have the genes to make beta-carotene. They do not express proteins along the biochemical pathway to make this vitamin precursor that we need. As a result, about 250,000 children go partially blind each year because they are eating rice and they don't get enough beta-carotene in their diet.

Other organisms have the genes coding for the enzyme that can complete this biochemical pathway. So you can envision rice has chemical A, which can be converted to B, to C, then to beta-carotene. So there are three enzymes along that pathway; other organisms have them. A scientist named Ingo Potrykus isolated DNA for each one of these enzymes. One of them was from a bacterium; the other two genes happened to be from a daffodil plant. One by one, over a period of almost a decade, he took each one of these genes and introduced it to rice plants along with a promoter that would stimulate gene expression in the developing rice grain. The idea would be, then, the rice grain will have the biochemical pathway to make beta-carotene.

The result is a rice plant that made grains with beta-carotene, and these grains are golden—they're more golden-colored than the translucent and white—because they have this higher beta-carotene content. They contain dietarily adequate amounts of beta-carotene. Thanks to this transgenic biochemical pathway—three new genes. These plants are now being crossed with local varieties all over the world to make the beta-carotene phenotype part of rice that is used in different regions of the world. So I've descried three well-known examples of plant biotechnology.

There is public concern about plant biotechnology. I mentioned before that at the start of the 1970s, there was concern about biotechnology in general when it first came up, and recombinant DNA work in particular. We just didn't know what we were doing, and we were worried. When this was shown to be safe, these concerns abated. But plant biotechnology and genetically modified foods; now these aren't necessarily the same. Not all plant biotechnology creates a modified food. For example, if you're wearing something made of cotton made in America, it's been made by a genetically modified plant; no question. Well, plant biotechnology that makes genetically modified food has been a public concern, especially in Europe.

The objections to biotechnology in agriculture are threefold. The first objection is that genetic manipulation is an unnatural interference with nature. This is what a philosopher calls the "yuck factor." Eating food from a plant that has genes from bacteria is just, in the minds of some people, going too far—there's just too much technology here. There's no real response to this emotional argument. Scientists will say, all major crops have been genetically manipulated, so that's okay. You'll accept the fact that corn has been extensively bred over the years. Why do you object to biotechnology? Biotechnology is really different. We're taking genes from all over the plant and animal world, and bacterial world, and splicing them together: the "yuck factor."

The second objection is that genetically modified foods might be unsafe to eat. Some modifications of proteins—for example, taking a soybean protein and modifying it, or taking the corn protein—may create a three-dimensional structure in the protein that some people might be allergic to. It turns out that in the examples I gave you, except for golden rice, most genetically modified plants grown now are not altered phenotypically in the food part of the plant. They've got some extra DNA sequences, but they're not being modified in the food part of the plant. But we've got to be careful about allergies. The third concern is that genetically modified plants are dangerous to the environment: Although a single gene—we were in control here—has been transferred to the crop plant from somewhere else, that gene for resistance to pesticides might be inadvertently transferred to neighboring plants in the field or adjacent to it, and this has been observed in some instances, but not in others. So there's a danger of creation of "super weeds" with resistance.

There's two ways to look at these public concerns. The one way is, let's proceed with caution. Let's do as many tests as we can to make sure that something doesn't cause harm, a new technology like this; and be careful, as we grow genetically modified plants, for genes that are escaping, or for allergies or other problems. Proceed with caution. The other way to look at it is the precautionary principle. The precautionary principle says if you can't prove that this will never cause a problem, don't do it. It's kind of like, you never know, over the long period of time, what's going to happen. That's the precautionary principle. So there are two sides to this argument, and it's especially one that is being made in Europe—less so in other parts of the world, and certainly not so in the less-developed parts of the world where biotechnology has become a major way to improve plants.

In this course, we've come from describing heredity, to understanding its mechanism, to controlling it. In the first lectures, I described what genetics is and how a scientist monk named Gregor Mendel, and others, described the rules of inheritance. This led to the identification of what a gene is, DNA, and how it works, expressing itself usually as protein in the cell. With these basics of descriptive genetics in hand, I described how this knowledge has been applied to human use in the biotechnology industry. From making products to solving crimes and cleaning up the environment, biotechnology is becoming increasingly important. Modern genetics is even rewriting the "book of life" as explained by Charles Darwin's theory of evolution by natural selection. We are finding out more about the amazing array of organisms and how they are related to one another, and even how we as humans may have evolved over time.

Genetics and DNA are having a growing impact on medicine. With precise molecular descriptions of genetic causes of disease in hand, we are now able to diagnose and screen for people with these particular diseases, and we are just beginning to design specific treatments. Things like gene therapy, cloning, and stem cells are at the leading edge of modern medicine and hold great promise for the future. I ended the course with agriculture, that other application of biology to human welfare, not just because it's important—you know, we have to eat—but because so many of us in the rich world take agriculture for granted. The applications of modern genetics and DNA to the problem of feeding the world are already profound, and an exciting future is possible. The genetic genie is out of the bottle. Thank you.

Timeline

B.C.

2500 .... Oral records of deliberate breeding for desirable characteristics of the date palm and the horse.

350 .... Aristotle, the Greek philosopher, proposes that the genetic material is carried in sperm and that the female menstrual fluid "organizes" this to form offspring.

A.D.

200 .... Report of the inheritance of hemophilia in the Babylonian Talmud, a biblical commentary.

1721 .... Zabdiel Boylston uses inoculation to prevent smallpox in Boston (Edward Jenner provides experimental evidence for the effectiveness of inoculation in 1796).

1766 .... The Dutch microscopist, Antonie Van Leeuwenhoek, observes human sperm under the microscope and "sees" tiny humans, as predicted by Aristotle.

1831 .... The naval survey ship *Beagle* leaves England for a round-the-world, five-year expedition with Charles Darwin aboard as naturalist. Darwin's careful observations lead him to propose a mechanism for evolution.

1852–1854 .... Gregor Mendel attends the University of Vienna, where he studies mathematics, chemistry, and biology.

1858 .... Publication of *On the Origin of Species* by Charles Darwin, explaining how natural selection of variations passed on genetically to offspring leads to the evolution of organisms through time.

1866 .... Gregor Mendel reports on his experiments on garden peas, showing the particulate nature of the genetic determinants.

1868 .... Friedrich Miescher isolates DNA.

1873 .... The term "intelligent design" is used to describe the origin of complex living systems.

1895 .... Albrecht Kossel finds that DNA is a long polymer of nucleotides A, T, G, and C.

1900 .... Botanists Hugo DeVries, Carol Correns, and Erich von Tschermak independently verify Mendel's conclusions about genes and alleles— and then discover his paper that had been published 34 years previously.

1903 .... Chromosomes are identified in dividing cells as the probable carriers of genes.

1908 .... George Shull crosses two pure lines of corn, producing plants whose seeds are very high yielding, demonstrating hybrid vigor (heterosis).

1910 .... Peyton Rous discovers that the cause of a type of cancer in chickens is transmitted from one animal to another (he is awarded the Nobel Prize in 1966). Archibald Garrod describes the disease alkaptonuria as an inherited mutation that is expressed as a defective enzyme; the one gene–one enzyme idea is confirmed 40 years later.

1918 .... Tsar Nicholas II of Russia and most of his family are killed and buried (DNA forensics is used to identify the remains in 1992).

1928 .... Frederick Griffith discovers genetic transformation in bacteria, showing that nonliving extracts of one type can turn another type into the first one; this indicates a chemical nature for genes.

1934 .... Asbjorn Folling describes phenylketonuria as a genetic disease.

1935 .... Semi-dwarf, high-yielding wheat is developed in Japan by genetic selection and crosses.

1944 .... Oswald Avery shows that DNA causes genetic transformation in bacteria, pointing to DNA as the genetic material.

1948 .... The protein in hemoglobin is identified as the primary phenotype in sickle cell disease, pointing to protein as the expression of a gene.

1950 .... Ernst Wynder finds a linkage between smoking and lung cancer in careful population studies, confirming data that were first reported almost 300 years before.

1952 .... Alfred Hershey and Martha Chase show that DNA is the genetic material of a virus.

1953 .... James Watson and Francis Crick propose the double-helix structure of DNA.

1954 .... Sickle cell disease is described as a balanced polymorphism, existing in high frequency in some populations because it confers resistance to malaria.

1956 .... Arthur Kornberg describes DNA polymerase, the enzyme that catalyzes DNA replication.

1957 .... Semiconservative replication of DNA is demonstrated in bacteria, and later in eukaryotes.

1958 .... A carrot is cloned from a single specialized cell, thus showing that each specialized cell is totipotent.

1959 .... The roles of messenger RNA and transfer RNA in gene expression are described.

1960 .... The immunoassay is invented to test for tiny amounts of substances; it soon has wide applications, especially to detect hormones. An unusual chromosome called the Philadelphia chromosome is found to be diagnostic in chronic myelogenous leukemia. Forty years later, a drug is developed specifically for the gene product from this chromosome.

1961 .... The first codon is identified in the genetic code, relating the nucleotides in messenger RNA to an amino acid in a protein; the other codons are soon identified. High-yielding, semi-dwarf, adaptable wheat is developed by Norman Borlaug in Mexico. It soon results in bumper crops there and in India.

1962 .... A frog is cloned by nuclear transplantation from a specialized cell nucleus. This shows totipotency in animal cells. Werner Arber describes bacteriophage restriction and proposes specific restriction endonucleases made by bacteria that cleave incoming phage DNA at specific sequences. Newborn screening for the genetic disease phenylketonuria begins. Its public health success results in other screening programs.

1963 .... A high-lysine variety of corn is described from a screen of thousands of genetically different varieties. This leads to quality-protein maize and improvement in human nutrition.

1964 .... Robert Holley determines the first sequence of a nucleic acid.

1965 .... Nucleic acid hybridization becomes widely used to study relationships between nucleic acids.

1968 .... Motoo Kimura proposes evolution by accumulation of neutral mutations not subject to natural selection. The term "Green Revolution" is used to describe the impact of new wheat and rice varieties on poor regions of the world.

1970 .... Norman Borlaug is awarded the Nobel Peace Prize for breeding high-yielding varieties of wheat for use in the poor regions of the world.

1971 .... Daniel Nathans cuts and maps a viral genome using a restriction enzyme, showing the potential use of these enzymes for manipulating DNA in the lab. The two-hit model for cancer involving tumor suppressor genes is proposed. This leads to the discovery of these genes and their control of cell division.

1973 .... First report of genetically functional recombinant DNA, as genes from different bacteria are spliced together in the lab and then put into a single cell. Soon, human genes are put into bacteria and expressed.

1976 .... Recombination of alleles explains the diversity of antibodies.

1977 .... DNA sequencing methods are developed and soon automated. This ultimately leads to genome sequencing projects.

1979 .... The human insulin gene is expressed in bacteria. This is first drug made by DNA biotechnology, and a new industry is born. Smallpox is eradicated through vaccination.

1982 .... A genetically modified bacterium is patented; upheld by the U.S. Supreme Court, this leads to many more patents of organisms and genes.

1983 .... The polymerase chain reaction is invented.

1984 .... The Human Genome Project is first proposed.

1985 .... Instruments are invented to make DNA sequences in the lab; custom DNA is now possible. The dystrophin gene that is defective in Duchenne muscular dystrophy is isolated. DNA identification by repeated sequences is invented by Alec Jeffreys. It soon has many applications in forensics.

1989 .... Bacteria with genes for digesting oil are used in bioremediation of the oil spill from the tanker *Exxon Valdez*.

1990 .... The novel *Jurassic Park* brings DNA technology to public attention.

Functional human antibodies are made in transgenic plants. Gene therapy is successfully done on a patient with immunodeficiency, leading to much hope and hype. A transgenic cow makes a human protein in its milk; this leads to "pharming." Preimplantation genetic diagnosis is done on an eight-celled embryo to screen for mutant alleles for cystic fibrosis. None are found, and a normal baby is born.

1994 .... Quality-protein maize is developed by plant geneticists. It becomes widely used and improves human nutrition as well as crop production.

1995 .... The first genome of an organism is sequenced: a bacterium that causes meningitis. New genes are found and other sequences rapidly follow. First gene expression analysis by DNA microarray is performed, leading to many applications for basic science and medical diagnosis, as well as the development of computing tools to analyze a mass of data.

1996 .... Dolly the sheep, the first cloned mammal, is born. Other mammals are soon cloned.

1998 .... Human embryonic stem cells are grown in the laboratory, making possible their use in medicine. The RNAi mechanism is explained to shut off specific gene expression. Many applications from basic research to drug development follow. Gleevec, the prototype drug in molecular medicine, enters clinical trials for a type of leukemia and is very successful.

1999 .... The first death due to a gene therapy clinical trial temporarily halts all such therapies in the U.S. Golden rice, rich in beta-carotene, is made by genetic modification of rice plants. Debate continues on the possible dangers of genetically modified crops.

2000 .... Drafts of the entire human genome sequence are completed (the final sequence is announced in 2003).

2001 .... Salt-tolerant tomato plants are made by genetic modification, opening up the possibility of genetically adapting crops to the environment.

2002 .... Stem cells are isolated from fat, one of several non-embryonic stem cells that can be used to develop specialized cells for medicine.

2005 .... The chimp genome is completed, leading to comparisons with the human genome to find differences.

2006 .... Gene therapy augments the immune system rejection of a melanoma tumor in a patient.

Glossary

adeno-associated virus: A small virus that infects human cells, incorporates its DNA into the human genome, but does not cause disease. It is used as a vector for human gene therapy.

adenovirus: A DNA virus that causes the common cold; when disabled from reproducing, it is used as a vector for human gene therapy. It does not incorporate its DNA into the human genome.

allele: One of the different forms of a particular gene. Alleles have different DNA sequences.

amino acid: A chemical building block for proteins. There are 20 different amino acids, and their chemical properties determine the properties of proteins.

anabolism: The chemical conversions in biochemistry in which energy is used to make more complex molecules from simple ones. The assembly of proteins from individual amino acids is an example.

angiogenesis: The formation of new blood vessels, which occurs when organs form in development, and when tumors and metastases form in cancer.

annotation: The assignment of amino acid sequences and functions to proteins from DNA sequence data.

antibody: A protein made by immune system cells that can bind specifically to an antigen, or nonself chemical grouping.

antigen: A chemical grouping whose three-dimensional structure marks it as nonself and so provokes an immune response.

B cell: A type of white blood cell that makes an antibody.

bacteriophage: A virus that infects and reproduces in bacteria.

bacterium: A single-celled prokaryotic organism. This classification excludes a special group of prokaryotes called the Archaea.

balanced polymorphism: A gene with alleles such that an allele is maintained in a population despite its disadvantage for reproduction because it provides an overriding advantage as well. For instance, the sickle cell allele for hemoglobin is disadvantageous because it can result in sickle cell disease but advantageous because it can result in resistance to malaria.

base pairs (nucleotides): Chemical interactions between nucleotides in the same or opposite strands of nucleic acids. A pairs with T or U; G pairs with C.

bioinformatics: The use of computing to analyze information in biological systems, especially extensive data from DNA and protein sequences.

bioremediation: The use of organisms, especially bacteria, to remove pollutants from the environment. For example, bacteria that digest oil are used to clean up accidental oil spills.

biosensor: The use of an organism or cells to provide information about another organism or cell or environmental condition.

biotechnology: The use of organisms to perform functions useful to people.

blending inheritance: The idea that when hereditary determinants from two parents come together after fertilization of the egg by sperm, the individual determinants disappear and do not have a separate existence but are irreversibly blended. Mendel's experiments led to a rejection of this idea.

blood typing: The use of genetically inherited allele coding for molecules on the surface of the red blood cell to identify people. The ABO blood groups are an example.

carrier: In genetics, an organism with a normal phenotype that is heterozygous for a recessive allele that determines an unusual phenotype. For example, the parents of a child born with sickle cell disease are often carriers for the allele that causes this disease.

catabolism: The biochemical pathways that involve breaking down complex substances into simpler ones, releasing stored chemical energy. Digestion of proteins into amino acids is an example.

catalyst: A chemical that speeds up a conversion of other substances but is not changed after the conversion.

cell: The basic unit of biological structure, function, and continuity. It contains the genome, as well as the chemical components for biochemistry.

cell cycle: The sequence of events by which a cell reproduces (divides).

chemotherapy: The use of drugs to treat a disease; used most commonly with cancer and some infectious diseases.

chromosome: A DNA molecule containing all or part of the genome of an organism, which has the ability to replicate.

cloning: In organisms, producing genetically identical copies of a cell or organism; in molecular genetics, isolating a gene and making multiple, identical copies of it by insertion into an organism.

DNA: Deoxyribonucleic acid, a polymer of nucleotide building blocks (A, T, G, and C) that acts as the genetic material in most living things.

DNA microarray: A collection of many gene sequences, usually affixed to a glass slide, that act as probes for hybridization in studies of gene expression.

DNA polymerase: An enzyme that catalyzes the polymerization of DNA from nucleotide monomers.

dominant: An allele whose phenotype is expressed in an organism that is either homozygous or heterozygous for the allele.

double helix: A molecule, usually DNA, that contains two interacting strands that curl into a helical form.

enzyme: A biological catalyst that speeds up a biochemical transformation without emerging changed by the process; most enzymes are proteins, although some are RNAs.

essential amino acids: Building blocks of protein that an organism cannot synthesize and that must be taken in the diet; humans must eat 8 essential amino acids and can make the other 12.

eukaryotic cell: A cell with a nucleus and other cell components that are each enclosed within membranes; these cells make up animals and plants.

expression vector: A DNA carrier for molecular cloning that contains sequences for the transcription and translation of the gene to be cloned.

extremophiles: Organisms that can live in environments that would be highly unsuitable for almost all other forms of life; these environments include very high temperature and high salt concentration.

fermentation: The breakdown of carbohydrates by organisms in the absence of oxygen gas, usually to alcohol or lactic acid. More generally, in biotechnology, fermentation is the use of microorganisms or their enzymes to form products from the breakdown of carbohydrates.

gene: The unit of heredity; a sequence of nucleotides on a chromosome that is expressed as a product that is part of the phenotype.

gene library: A collection of the DNA fragments from an organism's genome carried on vectors; these vectors are usually used to clone the library fragments in bacteria.

gene therapy: In medicine, the introduction of new genes into cells for improvement of the symptoms of a disease.

genealogy: The study of family pedigrees for the purpose of tracing ancestors.

genetic code: The sequence of nucleotides along mRNA that is used to translate the genome into amino acids in protein. The code is virtually the same in all organisms.

genetics: The science of heredity.

genome: The complete nucleic acid (usually DNA) sequence of an organism.

golden rice: Rice that has been genetically engineered to make beta-carotene, a precursor to vitamin A.

green fluorescent protein: A protein from certain jellyfish that gives a bright green, visible glow under ultraviolet light; the gene for this protein has been used as a marker in gene cloning.

growth factor: A protein made in mammals by one tissue that stimulates cell division in a target tissue.

herbicide tolerance: The ability of a plant to be resistant to the effects of an herbicide, a property sometimes conferred by genetic engineering.

heterozygous: An organism with two different alleles for a particular gene.

homozygous: An organism with two identical alleles for a particular gene.

human leukocyte antigen (HLA): A set of human genes coding for cell surface proteins that are involved in cellular immunity; HLA proteins mark an individual as unique.

hybridization: In genetics, the mating of two individuals homozygous for different alleles to produce heterozygous offspring. In molecular biology, the binding by complementary base pairing (A with T/U and G with C) of nucleic acids from different sources.

hypothyroidism: A disease caused by inadequate production of thyroid hormone. There are both genetic and nongenetic causes; genetic hypothyroidism is screened for in newborns.

independent assortment: The independent segregation of genes on different chromosomes during the formation of gametes in sexual reproduction.

locus: The location of a gene on a chromosome.

metabolism: The sum total of all of the chemical transformations in an organism.

metastasis: The ability of a tumor to break off cells that travel in the blood or lymphatic system to a new location in the body and grow to a satellite tumor.

minimal genome: The genes absolutely necessary for life as deduced by serial inactivation of all genes and testing of an organism for survival.

mitochondrion: The membrane-enclosed "powerhouse of the cell" that releases chemical energy in usable form and contains a small DNA chromosome coding for some of its proteins.

molecular clock: If a DNA sequence mutates at a constant rate over time, and the mutations are not selected by natural selection, comparing the difference of that DNA sequence in two organisms can give an estimate of the time they last had a common ancestor.

mRNA: Messenger RNA is transcribed from one of the two strands of DNA in a gene and carries coding information to the ribosome, where its information is translated to amino acids in protein synthesis.

mutation: A change in the genetic material that is passed on to both daughter cells after cell division. If the cell is a germ line cell, the change can be passed on to offspring and is inherited. If the change is in a somatic cell, it is passed on only to the cells deriving from the original changed cell.

natural selection: The process by which the changing environment causes some individuals with more favorable genes and alleles to have more offspring and pass those alleles to the next generation. This leads to the organism changing through time, or evolving.

neutral mutation: A genetic change that is not subject to natural selection but is nevertheless passed on to the next generation.

nucleic acid: A large molecule or DNA or RNA made up of nucleotide building blocks.

nucleotide: The building block of a nucleic acid. Each nucleotide has an identical sugar and phosphate group and one of five different bases: A, G, C, T, and U.

oncogene: A cellular gene that stimulates cell division and tumor formation when activated. Active oncogenes can be brought into cells by certain tumor viruses.

one gene–one protein: The hypothesis that each gene is expressed by a unique protein that is responsible for its phenotype at the biochemical level.

open reading frame: A sequence of DNA in a chromosome that codes for a protein.

pesticide: A substance that is used by people to kill unwanted organisms (pests). For example, insecticides are used to kill insect pests.

phagocyte: A white blood cell that surrounds, ingests, and digests foreign substances.

pharming: The use of animals to express and produce human proteins for use as drugs in medicine. Expression is usually in the animals' milk.

phenotype: The outward appearance of genes. It can be influenced by the environment.

phenylketonuria (PKU): A genetic disease in which affected individuals lack an active enzyme called phenylalanine hydroxylase. This causes mental retardation if untreated. Newborns are screened for PKU and if it is found are put on a special diet that results in normal development.

pluripotent: The ability of a stem cell and its offspring to specialize into a few different cell types. For example, some pluripotent stem cells in bone marrow can specialize into red blood cells and several types of white blood cells.

polymerase chain reaction (PCR): A method of amplifying a DNA sequence in the test tube by adding DNA polymerase and other necessary components for replication. A sequence can be amplified a millionfold in a few hours.

polymorphism: A difference in a particular DNA sequence between individuals.

population bottleneck: A severe reduction in a population, followed by an expansion by the few remaining individuals. The new population's frequencies of alleles will be a reflection of these few individuals, and this is probably different from the larger, original population.

prokaryotic cell: A cell that lacks a nucleus or other membrane-enclosed components.

promoter: A DNA sequence adjacent to the coding region of a gene, to which RNA polymerase binds to initiate gene expression. The events at the promoter are highly regulated in location and time.

protein: A large molecule composed of amino acid building blocks linked together.

pure-line selection: In crop plant genetics, the repeated selection of a genetically diverse plant population for a specific characteristic. Pure lines are generally homozygous.

quality-protein maize: A variety of corn (maize) that was developed in Mexico during the 1990s that has increased crop yield and more and better protein for human nutrition.

recessive: An allele that is expressed only when homozygous and not expressed when heterozygous (in which case the dominant allele is expressed).

recombinant DNA: DNA molecule made from DNA of two different organisms spliced together in the laboratory.

restriction enzyme: An enzyme made by a microorganism that catalyzes the cleavage of DNA at a specific nucleotide sequence.

reverse genetics: The process by which a gene coding for a phenotype is isolated first, and then the protein involved in that phenotype is isolated.

ribosome: A particle in the cell that acts as the "workbench" and catalyst for protein synthesis.

RNA: Ribonucleic acid, a polymer of the nucleotides A, G, C, and U. There are several types of RNA in the cell, such as transfer RNA and messenger RNA.

RNA polymerase: An enzyme that catalyzes the formation of RNA from nucleotides, using base pairing to DNA as a template.

RNAi: The use of double-stranded RNA to inhibit the translation to protein of a specific mRNA. A cellular mechanism cuts a larger RNAi into small, single-stranded fragments that actually do the inhibition.

screening: In medicine, the presumptive identification of an individual with a disease by the use of a rapid test that can be applied to large numbers of people.

segregation: In genetics, the separation of the two alleles for a gene into different cells during gamete formation.

semiconservative replication: The mechanism of duplication of DNA whereby each of the two strands in the parental DNA acts as a template for a new strand by complementary base pairing so that each of the two DNA molecules produced has one parental and one new strand.

sex determination: Primary sex determination is the genetically determined formation of either male or female gametes. Secondary sex determination is the outward appearance of the individual with regard to male and female characteristics.

short tandem repeat: A DNA polymorphism in which a sequence of 2–10 base pairs is repeated a number of times, in an inherited manner.

shotgun sequencing: DNA sequencing in which a large DNA is fragmented into many smaller pieces, each piece sequenced, and the sequences aligned by computer analysis.

single nucleotide polymorphism: A DNA sequence that varies between individuals of species by a single base pair.

stem cell: A cell in the body that replicates continuously and can form certain specialized cells.

substrate: In biochemistry, a molecule that is acted upon by an enzyme to make a product.

synthetic biology: The attempt to use knowledge of the minimal genome to synthesize a DNA genome in the laboratory and put it inside an enclosed space to custom-make a cell.

synthetic DNA: DNA artificially made in the laboratory by nonbiological methods.

T cell: A white blood cell involved in cellular immunity.

therapeutic cloning: The use of cloning by donor nuclear transplantation to produce an embryo and then embryonic stem cells that can provide specialized cells for therapy on the nuclear donor.

totipotent: A cell able to produce all other cells of an organism. For example, a fertilized egg is totipotent.

transcription: The expression of a gene by the production of RNA from a DNA template, catalyzed by RNA polymerase.

transformation: The introduction of DNA from an outside source to a cell, causing it to become genetically different.

transgenic: A eukaryotic organism, usually an animal, that has received and integrated DNA from a different organism.

translation: The synthesis of a chain of amino acids as a protein in response to the information of nucleotide sequence in a gene as appearing in mRNA.

tumor suppressor gene: A gene in mammals that inhibits cell division and therefore cancer formation.

vector: A DNA molecule that is used as a carrier to bring a foreign gene into a recipient cell.

virus: An infectious particle usually composed of DNA and protein that requires a host cell to replicate.

X-ray diffraction: A physical method that involves measuring the changes in orientation of X rays as they pass through a crystal. It gives information on the three-dimensional arrangement of atoms in the crystal.

Biographical Notes

Allison, Anthony: A British geneticist who found in the late 1940s that the frequency of the allele for sickle cell hemoglobin was highest in Africa in regions where the incidence of malaria was highest. He proposed that the sickle allele was an example of a balanced polymorphism, where the selective advantages of having the allele outweighed the disadvantages.

Arber, Werner: A Swiss biologist whose studies on how bacteria defend themselves against viral infection led to the discovery in 1962 of restriction endonucleases. These enzymes are tools for cutting DNA in the laboratory to prepare recombinant DNA. He was awarded the Nobel Prize in 1978.

Aristotle: A supreme philosopher in ancient Greece, he made careful observations of the natural world, including biology. His ideas on genetics, promulgated around 340 B.C., included one that an individual's inheritance was primarily from the father. He believed that sperm contained tiny humans that were then organized by the menstrual fluid during sexual intercourse.

Avery, Oswald: An American medical researcher, born in Canada, who found in 1944 that the active cellular ingredient that caused genetic transformation in bacteria was DNA. This was a key line of evidence for DNA as the genetic material.

Blumwald, Eduardo: An American plant biologist who studied the mechanisms of tolerance to salty soils. In the late 1990s, he found a gene in the model plant *Arabidopsis* that when active conferred salt tolerance, and when this gene was transferred to tomato plants, they too were salt tolerant. This gene is under active investigation for transfer into other crops that could then grow on salty soils.

Borlaug, Norman: Plant geneticist who led the team in Mexico that bred high-yielding strains of wheat that were adaptable for cultivation in poor regions. The adoption of these strains led to spectacular gains in food production in many areas of the world. In 1970, Borlaug was awarded the Nobel Peace Prize for his discovery, which staved off famines.

Boyer, Herbert: An American biochemist who, along with Stanley Cohen, made the first functional recombinant DNA in a test tube in 1973 by joining genes from two different bacteria and inserting them into a third strain. He then went on to be a founder of the biotechnology company Genentech.

Boyleston, Zabdiel: An American physician who followed the advice of minister Cotton Mather to inoculate people in Boston during a smallpox epidemic in 1721. Almost all of these people survived.

Brock, Thomas: An American microbiologist and author of a leading textbook on the subject, he studied the biochemistry of bacteria that tolerate the extreme heat of hot springs at Yellowstone National Park. In 1970, he discovered that they had a gene coding for a heat-tolerant DNA polymerase. This was later used for the polymerase chain reaction.

Cano, Raul: A Cuban American microbiologist, he and his students isolated and amplified in the late 1980s DNA from insects preserved in amber millions of years ago. This became the scientific basis for a fictional story of cloning dinosaurs in the novel and film *Jurassic Park*.

Chakrabarty, Ananda: A biologist working for General Electric who isolated a genetically modified bacterium capable of breaking down oil. He applied for a patent, and the case went to the U.S. Supreme Court, which in 1980 ruled that his patent was valid. This led to many more patents of organisms and DNA.

Chargaff, Erwin: An American biochemist who studied the chemical composition of DNA and found in 1951 that the ratios of the bases A:T and G:C were always about one and that every species had its own unique composition of the bases. "Chargaff's rules" were important evidence used by Watson and Crick to decipher the double-helical structure of DNA.

Chase, Martha and Hershey, Alfred: In 1952, these American geneticists performed a key experiment that showed that DNA is the genetic material of viruses. Hershey was awarded the Nobel Prize in 1969.

Cohen, Stanley: An American geneticist who worked with Herbert Boyer to make the first functional recombinant DNA in 1973, ushering in a new era of biotechnology.

Collins, Francis: An American physician-geneticist, he led the publicly funded effort to sequence the entire human genome. A draft sequence was announced in 2000 and a final sequence in 2003.

Crichton, Michael: An American novelist trained as a physician, he has written several books with themes related to genetics, notably *Jurassic Park* (1990), in which dinosaurs are cloned using DNA extracted from fossil insects. He is also one of the creators and a producer of the television series *ER,* which often has themes related to genetics.

Crick, Francis: An English physicist and biologist, he was the codiscoverer of the structure of DNA in 1953. In 1959, he proposed a role for RNA in gene expression and predicted the triplet genetic code. He was awarded the Nobel Prize in 1962.

Darwin, Charles: The English naturalist whose theory of evolution by natural selection, proposed in 1858, unified biology and still does. Darwin's idea was that there is a lot of genetic variation among individuals of a species, and those variants best adapted to the environment for reproduction are passed on to the next generation. Thus, species evolve.

DeVries, Hugo: Dutch botanist who, with Carl Correns and Erich von Tschermak, independently verified Gregor Mendel's conclusions about genes and alleles and then discovered Mendel's paper that had been published 34 years previously.

Doll, Richard: English epidemiologist who showed in 1950 that lung cancer is linked to cigarette smoking. His study led to further investigations linking smoking to heart disease.

Druker, Brian: American physician who led the team that developed the drug Gleevec to treat chronic myelogenous leukemia. His 2001 study showing the effectiveness of this targeted drug is a landmark in molecular medicine.

Dulbecco, Renato: Italian-born American virologist whose studies in the late 1950s and 1960s of the molecular genetics of tumor viruses laid the foundation for work on other viruses, including HIV. He was an early proponent of the Human Genome Project. He was awarded the Nobel Prize in 1975.

Fire, Andrew: American geneticist who, along with Craig Mello, discovered the mechanism of RNA interference (RNAi) in 1998. He was awarded the Nobel Prize in 2006.

Folling, Asbjorn: Norwegian physician and chemist who in 1934 discovered the genetic disease phenylketonuria in two children with mental retardation. Newborn screening for phenylketonuria and dietary control since 1963 have led to a significant reduction in these symptoms in affected individuals.

Franklin, Rosalind: British physical chemist whose studies in 1952 of DNA using X-ray diffraction provided clear evidence for the helical nature of the molecule and were a key line of evidence used by Watson and Crick in developing the double-helical structure for DNA.

Garrod, Archibald: British physician who in 1910 proposed that the disease alkaptonuria is due to a genetically controlled absence of an active enzyme. The enzyme was specifically identified years later, and the genetic mutation in DNA in the 1990s.

Gehring, Walter: Swiss geneticist whose pioneering work on the molecular genetics of development led to his codiscovery in 1984 of a DNA sequence called the homeobox that is part of genes that control positional information in development. These genes were initially shown to occur in fruit flies, but similar genes occur throughout the animal world.

Griffith, Frederick: A British public health scientist, he accidentally discovered genetic transformation in bacteria in 1928. His studies laid the groundwork for the proof that DNA is the genetic material responsible for transformation.

Guthrie, Robert: An American pediatrician and microbiologist who developed a simple screening test for phenylketonuria in 1963 and then led a major study that proved its usefulness in early detection of the disease in newborns.

Hedrick, Marc: American surgeon who isolated stem cells from fat in 2001 and showed that they are pluripotent.

Henslow, John Stevens: An English geologist and botanist, he was the professor at Cambridge who most influenced Charles Darwin when he was a student there. In 1831, he helped get Darwin the position as naturalist on the survey ship *Beagle*.

Hershey, Alfred and Chase, Martha: In 1952, these American geneticists performed a key experiment that showed that DNA is the genetic material of viruses. Hershey was awarded the Nobel Prize in 1969.

Holley, Robert: An American chemist, he led a team that was the first to determine the sequence of a nucleic acid, an 80-base RNA, in 1964 after five years of work. It takes a machine minutes to do this today. He was awarded the Nobel Prize in 1968.

Itakura, Keiichi: A Japanese-born American chemist, he developed methods to make DNA molecules in the chemistry laboratory. In 1978, he synthesized the gene for human insulin, which was then put into bacteria in the first widespread use of recombinant DNA to produce a drug.

Itano, Harvey: An American pathologist who in 1948 discovered that abnormal hemoglobin is the molecular basis of the phenotype in sickle cell disease.

Jeffreys, Alec: A British geneticist, he developed the use of DNA markers to identify organisms in 1985. DNA analysis quickly became widespread in forensics.

Kimura, Motoo: A Japanese evolutionary geneticist, in 1968 he developed the mathematical and theoretic bases for the theory that evolution can occur through the accumulation of neutral mutations that are not subject to natural selection.

Knudson, Arthur: An American physician, his careful examination of a hereditary cancer led in 1971 to the "two-hit" hypothesis, in which he proposed that cancer was partially due to two mutations in alleles of a tumor suppressor gene. Later, these genes were shown to indeed exist, and his hypothesis has been borne out.

Kornberg, Arthur: An American biochemist, in 1956 he was the first to describe DNA polymerase, the enzyme that catalyzed DNA replication. This was a key line of evidence in support of the double-helix model for DNA proposed a few years earlier. He was awarded the Nobel Prize in 1959.

Kunkel, Louis: An American medical geneticist, he showed in 1985 that the phenotype in Duchenne muscular dystrophy, the most common form of this disease, is due to a minor muscle protein called dystrophin. He isolated this protein by reverse genetics, first describing its gene.

Mello, Craig: An American geneticist who, along with Andrew Fire, discovered the mechanism of RNA interference (RNAi) in 1998. He was awarded the Nobel Prize in 2006.

Mendel, Gregor: An Austrian monk whose careful studies of crosses he made on pea plants laid the foundations for the modern science of genetics. His work, published in 1866, was ignored for 35 years but is now revered.

Miescher, Freidrich: A Swiss biologist who was the first person to isolate DNA, which he called "nuclein" when he extracted it from white blood cells in 1868.

Mullis, Kary: An American biochemist, he invented the polymerase chain reaction in 1983. It was an instant hit and is widely used to amplify DNA. He was awarded the Nobel Prize in 1993.

Nathans, Daniel: In 1971, he used a restriction enzyme to cut and map a viral genome, showing the potential use of these enzymes for manipulating DNA in the lab. He was awarded the Nobel Prize in 1978.

Nirenberg, Marshall: An American biochemist, his 1961 experiment identifying the first genetic codeword (a specific triplet of nucleotides that gets translated to a specific amino acid) led to the complete description of the near-universal genetic code. He was awarded the Nobel Prize in 1968.

Pauling, Linus: One of the greatest chemists of the 20th century, in the 1940s and 1950s he described the structure of proteins and was instrumental in identifying the alterations in hemoglobin in sickle cell disease. He was awarded two Nobel Prizes: for chemistry in 1954 and for peace (for leading the opposition to atmospheric testing of nuclear bombs) in 1962.

Potrykus, Ingo: Swiss plant biologist who spent his career studying crop plants of importance to the poor regions of the world. Using DNA technologies, he developed golden rice in 1999 to help improve the diets of millions.

Riggs, Arthur: An American biologist who did important early work on chromosome replication in eukaryotes. In 1978, he inserted the gene for human insulin into bacteria in the first widespread use of recombinant DNA to produce a drug.

Rous, Peyton: An American physician who in 1910 discovered that the cause of a type of cancer in chickens is transmitted from one animal to another; it was the first demonstration of a tumor virus. He was awarded the Nobel Prize in 1966.

Sanger, Frederick: An English biochemist who developed the methods to determine the sequence of the amino acids in proteins, for which he was awarded the Nobel Prize in 1958. Then he developed a method to determine the sequence of nucleotides in DNA, for which he was awarded a second Nobel Prize in 1980. He has been a leader in the genome sequencing effort.

Shull, George: An American geneticist who in 1908 crossed two pure lines of corn and first described the hybrid vigor of heterosis. Hybrid corn varieties soon became the major ones planted.

Skorecki, Karl: An Israeli physician who in 1997 used DNA polymorphisms to show that Jewish priests in the Cohanim tradition were all descended in a male line from an ancestor of several thousand years ago.

Smith, Hamilton: An American physician and microbiologist who was one of the first scientists to characterize the chemistry of restriction enzymes and in 1978 was awarded the Nobel Prize. He has also been a leader in DNA sequencing efforts and in 1975 was in the team that sequenced the first bacterial genome.

Spiegelman, Sol: An American microbiologist and biochemist who used nucleic acid hybridization, a technique he pioneered in 1961, to show that only one of the two strands of DNA in a given region is expressed and transcribed into RNA.

Steward, Frederick: An American plant physiologist who cloned entire carrot plants from specialized cells, thus demonstrating totipotency in 1958.

Thomson, James: An American cell biologist who isolated human embryonic stem cells in 1998 and grew them in the laboratory, a major advance in potentially using them for therapy.

van Leeuwenhoek, Antonie: The Dutch founder of cell biology was the first person to report the existence of living cells that he observed under the recently-invented microscope.

van 't Veer, Laura: A Dutch physician and cancer researcher who used DNA microarrays to study gene expression in different breast cancers and in 2002 developed a gene expression signature to differentiate tumors with good from poor prognosis, a major event in molecular medicine.

Vasal, Surinder: An Indian geneticist and plant breeder who works in Mexico, he developed quality-protein maize (corn) in 1990; this variety has improved the diets of millions of people while yielding high amounts of grain.

Venter, Craig: An American biologist whose private industry team invented shotgun sequencing, a way to rapidly get the sequence of a large genome. This led to the sequences of bacteria, the fruit fly, and the human genomes. He has also been active in finding new organisms through genomics, and in synthetic biology.

Watson, James: An American biologist who was the codiscoverer of the double-helix model for DNA in 1953. He was awarded the Nobel Prize in 1962.

Wilkins, Maurice: An English physical chemist who did studies on DNA by X-ray diffraction in early 1953 that led to the double-helix model. He was awarded the Nobel Prize in 1962.

Wilmut, Ian: An English biologist who with Keith Campbell led the team that in 1996 cloned Dolly the sheep by nuclear transplantation into an egg. Dolly was the first mammal to be cloned.

Yalow, Rosalyn: An American medical physicist who in 1960, with colleague Sidney Berson, invented immunoassay—a way to determine tiny quantities of substances. The ability to measure hormones revolutionized medicine. She was awarded the Nobel Prize in 1977.

Bibliography

Essential Reading:

Acquah, George. *Understanding Biotechnology.* Upper Saddle River, NJ: Pearson Prentice-Hall, 2004. A self-testing, internet-based outline.

Altieri, Miguel. *Genetic Engineering in Agriculture: The Myths, Environmental Risks and Alternatives.* Oakland, CA: Food First, 2005. Makes the case that genetically modified crops might not be a good thing.

Barnum, Susan. *Biotechnology: An Introduction.* Belmont, CA: Thomson Brooks-Cole, 2005. A somewhat advanced, but accessible, textbook for college-level courses.

Bellomo, Michael. *The Stem Cell Divide.* New York: AOMCOM Press, 2005. A balanced view of the science and the controversy.

Berg, Jeremy M., John Tymoczko, and Lubert Stryer. *Biochemistry.* 6th ed. New York: W. H. Freeman, 2006. Elegantly written and illustrated, this is an authoritative and comprehensive textbook.

Brookes, Martin. *Fly: The Unsung Hero of 20th-Century Science.* New York: HarperCollins, 2001. The history of genetics through its most popular organism of study.

Brooks, Gavin. *Gene Therapy: Using DNA as a Drug.* London: Pharmaceutical Press, 2003. Comprehensive introduction to the strategies and pitfalls of human gene therapy.

Cain, Michael, Hans Damman, Robert Lue, and Carol Yoon. *Discover Biology.* 3rd ed. New York: W. W. Norton, 2007. An excellent and interesting approach to general biology for the nonspecialist.

Carlson, Elof Axel. *The Unfit: A History of a Bad Idea.* Woodbury, NY: Cold Spring Harbor Laboratory Press, 2001. A very readable and fascinating account of the history of eugenics.

Chrispeels, Maarten and David Sadava. *Plants, Genes and Crop Biotechnology.* Sudbury, MA: Jones and Bartlett, 2003. A comprehensive introduction to plant biology in an agricultural context, with extensive coverage of applied genetics.

Crick, Francis. *What Mad Pursuit: A Personal View of Scientific Discovery.* New York: Basic Books, 1988. The discovery of the structure of DNA through the eyes of one of the scientists involved. See also Watson, James D.

Darwin, Charles. *The Origin of Species*. New York: Random House, 1979. Originally published in 1859. If there is one biology book that everyone should read, this is it.

Davies, Kevin. *Cracking the Genome: Inside the Race to Unlock Human DNA*. New York: The Free Press, 2001. The story of how publicly- and privately-financed groups sequenced the human genome, finishing at the same time.

Dawkins, Richard. *The Selfish Gene: 30th Anniversary Edition.* Oxford: Oxford University Press, 2006. What if genes use organisms to propagate themselves, instead of the other way around? This book and its author revolutionized the way some biologists think about evolution and genetics.

Denniston, Katherine and Joseph Topping. *Introduction to General, Organic and Biochemistry.* 4th ed. New York: McGraw-Hill, 2003. In one compact and well-illustrated volume, this text delivers what the title says: three college courses.

DeSalle, Rob and Michael Yudell. *Welcome to the Genome: A User's Guide to the Genetic Past, Present and Future.* Hoboken, NJ: John Wiley and Sons, 2005. An easy-to-read, fascinating summary of what genome studies mean.

DeVita Jr., Vincent, Samuel Hellman, and Steven Rosenberg. *Cancer: Principles and Practice of Oncology.* Philadelphia: Lippincott Williams and Wilkins, 2005. The authoritative book on cancer in all of its aspects.

Devlin, Thomas. *Textbook of Biochemistry with Clinical Correlations.* 6th ed. Hoboken, NJ: Wiley-Liss, 2006. Excellent, in-depth treatment of medical biochemistry, with many examples of genetic diseases.

Entine, Jon. *Let Them Eat Precaution: How Politics is Undermining a Genetic Revolution in Agriculture.* Washington, DC: AEI Press, 2006. Makes the case that genetically modified crops are a good thing.

Evans, Gareth and Judith Furlong. *Environmental Biotechnology: Theory and Application.* West Sussex, England: John Wiley and Sons, 2004. Although written for specialists, this collection of articles is surprisingly accessible and comprehensive.

Federoff, Nina and Nancy Brown. *Mendel in the Kitchen.* Washington, DC: National Academies Press, 2004. Excellent overview of genetics and plant breeding.

Fisher, Barry, David Fisher, and Jason Kowolski. *Forensics Demystified.* New York: McGraw-Hill, 2007. An excellent, readable, and well-illustrated introduction to the use of genetics and DNA technology in forensics.

Futuyma, Douglas. *Evolution.* Sunderland, MA: Sinauer Associates, 2005. A comprehensive textbook on the subject, with excellent chapters on DNA studies.

Goldsby, Richard, Thomas Kindt, and Barbara Osborne. *Kuby Immunology.* 6th ed. New York: W. H. Freeman, 2006. An excellent, well-illustrated, and comprehensive text, with medical applications throughout.

Gralla, Jay and Preston Gralla. *The Complete Idiot's Guide to Understanding Cloning.* New York: Penguin, 2004. Don't let the title repel you: This is a solid book written by a professor-scientist and journalist.

Griffiths, Anthony, Susan Wessler, Richard Lewontin, William Gelbart, David Suzuki, and Jeffrey Miller. *An Introduction to Genetic Analysis.* 8th ed. New York: W. H. Freeman, 2007. An excellent, comprehensive text written for undergraduates.

Henig, Robin. *The Monk in the Garden: The Lost and Found Genius of Gregor Mendel, the Father of Genetics.* Boston: Houghton-Mifflin, 2001. A vivid portrayal of Mendel and his times.

Judson, Horace Freeland. *The Eighth Day of Creation: Makers of the Revolution in Biology.* Woodbury, NY: Cold Spring Harbor Laboratory Press, 1996. If you ever wanted to know how science is really practiced and how real people laid the foundations of the revolution in molecular biology, read this book.

Lewin, Benjamin. *Genes VIII.* Upper Saddle River, NJ: Pearson Prentice-Hall, 2005. A well-written, authoritative textbook of DNA and molecular biology. Assumes knowledge of university-level general biology.

Lewis, Ricki. *Human Genetics.* 7th ed. New York: McGraw-Hill, 2006. A superb, readable textbook aimed at nonscientists and written by a talented science writer–biologist.

Lindee, Susan. *Moments of Truth in Genetic Medicine.* Baltimore: Johns Hopkins, 2005. A historian uses several well-known cases to show how far we have come as a society in dealing with human genetic diseases.

Litwack, Gerald. *Human Biochemistry and Disease.* New York: Academic Press, 2007. Using human diseases as a starting point, this book has an innovative and interesting approach to a complex subject.

Lodish, Harvey, Arnold Berk, Paul Matsudaira, Chris Kaiser, Monty Krieger, Matthew P. Scott, Lawrence Zipursky, and James Darnell. *Molecular Cell Biology.* 5th ed. New York: W. H. Freeman, 2005. The authoritative text of cell biology and biochemistry.

Maddox, Brenda. *Rosalind Franklin: The Dark Lady of DNA.* New York: HarperCollins, 2002. The riveting story of the scientist whose role in the discovery of the structure of DNA was long underappreciated.

Massie, Robert. *The Romanovs: The Final Chapter.* New York: Random House, 1995. The fascinating story of the remains of the Russian royal family, and how DNA technology was used to identify them.

McCabe, Linda L. and Edward E. R. B. McCabe. *DNA: Promise and Peril.* Berkeley: University of California Press, 2008. Two leading human geneticists look at how the exploding knowledge of the human genome impacts medical practice and how we look at ourselves.

McConkey, Edwin. *How the Human Genome Works.* Sudbury, MA: Jones and Bartlett, 2004. Excellent, concise coverage of the genome, written for the nonscientist.

Meyer, Anna. *The DNA Detectives: How the Double Helix is Solving Puzzles of the Past.* New York: Avalon Publishing, 2005. A readable account of the use of DNA forensics in history and human evolution.

Mullis, Kerry. *Dancing Naked in the Mind Field.* New York: Vantage Books, 2000. How an iconoclastic scientist discovered the polymerase chain reaction (PCR), won the Nobel Prize, and revolutionized DNA studies.

Panno, Joseph. *Gene Therapy: Treating Disease by Repairing Genes.* New York: Facts on File, 2005. A readable account of how gene therapy can be done and the challenges it faces in medicine.

Pasternak, Jack. *An Introduction to Human Molecular Genetics.* 2nd ed. Bethesda, MD: Fitzgerald Science Press, 2005. An authoritative text that is well organized and is a useful reference.

Pierce, Benjamin. *Genetics: A Conceptual Approach.* New York: W. H. Freeman, 2005. An excellent textbook for undergraduates with a modest background in biology.

Reilly, Philip. *Abraham Lincoln's DNA and Other Adventures in Genetics.* Woodbury, NY: Cold Spring Harbor Laboratory Press, 2000.

———. *Is It in Your Genes? How Genes Influence Common Disorders and Diseases That Affect You and Your Family.* Woodbury, NY: Cold Spring Harbor Laboratory Press, 2004. One of the best and liveliest books written for the general public on human genetics.

———. *The Strongest Boy in the World and Other Adventures in Genetics.* Woodbury, NY: Cold Spring Harbor Laboratory Press, 2006. Fascinating stories on how the human genome is changing medicine, written by a physician-lawyer.

Ridley, Mark. *Evolution (Oxford Readers).* Oxford: Oxford University Press, 2005. A compact yet in-depth discussion of what the great thinkers on the science of evolution thought.

Ridley, Matt. *Genome: The Autobiography of a Species in 23 Chapters (P.S.)* New York: HarperCollins, 2006. A science writer delves into the human genome in a lively and interesting way.

Robbins-Roth, Cynthia. *From Alchemy to IPO: The Business of Biotechnology.* Cambridge, MA: Perseus Group, 2001. How discoveries of DNA manipulation led companies listed on the stock exchange.

Sadava, David, Craig Heller, Gordon Orians, William Purves, and David Hillis. *Life: The Science of Biology.* 8th ed. Sunderland, MA: Sinauer Associates; New York: W. H. Freeman, 2008. An introductory biology text at the college level, with many illustrations of classic experiments and extensive coverage of genetics and DNA.

Scott, Christopher Thomas. *Stem Cell Now: From the Experiment That Shook the World to the New Politics of Life.* New York: Penguin, 2005. Written by a molecular biologist–journalist, this balanced treatment of a controversial subject is scientifically accurate and presents the ethical issues dispassionately.

Smith, John. *Biotechnology.* 4th ed. Cambridge: Cambridge University Press, 2004. An excellent textbook on genetic manipulation and its social consequences.

Sompayrac, Lauren. *How Cancer Works.* Sudbury, MA: Jones and Bartlett, 2004. Excellent, concise coverage of cancer, written for the nonscientist.

———. *How the Immune System Works.* Malden, MA: Blackwell Sciences, 2002. Readable, well-illustrated, and compact, this is a remarkable book for the nonscientist on a complicated subject.

Stone, Linda, Paul Lurquin, and Luca Cavalli-Sforza. *Genes, Culture and Human Evolution: A Synthesis.* Malden, MA: Blackwell, 2007. Lucidly written by leaders in the field, the book examines how DNA studies of human groups relate to anthropology.

Tannock, Ian, Richard Hill, Robert Bristow, and Lea Harrington. *The Basic Science of Oncology.* 4th ed. New York: McGraw-Hill, 2005. Although written by authorities for advanced readers, this text is highly accessible and provides clear explanations of many phenomena in cancer.

Thieman, William and Michael Palladino. *Introduction to Biotechnology.* San Francisco: Benjamin-Cummings, 2004. A readable text for nonscientists, including issues for discussion.

Venter, J. Craig. *My Life Decoded: My Genome.* New York: Viking Press, 2007. A lively view of the present and future of genome sequencing by a leader in the field.

Walker, Sharon. *Biotechnology Demystified.* New York: McGraw-Hill, 2007. A short, self-paced textbook with learning guides that skims the subject well.

Watson, James D. *Avoid Boring People: Lessons from a Life in Science.* New York: Oxford, 2007. An inside view of how science really works, by one of the codiscoverers of the model of DNA.

―――. *The Double Helix.* New York: Athenaeum, 1968. The discovery of the structure of DNA through the eyes of one of the scientists involved. See also Crick, Francis.

―――, Jan Witkowski, Richard Myers, and Amy Caudy. *Recombinant DNA: Genes and Genomics.* 3rd ed. New York: W. H. Freeman, 2007. A detailed guide to the major discoveries of molecular biology.

Weinberg, Robert. *The Biology of Cancer.* New York: Garland Science, 2007. Written by a leading cancer researcher, an up-to-date, well-illustrated, and beautifully written textbook of the science behind cancer. For readers with a desire for advanced knowledge.

Zaikov, George. *Biotechnology and Environment.* Haupaugge, NY: Nova Science, 2005. A short, accessible volume from experts on using microbes in environmental cleanup.

Notes

Notes

Notes

Notes

Notes

Notes